FREE
Yourself
from
Chronic Pain
and Sports Injuries

**How Prolotherapy
Regenerative Medicine Can
Help You Become PAIN FREE**

SECOND EDITION

FREE
Yourself
from
Chronic Pain
and Sports Injuries

**How Prolotherapy
Regenerative Medicine Can
Help You Become PAIN FREE**

SECOND EDITION

Donna D. Alderman, D.O.
Osteopathic Physician and Surgeon

FAMILY DOCTOR PRESS

www.FamilyDoctorPress.com

Free Yourself from Chronic Pain and Sports Injuries

Publisher's Cataloging-in-Publication data

Alderman, Donna D.
   Free yourself from chronic pain and sports injuries : how prolotherapy regenerative medicine can help you become pain free, second edition / Donna D. Alderman, D.O.

   p.: cm.

   Includes bibliographical references and index. | Valencia, CA: Family Doctor Press, 2018.
   ISBN 978-0-9815242-1-4

1. LCC Pain--Therapy.   2. Chronic Pain--Treatment.   3. Regenerative medicine.   4. Osteoarthritis--Treatment.   5. Osteoarthritis--Alternative Treatment.   6. Musculoskeletal disease--Treatment. 7. Sports injuries--Treatment. 8. Sports injuries.   9. Stem cells--Therapeutic use.   10. Orthopedic procedures.   11. Integrative Medicine.   12. Complementary Therapies.   13. BISAC MEDICAL--Orthopedics   14. MEDICAL--Alternative & Complementary Medicine   15. MEDICAL--Pain Medicine

LCC RB127 .A44 2018
DDC 616/.0472--dd23
LCCN 2018902227

Book designer: Pamela Terry, Opus 1 Design, www.opus1design.com
Illustrations including cover art: Steve Tatman, www.stevetatman.com
Book consultants: Brookes Nohlgren, www.booksbybrookes.com;
Melissa Brown Levine, www.melissabrownlevine.com

Special thanks to Mitzi Killeen, MLS, Special Collections Librarian, Philadelphia College of Osteopathic Medicine, and to my student helpers: Danielle Villaruz, Monique Gudino, and Justin Schmidt.

Printed in China

This book is dedicated to Earl H. Gedney, D.O. and George S. Hackett, M.D., whose "outside the box" thinking resulted in the birth of Prolotherapy; to Gustav A. Hemwall, M.D., for his work in the field and his courage to explore new ways to help his patients; to Andrew T. Still, M.D., the father of osteopathic medicine, for his insight into the importance of the musculoskeletal system and a total approach to health care; and to Robert W. Alexander, M.D., for his invaluable contributions to Biocellular Prolotherapy and the entire field of regenerative medicine.

About the Author

Dr. Donna Alderman is an osteopathic physician and an expert in orthopedic regenerative medicine. She is a graduate of Cornell University and Western University of Health Sciences, and board certified in Prolotherapy as well as integrative medicine. Dr. Alderman has authored multiple medical journal articles and textbook chapters on traditional Dextrose Prolotherapy, Platelet-Rich Plasma (PRP) and Biocellular (Stem Cell–Rich) Prolotherapy—all nonsurgical, regenerative treatments for musculoskeletal pain and sports injuries. She has practiced this medical specialty since 1996 and is a frequent lecturer for several physician teaching organizations and colleges. Dr. Alderman is medical director at the Hemwall Center for Orthopedic Regenerative Medicine, with two offices in California. For more information, visit her website: www.prolotherapy.com.

Contents

List of Illustrations

DISCLAIMER

The information presented in this book is based on the experiences of Donna D. Alderman, D.O., and is for educational and informational purposes only. In no way should this book be used as a substitute for your own physician's advice. It is offered with the understanding that the publisher and author are not rendering medical or other professional services. This book does not constitute a doctor-patient relationship. Do not rely on the information in this book without seeking independent professional medical advice.

Traditional Dextrose Prolotherapy, Platelet-Rich Plasma (PRP) Prolotherapy, and Biocellular (Stem Cell–Rich, also known as Stem/Stromal, Lipoaspirate, Bone Marrow Aspirate, or, simply, Stem Cell) Prolotherapy (hereinafter collectively referred to as "Prolotherapy") are medical techniques. As with any medical technique, results will vary among individuals, and there are risks involved. All potential results and risks should be discussed with a qualified health-care professional to determine if Prolotherapy is right for you prior to receiving any such treatment.

Patient stories in this book are the personal experiences of individual patients and are intended to inform, educate, and entertain. However, since responses to any medical treatment are individual, there is no guarantee that you or anyone else will experience the same outcome that these patients, or others, have experienced. Anyone considering Prolotherapy should seek a formal evaluation performed by a physician who is competent in treating musculoskeletal pain with Prolotherapy. Those desiring treatment should make medical decisions with the aid of their personal physicians. No medical decisions should be made based solely on the contents of this book or on any general recommendations made herein.

Physicians should use and apply the technique of Prolotherapy only after they have received extensive training and have demonstrated the ability to administer Prolotherapy treatment safely. The author, publisher, and publishing agents shall have neither liability nor responsibility to any person or entity with respect to any loss or damage caused or alleged to be caused directly or indirectly by the information contained in this book.

FOREWORD

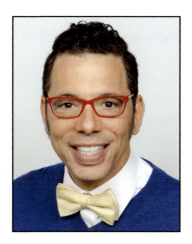

Ross A. Hauser, M.D.

Dr. Hauser is medical director for Caring Medical Regenerative Medicine Clinics, specializing in Prolotherapy Regenerative Medicine. Dr. Hauser has written multiple books on Prolotherapy, including *Prolo Your Pain Away!* and *Prolo Your Sports Injuries Away!* He has also published over 30 scientific journal articles on Prolotherapy and chronic pain.

The consummate physician does what is best for the patient, no matter the circumstances. For physicians who dare tackle the chronic pain sufferer, this may mean using the treatment known as Prolotherapy. I was fortunate to write one of the early books on the subject, *Prolo Your Pain Away!* As I promoted the book, I was able to meet some of the doctors around the country who were using this technique. At a meeting of the American College for Advancement in Medicine in the 1990s, I first came across the enthusiasm and energy of Dr. Donna Alderman. When she saw my table, she cried out, "I love Prolotherapy! I just learned it, and it's wonderful!" She grabbed up several copies of my book, and we struck up an enduring bond of friendship. She received additional training in Prolotherapy from the grandmaster, Dr. Gustav Hemwall, and was a volunteer at Beulah Land Natural Medicine Clinic in rural Illinois, using her skills as a prolotherapist to relieve the chronic pain and suffering of many people. Not only have I had the opportunity to help train Dr. Alderman but I have also been fortunate to work beside her and to see her compassion for patients and passion for Prolotherapy. Dr. Alderman is the consummate physician in her desire to get to the root cause of a patient's problems.

In 2008, Dr. Alderman utilized her interest in Prolotherapy in a most important way by putting her knowledge into the first edition of her book, *Free Yourself from Chronic Pain and Sports Injuries*. In this expanded and updated second edition, she again explains in easy-to-understand language the central tenets of Prolotherapy, as well as why connective tissue (ligament and tendon) weakness is the most common cause of chronic musculoskeletal pain, why these structures don't always heal organically, and how Prolotherapy can strengthen them. She goes on to explain the newest technology and how advanced formulas such as platelet-rich plasma, adipose (fat), and bone marrow concentrates are being used to take on more severe cases of chronic pain and joint degeneration. As a leader in the field, Dr. Alderman shares her expertise in explaining how even bone-on-bone osteoarthritis can be helped with these advanced Prolotherapy injections. Dr. Alderman explains how, with the use of modern diagnostic musculoskeletal ultrasound, a physician can more effectively diagnose and then guide these Prolotherapy formulas to their target locations.

This new edition has many updated illustrations that make it very user-friendly for both patients and physicians who are interested in the regenerative medicine field. You do not need to know anything about medicine to read Dr. Alderman's book. She understands that as people search the Internet in the hope of finding a solution for their musculoskeletal pain, they will need resources. One of the best resources they will find is this book. Dr. Alderman accomplishes her goal of making an accessible, yet thorough, reference work that explains the regenerative power of Dextrose, as well as the advanced formulas of Platelet-Rich Plasma, and Biocellular (Stem Cell–Rich) Prolotherapy. The advanced formulas enhance the healing power of Prolotherapy by directly injecting platelets, which contain repair-stimulating growth factors, and/or stem cell sources such as fat and bone marrow, which have the potential to regenerate cartilage, labrum, and meniscal cells, into injured tissues that are often depleted in advanced degenerative joint disease cases. Dr. Alderman has found great success using these formulas, even in cases where patients were told that surgery or joint replacement was their only option.

Do you have musculoskeletal or joint pain and want to be free of it? What are you going to do? Dr. Alderman puts it best when she says, "You may not have chosen to be in a motor vehicle accident that left you with years of neck and back pain, or to twist an ankle while playing basketball that never quite healed. *But you can choose what to do about it.*"

It is my hope that by reading this book you will come to the same conclusion as Dr. Alderman. She has learned, as you will by reading her book, that there is a way to set yourself free from chronic musculoskeletal and joint pain, and that way is Prolotherapy Regenerative Medicine.

PREFACE

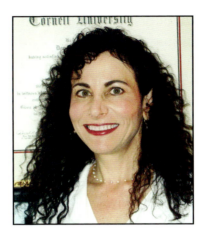

Donna D. Alderman, D.O.

Musculoskeletal pain is the most common medical complaint in the United States, as well as one of the most frequent reasons for primary care physician visits. In fact, the American Academy of Orthopaedic Surgeons estimates that one in two adults is affected by a musculoskeletal condition. That's over 126 million people in the United States alone! Injury and pain related to regular physical activity is a common occurrence, as are sports-related injuries, both causing ligament, tendon or muscle sprains, strains, tears and other joint injury. Osteoarthritis is also a major health issue and the most frequent joint disease. Unfortunately, the typical medical recommendations for these conditions may not always be effective, and often they have unwanted side effects. In some cases, surgery is considered, but that too may not always be effective—while also posing additional risk. In fact, today, many surgeons themselves are questioning whether surgery is necessarily always the best option for these conditions.

Clearly, there is a need for a safe and effective non-surgical treatment for musculoskeletal pain and osteoarthritis. Fortunately, we live in an age of possibilities where medicine is ever evolving and advancing. In the 1930s, forward-thinking physicians discovered that injections of natural, but irritating, substances to injured joint areas can stimulate the body's ability to heal these sites, reducing or eliminating pain. This procedure was named Prolotherapy, short for "proliferation therapy," because of its ability to stimulate the growth (proliferation) of new tissue.

Since the first edition of this book over ten years ago, there have been remarkable advances in Prolotherapy methods and technology. In addition to treatments involving traditional natural formulas, we have seen extensive positive results from using biologically active formulas such as platelet-rich plasma and/or adult stem cell sources taken from a patient's own body. With the increased use of these more advanced formulas, Prolotherapy has evolved into "Prolotherapy Regenerative Medicine." In this book, unless a particular formula is specified, the terms *Prolotherapy* and *Prolotherapy Regenerative Medicine* are used interchangeably to include all available formulas. Another huge development in the field is advancements in ultrasound imaging technology, resulting in increased use and availability of portable, high-resolution machines.

This means a doctor can use these machines in his/her office to almost immediately see what's going on in painful ligaments, tendons, and joints. This advancement not only improves diagnosis; ultrasound guidance can also help the doctor accurately place injections, improving results.

A modern version of the Hippocratic Oath states, "I will respect the hard-won scientific gains of those physicians in whose steps I walk, and gladly share such knowledge." My hope is to not only share this information but also "translate" scientific verbiage into easy-to-understand concepts so that anyone can grasp how and why Prolotherapy works. Thanks to the Internet, where a vast amount of information is available at one's fingertips, our society has shifted from one in which patients are dependent solely on their doctor's opinion to one in which patients can do their own research and take a more active role in making decisions about their medical treatments. The more patients know about their options, the better equipped they are to make informed choices. That is the purpose of this book: to provide the information to help you make the informed choice that's right for you. Like any medical approach, Prolotherapy is not for everyone, or for every condition. However, it has helped hundreds of thousands of people who might otherwise still be in pain.

ACKNOWLEDGMENTS

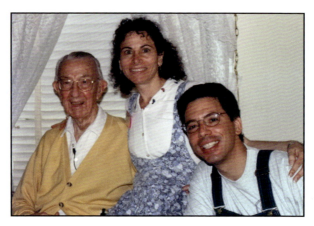

Dr. Alderman (center) with Dr. Gustav Hemwall (left) and Dr. Ross Hauser (right) at the First Annual Prolotherapy Injection Seminar in Thebes, Illinois, 1998

In the early 1990s, when I first heard about Prolotherapy, I thought, "This is too good to be true—a natural, nonsurgical treatment for musculoskeletal pain!" I discovered it *was* true, but little did I know, it would become my life's mission to learn about, practice and teach Prolotherapy, as well as to advance it into the new millennium. Had it not been for my instructors and colleagues in Prolotherapy, I would not have made it to this point. I want to thank Ross Hauser, M.D., who has always shared generously of his time and expertise, and who has contributed immensely to the field by way of his books for the general public, starting with *Prolo Your Pain Away!* and his many online videos to educate patients (even before there was YouTube!). I also want to acknowledge Jeffrey Patterson, D.O., who dedicated his life to forwarding Prolotherapy through his work at the

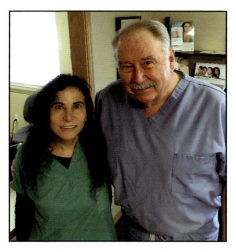

Dr. Alderman (left) and Dr. Robert Alexander (right),
Stevensville, Montana, 2015

University of Wisconsin School of Medicine and the
Hackett Hemwall Patterson Foundation until his
untimely passing in 2014. Other acknowledgments go
to William Faber, D.O., who, in 1990 wrote *Pain, Pain,
Go Away*, as well as Tom Raven, M.D.; Mark Cantieri,
D.O.; and George Pasquarello, D.O., who for years faith-
fully instructed the Prolotherapy course given at the
campus of the University of New England College of
Osteopathic Medicine, and who collectively authored
the first color Prolotherapy injection textbook for physicians. And last but not least, I want to thank Robert
Alexander, M.D., who has become a cherished friend
and mentor after I showed up in his Montana office
many years ago asking him to please "teach me stem
cell"—and that he did! I could not have wished for a
better, kinder, or more intelligent colleague to bring
me to the next level in my understanding of stimulated
healing.

PART I: BACKGROUND

Imagination is more important than knowledge.
Knowledge is limited. Imagination encircles the world.

—Albert Einstein

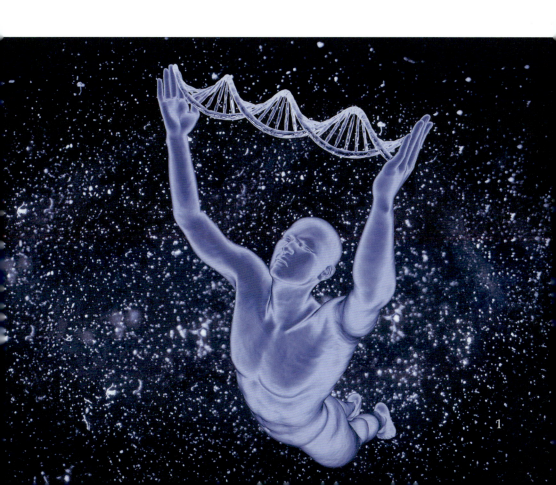

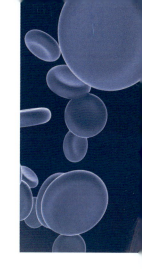

CHAPTER 1

The Exciting Possibilities of Regenerative Medicine

Years ago, a friend told me a story about his coworker, a woman named Sally. Sally had a 2-year-old son whom she brought with her to the office from time to time. My friend described this child as a "monster," always in a terrible, mean mood, smashing things, and continually screaming and crying. This went on for some time, with Sally regularly apologizing for her child's poor behavior, until one day when her child arrived at the office happy, well-behaved, and affectionate. Surprised by this dramatic change, my friend asked Sally, "What happened?" As it turned out, her son had been suffering from a very severe, but hidden, ear infection that had been going on for months. The doctor said it was the worst ear infection he had ever seen, almost resulting in hearing loss. Although Sally and her son had seen several other doctors over the previous months, delays in diagnosis or ineffective treatments had continued until this infection was finally found and successfully treated. Once the infection was resolved, and the continual pain this poor child had been experiencing was gone, his true personality was restored—a personality not even his mother knew at that point—and both he and his mother got their lives back. This is what can happen to an individual in chronic pain. Indeed, chronic musculoskeletal pain can be nagging, continual, and exhausting to the individual and his/her family. It was summed up best by a patient who told me, "Being in chronic pain is worse than being in prison; at least in prison you have a parole date." For the person with musculoskeletal pain, often many doctors have been consulted, but ineffective or only temporary solutions given, or no diagnosis is found, and the problem continues. Fortunately, Prolotherapy, and the exciting field of regenerative medicine, can often help.

What exactly is "regenerative medicine"? This term applies to a branch of medicine that focuses on ways to, repair, replace, or regenerate damaged human tissue. Prolotherapy is a regenerative medicine technique used to stimulate the repair of painful ligaments, tendons, and joints, including osteoarthritis and sports injuries. This technique has been around for many years, since before the term "regenerative medicine" even existed, and has a very interesting history (discussed in more detail in Chapter 3: "The History of Prolotherapy Regenerative Medicine"). Prolotherapy has advanced over the years and now includes the use of one's own blood platelets (high in growth factors) and/or stem cell–rich tissue as treatment formulas, further enhancing its remarkable ability to stimulate repair, reducing or eliminating pain.

I believe this is just the beginning and that some-day injuries or painful joint conditions will be rou-tinely treated with regenerative techniques as a first treatment. Imagine the possibilities this offers. Almost everyone has heard of, or knows, a person complaining about a "football injury" sustained years ago in high school or college. What if these types of injuries were treated immediately with regenerative techniques, and encouraged to fully heal from the get-go? Of course, years later, these injuries can often still be helped to heal "retroactively" with Prolotherapy; however, early inter-vention would avoid years of pain and suffering, and prevent structural changes or additional injury to other compensating joints. The use of one's blood or stem cell–rich tissue is an exciting possibility, which not only stimulates healing, but when used early in an injury encourages it to heal potentially *without* scar tissue![1] Times are changing; the age of regenerative medicine is here. While we are not there yet, treatment pathways are changing towards regenerative approaches. Just as antibiotics revolutionized the way infections could be treated, regenerative medicine is destined to change the long-term outcomes of painful injuries, improving the quality and length of our active lives.

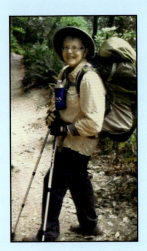

Government Employee

My first date with my husband, 25 years ago, was a lovely day hike in the Berkeley Hills. Our wedding vows two years later were, "Grow old along with me! The best is yet to be," from a poem by Robert Browning. Our intention was to hike into our 80s. This would turn out to be a challenge for me.

I have a long history of low back and knee injuries. At age 16, I threw out my right knee doing the twist. At 21, I threw out both knees landing my first parachute jump. At 24, I had to stop taking ballet lessons due to chronic back pain, which continued and worsened with age. By 40, I suffered from major back spasms, which made it difficult to even go to the bathroom in the morning. Some back seizures put me in bed for a week at a time. Over the years, I tried everything: acupuncture, chiropractic treatments, daily back exercises, months of physical therapy, hypnosis, reading John Sarno's *Healing Back Pain: The Mind-Body Connection*, massage, yoga, tai chi. You name it, I tried it. Some helped a little, some temporarily, but the pain and spasms continued.

I heard about Prolotherapy through a friend who'd had positive results after two failed surgeries for carpal tunnel syndrome. I had my first Prolotherapy when I was in my mid-50s, Dextrose Prolotherapy on my low back. I experienced immediate relief from my back spasms. After a short course of treatment, I was pain free and able to resume the active life I enjoyed.

Ten years later, my knee began to bother me, and an MRI confirmed a torn meniscus. I was scheduled for surgery, but really wanted to avoid that if possible. I decided to receive Biocellular (Stem Cell–Rich) Prolotherapy on my knee. Five weeks later, I was in Aspen on a week's vacation, hiking five to ten miles a day, pain free.

At the time of this writing, two years after my knee treatment, at age 66, I am still pain free and going strong. And I've taken up backpacking!

Mary Alice Lynch
Government Employee

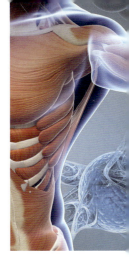

CHAPTER 2

Osteopathic Medicine and What Is a D.O.?

B efore going further, I want to address a question I have been asked at times during my career: "What is a D.O.?" Many people have heard or seen this abbreviation used, but may not fully understand what it is, or how it differs from an M.D..

D.O. versus M.D.

There are two types of fully licensed medical doctors in the United States: one receives an M.D. degree, "doctor of medicine," and the other receives a D.O. degree, "doctor of osteopathic medicine." The licenses to practice medicine held by both are legally and professionally equivalent.[1] Medical school education for M.D.s and D.O.s is also similar: both receive training in anatomy, physiology (how the body functions), pharmacology (prescribing medication), basic medicine, and surgery. After basic medical training is completed, both D.O.s and M.D.s can choose to become, for instance, a dermatologist, surgeon, pediatrician, gynecologist—essentially a practitioner of any specialty. The difference lies in the fact that D.O. medical schools require additional training hours in the musculoskeletal system, physical medicine, and osteopathic philosophical principles. To get a deeper sense of what that involves, let's take a look at both the philosophy of osteopathic medicine and the history of medicine in this country.

THE EVOLUTION OF OSTEOPATHIC MEDICINE IN THE UNITED STATES

In the early 1800s, modern medicine was in its infancy and, in some ways, barbaric. Medical doctors readily employed "treatments" that at best didn't help and at worst did great harm. For example, to treat many conditions, including fevers, doctors employed "bloodletting," opening a vein and letting it bleed to allow disease to "escape the body"—often with detrimental results. Other medical mainstays involved arsenic, lead, and mercury—all of which we now know to be poisonous. Sadly, one M.D. practicing in the mid-1800s, Dr. Andrew Taylor Still, watched helplessly as two of his young children died of meningitis. This traumatic event was a turning point for him in working toward a "better way" to treat and prevent disease. For the next ten years, he studied the human body and developed a philosophy of healing.

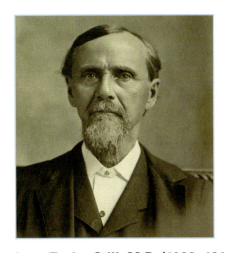

Andrew Taylor Still, M.D. (1828–1917)

Photo courtesy of Museum of Osteopathic Medicine, Kirksville, MO [2010.87.37]

Dr. Still's philosophy was both simple and profound: "To find health should be the object of the doctor. Anyone can find disease."[2] In addition to being a critic of the day's therapeutic "remedies," Dr. Still was also a forward thinker and realized that improvements in health care were greatly needed. He believed that the physician's role was not to just dictatorially prescribe remedies, but to help the patient reach a healthier condition. To enhance the body's natural healing ability, Dr. Still stressed preventive medicine, good nutrition, and exercise, as well as the importance of a properly functioning musculoskeletal system—a major component of the human body. He introduced techniques to improve blood flow and musculoskeletal balance, which included correcting the alignment of bones. This system of treating the musculoskeletal system led to the use of the term osteopathic, from the Greek osteo, meaning "bone," and the Latin pathic, meaning "suffering."

Dr. Still established these osteopathic principles in 1874 and implemented them into his own practice. He emphasized that the goal of the osteopathic profession was "to improve and advance our present systems of surgery, obstetrics, and treatment of general diseases to a more satisfactory position than they now hold."[3] In 1892, Dr. Still founded the first osteopathic medical college, the American School of Osteopathy, in Kirksville, Missouri. By then, general medical knowledge had made large strides forward with the development of the germ theory of disease, which was incorporated into osteopathic medical education. Later, in the early 1900s, the discovery and use of antibiotics was also integrated into standard osteopathic medical training, as were continued advancements in surgical and medical science over the ensuing years. Today, the medical education of D.O.s and M.D.s are considered to be equivalent, except that D.O. medical students continue to receive extra training in the musculoskeletal system, osteopathic physical medicine techniques and osteopathic philosophy.

THE OSTEOPATHIC PROFESSION IN CALIFORNIA

While I was a medical student in California, I traveled to the Midwest one summer for a special medical rotation. While there, I noticed several osteopathic hospitals, and a better understanding by the general public of what a D.O. is than I had observed in California.

The reason for this, I discovered, was because of a political event that occurred in California in the 1960s. By then, the standards of practice for D.O.s and M.D.s had grown very close together. Indeed, medical residency programs had long been mixed, with D.O.s and M.D.s studying and working side by side. With sentiment increasing that the two professions should unite, M.D.s and D.O.s constructed an agreement whereby, for a minimal fee, a D.O. could trade in his/her D.O. diploma for an M.D. diploma. Existing California osteopathic medical students also received an M.D. degree upon graduation, rather than the D.O. degree. As a result, thousands of D.O.s simply "vanished" behind M.D. degrees. While this might have simplified some aspects of health care, it was a step backward for the osteopathic profession in California.

Fortunately, in 1974, this California merger was reversed, and the osteopathic profession once again became visible in California.[4] Then, in 1977, a new osteopathic medical school, the College of Osteopathic Medicine of the Pacific, opened in Pomona, California. This top-notch osteopathic medical school is now included within the expanded Western University of Health Sciences, which also includes colleges of pharmacy, optometry, dentistry, podiatry, veterinary medicine, graduate nursing, and graduate biomedical science, as well as allied health professions for physical therapy, physician's assistant studies, and health professions education—all embraced within the osteopathic umbrella. Because of this, and the subsequent opening of other osteopathic medical schools in the Western states, many more patients are now aware of the osteopathic difference and its unique approach to health care. I chose to study osteopathic medicine because it aligns with my own concept of the art of medicine, where the doctor and patient work together toward the common goal of excellent health. Being an osteopathic physician has also given me tremendous insight into the musculoskeletal system and regenerative medicine, which ultimately led me to Prolotherapy.

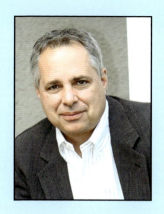

Architect

I am 57 years old, and have been a very active, athletic person all my life. I worked heavy construction for many years before becoming an architect as well as played sports, mostly basketball. By the time I reached my early 50s, a mere three hours per week of basketball caught up to me, and my knees became so painful, I couldn't play. Or if I did, I would be so sore for days that I could not walk without terrible pain.

I heard about Prolotherapy and thought the concept was simple, yet brilliant: trick the body into going into healing mode and then give it building blocks to assist in the process. Still, I saw medical treatments as most men do (as a last resort!), and I thought I would just wait it out instead. But then I tore a hamstring muscle so badly I went on an official "injured list." This was five years ago, when I was 52. Since I was now going to be out a while, I decided I would take the time to check out Prolotherapy.

After an evaluation, and an ultrasound that determined my hamstring was torn and I had osteoarthritis in my knees, the option of either Platelet Rich Plasma (PRP) or Biocellular (Stem–Cell Rich) Prolotherapy was recommended. I preferred the more aggressive treatment, using the stem cell source from my fat. I figured, if I was going to do this, I would rather go all out, so I had a Biocellular treatment done on my hamstring and knees. Instantly, I knew something was different—better. I wasn't immediately walking any better, but something in my gut told me this was working. I was a believer right then. In a week, I could jump without pain. Though I waited five weeks to start playing basketball again, I felt good enough to play in only three. I can't say I enjoyed the Prolotherapy treatment, but it didn't really hurt—I simply didn't like the idea of shots! However, the results have been life changing, and five years later, I am still going strong.

Since my original treatments, I have had Prolotherapy done on a few more areas: my neck and my plantar fascia. After one treatment of Dextrose Prolotherapy, the neck pain was gone and hasn't come back. Also, while playing basketball, I injured my foot, tearing my plantar fascia so severely it stopped me in my tracks; I could see bruising as well as blood pooling at the bottom of my foot. My regular doctor told me I could wait or have surgery, but with that type of injury, it could take months, if not years, to heal, and would form scar tissue and be weaker. Instead, I tried Biocellular Prolotherapy within a few days of the injury—the idea being that putting repair stem cells there would allow it to heal normally without scarring. I had a treatment; five weeks later, I was playing basketball again, and I have been pain free ever since.

Without Prolotherapy, I would have had to reduce my level of activity to merely walking, with no sports. Though I realize I am getting older, I am just not ready to act old. These treatments have kept me active and young.

Curt V. Schultz
Architect

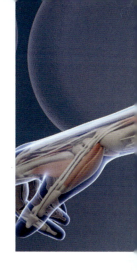

CHAPTER 3

The History of Prolotherapy Regenerative Medicine

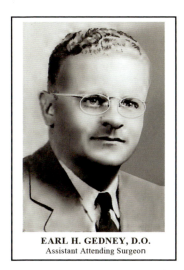

EARL H. GEDNEY, D.O.
Assistant Attending Surgeon

Photo from 1936 yearbook, Philadelphia College of
Osteopathic Medicine, courtesy of Special Collections Library

Prolotherapy was born from the work of several forward-thinking physicians, beginning in the 1930s. The earliest report of its use was around 1936 when Earl Gedney, D.O., a general surgeon at the Philadelphia College of Osteopathic Medicine, caught his thumb in closing operating room doors, which badly stretched that joint. After suffering several months of thumb pain and instability, colleagues told him nothing else could be done. He was advised to just "live with it" and to change professions since that injury prevented him from working effectively as a surgeon. However, Gedney was not of the mind-set to agree with this, so he started thinking outside the box and researching other options.

He remembered attending a lecture about using irritating solutions to treat abdominal hernias (a hernia is a muscle tear resulting in an opening or defect). In the 1930s, the risks associated with surgery were high, and so a nonsurgical approach to hernia repair was quite popular. Gedney knew about a group of physicians, called "herniologists," who had been using a nonsurgical technique for years. The idea behind the herniologists' treatment was that injections of irritating substances at the hernia muscular opening stimulated repair and the formation of thicker, denser tissue that closed this defect. These irritating solutions were said to cause "sclerosing" (thickening or hardening), and the technique was called "hernia sclerotherapy." The first organization devoted to hernia repair using this method was formed in 1923, and by the early 1930s, such procedures were widely accepted as very effective in the treatment of hernias.

THE LEAP TO JOINT PROLOTHERAPY

Gedney applied this knowledge of nonsurgical hernia repair to the nonsurgical repair of joints, ligaments, and tendons (connective tissue). He concluded that ligament or tendon injury around a joint causes instability, which then results in pain and weakness. He reasoned that if instability could be improved by strengthening the joint connective tissue—similar to what was being done with hernia defects—increased stability and decreased pain would result. Figuring that he had little to lose by being a guinea pig for his own theory, he started injecting his thumb with these irritating solutions. The effect was dramatically successful. Before long, he was back working as a surgeon. Excited about his results, he began a lifelong career of exploring this technique, which he named "joint sclerotherapy."

In June 1937, Gedney published the first journal article on the topic titled "Special Technique: Hypermobile Joint, a Preliminary Report." His article included a protocol and two patient treatment reports—one for knee pain and the other for low back pain—both successfully treated with this technique.[1] The next year, Gedney gave a presentation at the meeting of the Osteopathic Clinical Society of Philadelphia, where he outlined the theory of using irritating solutions to heal stretched, painful ligaments, tendons, and joints. He started working with different treatment solutions and perfecting this method with a colleague, David Shuman, D.O.. Both men began using it in the treatment of unstable joints, especially knees, lumbar spines, and sacroiliac joints. In 1949, Shuman published an article in the *Osteopathic Profession* titled "Sclerotherapy: Injections May Be Best Way to Restrengthen Ligaments in Case of Slipped Knee Cartilage."[2] Both Gedney and Shuman continued to do research and publish reports throughout the 1950s and '60s. They studied the microscopic effects of various formulas on ligaments and tendons to establish workable protocols for different joint treatment areas. They also traveled to medical centers and physician groups to discuss and demonstrate injections.

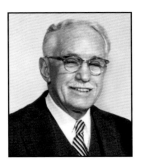

George S. Hackett, M.D. (1888–1969)

During this same time period, George Hackett, M.D., a trauma surgeon, made an interesting observation while performing surgery on patients who had previously received sclerosing treatment for muscular abdominal hernias. When done properly, the sclerosing solutions would have been placed only into the muscular defect; however, sometimes the solution was inadvertently placed deeper, at the junction of the ligament and bone. During his surgeries, Hackett noted this and is quoted as saying, "Injections made (in error) at the junction of ligament and bone resulted in profuse proliferation of new tissue at this union."[3]

In 1939, after 20 years of patient care, Hackett concluded that low back pain had a strong relationship to weakened (relaxed/stretched) spinal ligaments.[4] He proposed that injections of proliferating solutions could help strengthen weakened ligaments or tendons, and coined the word prolotherapy, short for "proliferation therapy" because of the treatment's ability to stimulate repair and "proliferation" (growth) of new tissue at joint injury sites. In 1956, he published the first formal physician's textbook on the subject titled: *Ligament and Tendon Relaxation Treated by Prolotherapy.* Hackett is also known for the statement, "A joint is only as strong as its weakest ligament."

Hackett, like other pioneers of Prolotherapy, went on to teach these techniques to fellow physicians, including Gustav Hemwall, a family physician in Illinois. (The two men appear together in the following photograph from the Minneapolis Morning Tribune.)

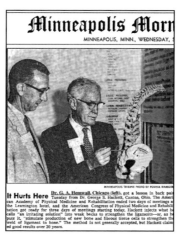

Minneapolis Tribune photo taken at the American Congress of Physical Medicine and Rehabilitation annual meeting in Minneapolis, Minnesota, in the 1960s

(Photo courtesy of Ross A. Hauser, M.D., Caringmedical.com)

It is interesting that in 1937, an article by another physician, Louis Schwartz, appeared in the *Journal of the American Medical Association,* reporting on the successful treatment of temporomandibular joint instability (TMJ: a joint in the jaw), using a proliferant solution.[5] There is no evidence of direct collaboration between these different groups of doctors, so it would appear that all these physicians arrived at the same conclusion independently: Prolotherapy had the potential to resolve joint instability and pain.

Books directed towards educating the general public started emerging in 1960 when David Shuman published the first layperson's book on joint Prolotherapy entitled *Your Aching Back and What You Can Do About It.* Then, in 1990, William Faber, D.O., and Morton Walker, D.P.M, published *Pain, Pain, Go Away.* In 1998, Ross Hauser, M.D., a protégé of Dr. Hemwall, began publishing multiple books, starting with *Prolo Your Pain Away!* In writing the preface to that book's first edition, C. Everett Koop, M.D., the former United States Surgeon General, publicly endorsed Prolotherapy as a viable, effective treatment of ligament, tendon, and joint injuries.[6]

PHYSICIAN EDUCATION

Formal, large-scale physician education began in 1954 with the creation of the American Osteopathic College of Sclerotherapy. In 1956, this group became recognized and chartered by the American Osteopathic Association (AOA), and offered the first official training for Prolotherapy techniques. This AOA affiliate group is known today as the American Osteopathic Association of Prolotherapy Regenerative Medicine (AOAPRM). Other groups, such as the Hackett Hemwall Patterson Foundation and the American Association of Orthopedic Medicine (AAOM), also continue to educate physicians in traditional as well as newer forms of Prolotherapy. The collective knowledge of 80 years of outside the box, creative thinking in how to stimulate healing has resulted in modern-day Prolotherapy Regenerative Medicine. It is likely that the original pioneers of Prolotherapy—Drs. Gedney, Shuman, Hackett, Schwartz, and Hemwall—would be truly amazed and proud of how far this amazing therapy has come.

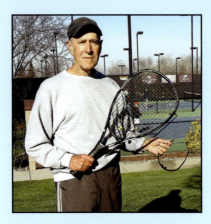

Tennis Player

About six years ago, I was told I needed a shoulder replacement. I had played tennis several days a week for 35-plus years and prior to that had spent many years pitching baseball. In short, I had worn out my left shoulder and had several things wrong with my right shoulder as well. On a scale of one to ten, where ten is the worst, the pain in my left shoulder was almost constantly a nine with any use, and my range of motion was reduced to about only 10 to 20 percent of normal. So I put myself on the waiting list to have the replacement surgery. In the meantime, I decided to try Prolotherapy.

After five PRP Prolotherapy treatments on my left shoulder, spread out over eight months, I was pretty much pain free, with my range of motion back to 98 percent. Since then, I have continued to improve. I have gone back to playing tennis and am enjoying the game more than I did before. It has now been over four years since my last PRP Prolotherapy treatment, and I am still pain free and doing well!

I am grateful for Prolotherapy. It allowed me to play tennis again and avoid shoulder replacement surgery. That is remarkable, especially given the severity of my injury and long-term damage to my shoulder.

Richard Vizzusi
Tennis Player

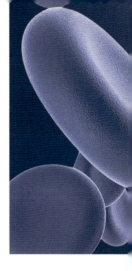

CHAPTER 4

Why Don't More Doctors Know About Prolotherapy?

In 1998, at the First Annual Prolotherapy Injection Seminar, given in Thebes, Illinois, one of the attending student physicians quite abruptly, and with clear skepticism, asked Dr. Gustav Hemwall, the world's most experienced Prolotherapist at the time, "If Prolotherapy is so great, why don't more doctors know about it?" Dr. Hemwall paused a moment and then calmly answered, "Because it's too simple."

I was the brash young doctor who asked that question back then, and, ironically, now I am asked the same question—though, I'm glad to say, not as often as when the first edition of this book was published in 2008. Since then, more and more doctors have been finding out about Prolotherapy, especially the more advanced forms such as platelet-rich plasma or stem cell–rich formulas. Nowadays, there is increased public awareness about regenerative approaches to healing, as well as many more training seminars and conferences. In fact, I have given many lectures to physician groups over the last ten years, and there is a huge interest in these therapies. In addition, some medical schools now give lectures on Prolotherapy, and some residency programs educate doctors in these techniques. Nevertheless, some physicians still don't know about Prolotherapy— or they don't understand how it works—and so dismiss its validity.

A patient of mine who'd experienced great results from Biocellular Prolotherapy on his knee told me he'd shared his excitement with a family friend, who happened to be a physician. The physician family member then proceeded to "pooh-pooh" the technique, saying that no studies demonstrated its effectiveness and that the only reason it had worked was because of the placebo effect. My patient shared with me how dismayed he felt about the doctor's dismissiveness. I explained that since Prolotherapy is not generally taught in medical schools, some doctors assume that no medical evidence supports it, which is simply not true, as Chapter 8: "Prolotherapy Regenerative Medicine Is Evidence Based" and the "Bibliography of Medical Studies, Research Articles, and Books regarding Prolotherapy Regenerative Medicine" in the appendix of this book vividly convey. As for the placebo effect, though it does exist in human medicine, Dextrose, PRP, and Biocellular Prolotherapy treatments have all been conducted on animals with excellent results. Although there is some controversy about the placebo effect in animals, most scientists generally agree that animals do not experience this phenomena since animals have no expectation with treatment. (If Tali, a playful Australian shepherd mix could speak, she'd attest to how effectively PRP and Biocellular Prolotherapy treated her front paws; see her story, immediately following this section).

Skepticism is healthy, especially in science and medicine. As noted earlier, I myself was skeptical when I first learned about Prolotherapy. That's why education and getting the facts and evidence is so important before drawing a conclusion. Understanding the scientific concepts, reviewing the medical literature, and hearing from reputable sources about the outcomes of a particular treatment is, in my opinion, the best way to decide on a treatment's validity. My goal with this book is to educate and inform by sharing scientific theories, concepts, and evidence. Parts of the book may be on the dry side, but I have tried to make it interesting and informative with drawings, combined with personal patient stories. My hope is that by the end of this book, you will reach your own conclusion about whether this is a therapy you wish to pursue, or not, in your journey towards becoming pain free.

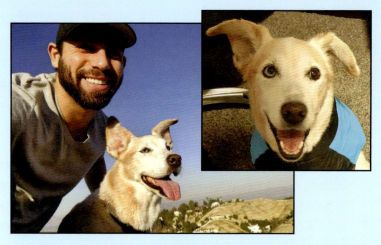

Tali, an active dog, now age 13, seen here
with her owner, Aaron Comis, after a hike

Active Dog

Tali is my very playful and happy Australian shepherd mix. In 2011, when Tali was just six years old, and I was still in college, Tali injured her right knee while playing with another dog. She began limping and was unable to put any weight on her right front paw. She just sat in the corner whimpering, looking unhappy and in pain. It was very sad for me to watch. Tali's veterinarian said she had ruptured her right knee ligament (equivalent in the human to the anterior cruciate ligament), which is common in this type of dog, and she would need major surgery if medication and rest didn't help.

We tried eight weeks of rest and anti-inflammatory medications, but Tali only got worse. I then asked my aunt Donna (Alderman) if she would be willing to treat Tali with PRP Prolotherapy since she had been doing this therapy successfully in humans for many years. In coordination with my veterinarian, Aunt Donna did PRP Prolotherapy on Tali's right knee. After a brief recovery, Tali began to put weight on her right paw again. Soon she was walking and then running—without a limp! This was just eight weeks after the

PRP Prolotherapy treatment. Tali recovered fully, became her old active self again, and never had another problem with that leg.

About a year later, a similar incident occurred with the other leg (left knee), and Tali was limping again. (The right knee, previously treated, was still doing well.) So once again, I asked Aunt Donna to help. She suggested we do Biocellular (Stem Cell–Rich) Prolotherapy on Tali's new injury using adipose from Tali's abdominal fat pad. Again, in conjunction with my veterinarian, Aunt Donna did the Biocellular treatment to Tali's left knee and also put a little into Tali's right knee so that they'd be equally treated. After a couple of months, Tali had fully recovered. That was almost seven years ago, and Tali has never had any other issues with either of her knees since; she is now 13 years old and as active as ever! We have gone on many hikes, often to the tops of heavy trails, as in the picture above, a recent trek running to the top of a mountain trail. Tali never hesitates to use her knees—running, jumping, and being happy as ever. I am a believer in this treatment because animals do not experience the placebo effect; I know there is really something to this. This treatment saved Tali, and both Tali and I are truly grateful.

Aaron Comis
NASA Engineer for Space Exploration
(on behalf of Tali Alderman-Comis)

PART II: THE SCIENCE

Nothing in life is to be feared,
it is only to be understood.
Now is the time to understand more,
so that we may fear less.

—Marie ("Madam") Curie
Scientist awarded the Nobel prize for her
pioneering research into radiation/X-ray

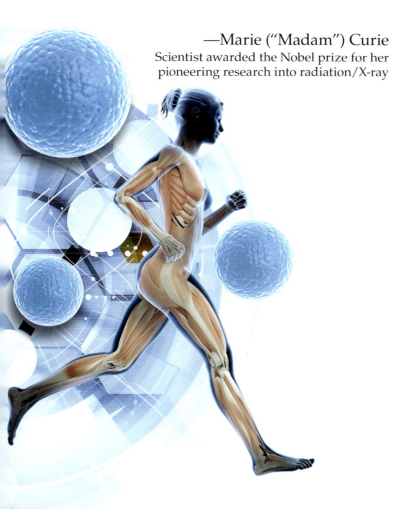

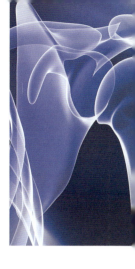

CHAPTER 5

Prolotherapy Basics

Prolotherapy is based on a very simple principle: *the body has the capacity to heal itself.* Let's say you get a paper cut. You first notice there is a rip in your skin and a little blood. Then the wound stops bleeding; it gets a little red and sore, but within a few days, it has healed. This example illustrates a stimulus-response system: you injure yourself (stimulus), which sets in motion a cascade of actions that result in healing (response). A healthy body routinely and automatically responds in this way—like a computer with "healing programs" installed.

With musculoskeletal and joint injuries, a similar "stimulus-response" process occurs. However, the healing time is much longer than with a simple paper cut, lasting weeks to months rather than days. Another difference is that, even for a healthy person, the body tends not to heal 100 percent from ligament, tendon, and joint injuries. In fact, it has been estimated that the usual best result of a ligament or tendon (connective tissue) repair cycle may be as little as 50 to 60 percent of preinjury strength.[1] The reasons for this will be discussed later in this chapter. To understand how Prolotherapy can help heal such unresolved injuries, it is important to understand some basics about the musculoskeletal system. Although my "Prolotherapy 101" may seem almost too simple, I have found that these basic concepts are often overlooked. Once grasped, the rest makes much more sense, so that is where I will start.

PROLOTHERAPY 101

Look at the diagram of the shoulder joint in Figure 5.1. Locate the red muscle on the arm. The whitish portion of the muscle is the *tendon*; it attaches muscles to bones. Notice that bones are connected to other bones by *ligaments*, which, like tendons, are composed of strong collagen fibers and are whitish in color. Ligaments and tendons are known as "connective tissue" because they connect the body's framework of bones, providing stability and allowing for motion.

Looking again at this picture, answer these basic questions:

> *Question:* Why do you think muscles appear red in color, while ligaments and tendons appear whitish? (If you're not sure, consider this: What might make muscles appear red?)
>
> *Answer:* Blood!

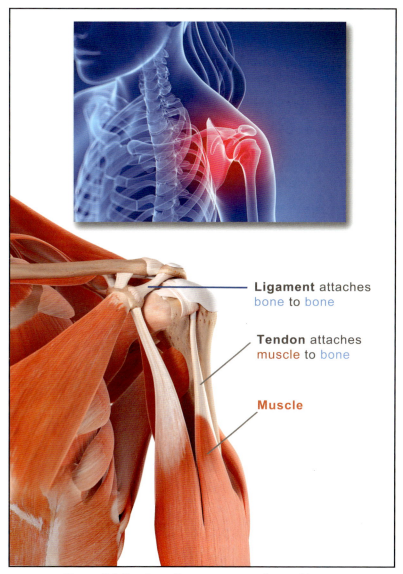

Figure 5.1: Tendons, ligaments, muscles and bones

Your body needs blood to heal. Blood brings oxygen, nutrition, healing factors, and cells to injured areas. Unfortunately, there is only a very small blood supply in ligaments and tendons, hence their whitish color. This also explains why a ligament or tendon injury takes a longer time to heal, once injured, than other areas of the body.

> *QUESTION:* Imagine someone has badly twisted and sprained his/her ankle (a sprain is overstretching or tearing of a ligament). What does that ankle look like an hour after being sprained?

> *ANSWER:* Swollen! You may even recall this happening if you have ever sprained an ankle. This is the body's immediate response to a ligament injury. A signal is sent to the brain: "Send blood!," since the ligament doesn't have much and needs it to heal. This injury has created a "stimulus," which then starts the "response" of healing. The body immediately tries to get blood to the area as a first response to begin repair, thus the swelling. This is also known as a "good inflammation."

CONNECTIVE TISSUE HEALS SLOWLY

Even under the best of circumstances, proper rest and good nutrition, ligaments and tendons heal slowly, and often incompletely. A typical ligament or tendon injury can take four to six weeks to heal, with most of the healing occurring in the first two weeks. You can probably recall someone being on crutches or hobbling around for several weeks after a bad ankle sprain. Unfortunately, after four to six weeks, the body's stimulus to heal diminishes significantly. In other words, if healing does not occur within the first four to six weeks after an injury, not much additional healing is likely to occur later, because the stimulus to heal is now so weak or gone. Even if an injury heals reasonably during the four to six week healing period afterwards, there is a risk that it may not return to 100 percent of where it was.[2] If connective tissue does not heal completely—even if healing is only at 95 percent rather than 100 percent—the joint becomes a little weaker and therefore more predisposed to another injury. Initially, the individual may not notice this small difference. However, injury to the same joint, followed by that joint's failure to heal completely, may occur over and over again, each time reducing the area's overall strength and stability. It can go from 100 percent to 95 percent, to 90 percent to 80 percent, etc., with repeated injuries. Each time this occurs, the ligaments and/or tendons become a little more injured and stretched, also known as "laxity." A person may experience this laxity as weakness or instability in the joint—and eventually as pain. If this happens enough times, or is severe enough, weakness, instability, and/or pain can become chronic, meaning the pain or instability does not go away even after several weeks. Note that injuries may be "acute," meaning occurring suddenly with rapid progression, and then improve after going through a healing period of six weeks. These injuries can also become "chronic," meaning if healing is incomplete, or there are repeated acute injuries that do not heal completely, the pain may not go away. Note that the medical definition of chronic is "persistent or long lasting," usually more than three months.[3]

Even disc herniations have been linked to connective tissue weakness. As early as 1952, Dr. P. H. Newman, a British surgeon with years of experience performing disc operations, concluded that torn or weakened ligaments around the spine **preceded** disc herniations, sometimes years in advance.[4] Dr. Newman believed the most common cause of chronic low back pain was strain in the spine area where ligaments had been weakened.[5]

THE VICIOUS CYCLE OF CONNECTIVE TISSUE INJURY

Ligaments and tendons are connective tissue composed of fibers—including collagen, a very strong protein—the purpose of which is primarily to provide strength to the joint connections. Therefore, while there is some flexibility, that flexibility has limits. Think about pulling on a rope; you can stretch it a little, but if you twist and pull it in unusual directions, or pull too hard, it will start to fray and eventually tear. Connective tissue can be overstretched, and sometimes this occurs gradually, as in repetitive motion injury, or all at once. If the injury is very severe, and the tendon or ligament has ruptured or been pulled off the bone, surgery may be needed. However that is rare, and, in most cases, the ligament or tendon has simply become lax (overstretched), with tears or micro-tears that have accumulated and not healed, resulting in weakness and eventually chronic pain[6] (see Figure 5.2: The vicious cycle of connective tissue injury).

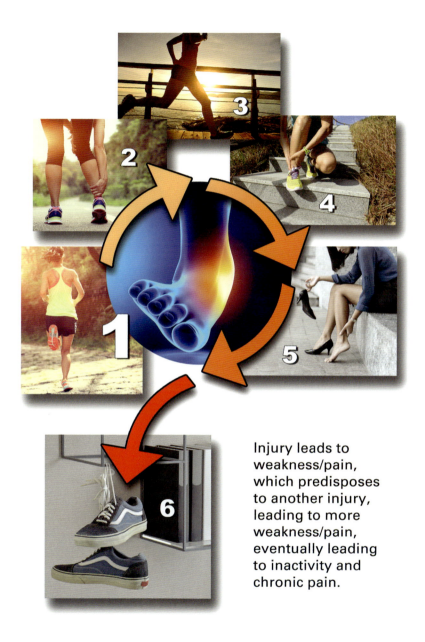

Injury leads to weakness/pain, which predisposes to another injury, leading to more weakness/pain, eventually leading to inactivity and chronic pain.

Figure 5.2: The vicious cycle of connective tissue injury

Unfortunately, the onset of chronic pain and weakness may start to limit the activities of an otherwise active or athletic person. This can be sudden, or it can be slow and progressive, until one day, the individual finds that he/she can no longer participate in his/her usual activities or sports without pain and may even give them up.

How Prolotherapy Regenerative Medicine Works

As discussed previously, the term *Prolotherapy* is short for "proliferation therapy," so named because it stimulates the proliferation (growth) and regeneration of injured ligaments, tendons, and joints. The body, like a very sophisticated computer, has the programming in place to heal; it just needs to be stimulated in that direction. Remember, after the typical four to six week healing cycle that connective tissue goes through when injured, the stimulus to heal is very small or gone. Prolotherapy is designed to be a stimulus that starts the healing response up again. In fact, you could say that Prolotherapy "tricks" the body into beginning a new, strong, and directed healing cycle for injuries that have not healed on their own.

Here's how it works. A trained medical practitioner injects a natural solution (either dextrose, platelet-rich plasma, or stem cell–rich sources taken from your own body) precisely at the site of an injury. Even though these substances are natural, their introduction into connective tissue or joints is irritating and triggers a strong healing response. The body reacts as it would if it were organically injured, but in a much more controlled, directed, and powerful fashion. There is also irritation caused by the needle itself. That, in combination with the Prolotherapy formula, stimulates increased blood flow to the area, resulting in a "sterile" (because it is done in a clean, sterile manner) "good inflammation." This response is designed to raise growth-factor levels and effectiveness to resume or initiate a connective tissue healing cycle that is incomplete, ineffective, or was never started.[7] Prolotherapy produces a controlled, concentrated "stimulus-response" healing cycle at areas that otherwise would not be stimulated to heal on their own, and it does this with low risk and few side effects. It has a high success rate in helping repair and strengthen injured and weak ligaments, tendons, and joints, reducing or eliminating pain.

PROLOTHERAPY FORMULAS

Different Prolotherapy formulas can be used depending on the nature of the injury. Traditional Prolotherapy uses concentrated dextrose (sterile sugar solution) as the main ingredient. Dextrose is an extract of corn, which is identical in composition to blood glucose; therefore, it is well tolerated. However, when concentrated dextrose is injected into connective tissue or joints, this causes a local irritation, which then brings on the desired good inflammation and healing response. In addition to dextrose, a local anesthetic is generally mixed in

Natural Growth-Factor Stimulation
for Tissue Repair

In 1955, Hackett and Henderson reported on Prolotherapy injections on rabbit tendons; see Figure 5.3, which is a photograph of the results showing an increase in size and strength for treated tendons. Over the years, tissue biopsies of ligaments and tendons treated with traditional Dextrose Prolotherapy have also shown increased texture and strength in both animal and human studies.[8] This is because Prolotherapy injections cause the natural increase of growth factors, and the ability of these growth factors to stimulate repairs.[9] Natural growth factor elevation has been shown to be effective in stimulating repair of even full-thickness cartilage defects in other animal injection studies.[10]

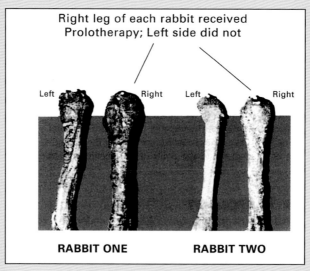

Figure 5.3: Early experiment with rabbit tendons (1955)

(Adapted from photo courtesy of Ross A. Hauser, M.D.. Caringmedical.com)

This picture represents two sets of rabbit tendons treated with Prolotherapy. The right tendon of each pair received three Prolotherapy treatments. The left tendon of each pair had no treatment. The tendons that received Prolotherapy show an increase in diameter of 40 percent; this increase is estimated to have doubled the strength of the tendon.

the formula and sometimes Sarapin (an extract of the pitcher plant) or other natural ingredients such as a small amount of zinc, manganese, or B12. Sometimes saline (salt water) is used as the main ingredient if the individual is sensitive to corn.

In addition to Traditional Prolotherapy formulas, more advanced Prolotherapy formulas are now used, specifically platelet-rich plasma and adult stem cell sources such as bone marrow or fat taken from one's own body. I will discuss these advanced formulas in more detail later in specific chapters dedicated to each. However, whichever formula is used, the mechanism is the same: getting the body to "wake up" and heal the injured area. As long as an individual is healthy, the body can be stimulated to heal, and Prolotherapy can be effective even years after the original injury, pain, or weakness occurred.

OTHER TERMS USED FOR PROLOTHERAPY

Other terms used for traditional Dextrose Prolotherapy are *Regenerative Injection Therapy, Reconstructive Therapy, Growth-Factor Stimulation Injection,* and *Nonsurgical Tendon, Ligament, and Joint Reconstruction.*[11] An older, inaccurate term, rarely used now is *Sclerotherapy* (from Greek *sclero* for "hardening")—a name based on the original theory that this treatment strengthens by means of the formation of harder scar tissue. However, biopsy studies over the years with current formulas used have demonstrated that it is not scar tissue formation that results from these injections.[12] Rather, studies have shown that Dextrose Prolotherapy stimulates proliferation of new, normal, thicker, stronger connective tissue.[13] Regarding the more advanced Prolotherapy formulas, these are also sometimes referred to by other terms. Platelet-Rich Plasma Prolotherapy is sometimes abbreviated *PRP Prolotherapy* or *PRPP*. It is also often referred to as just *platelet-rich plasma, PRP,* or *PRP Injection Therapy.* Biocellular (Stem Cell–Rich) Prolotherapy has several other names that are sometimes used, depending on where the stem cell–rich tissue is taken from. The umbrella term is "Biocellular" Prolotherapy, which includes all stem cell sources. However, if taken from fat, the term *Lipoaspirate Prolotherapy* is sometimes used (from *lipo* meaning "fat," and *aspirate* "to draw up"). Other terms used are *Stem/Stromal Cell Prolotherapy,* or, simply, *Stem Cell Prolotherapy.*

WHO IS A CANDIDATE FOR PROLOTHERAPY TREATMENT?

The guidelines for determining who is a candidate for Prolotherapy were published in 1956 in the first physician textbook on the subject. The authors in that text write,

Criteria for Injection Therapy in New Patients

1. Appropriate medical problem

2. Desire for recovery

3. No underlying medical conditions that would significantly interfere with healing

4. Ability and willingness to follow instructions

5. Willingness to report progress

6. Willingness to receive painful injections in an effort to recover from injury

These criteria still hold true today. Age is not a factor as long as the individual is healthy, and fits the other criteria. It also does not matter how long the person has been in pain, or how long ago he/she was injured, as long as the person is in good general health.[14] My youngest patient was 6, a very mature tennis player who just wanted to get better and was not afraid of injections. My oldest patient, Mary Faye LaBelle, was a healthy 100 years old at the time of her last treatment and did very well.

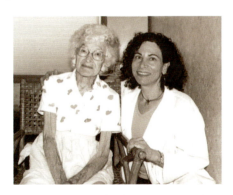

Mary Faye LaBelle, age 100, and
Dr. Donna Alderman, September 2000

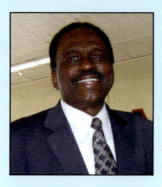

Former City Attorney

For years, in my capacity as city attorney for Compton, California, I headed the workers' compensation program. I am also a proponent of the use of natural remedies for physical illnesses. In 1999, I read an article in *Whole Life Times* about Prolotherapy: a treatment for the elimination of pain that avoided surgery or the use of drugs. At the same time, the *Glendale Gazette* published an article about Prolotherapy and Dr. Donna Alderman. I shared the article with a number of friends and relatives, and then invited my mother and brother—who had arthritic challenges—to accompany me to Dr. Alderman's office. My brother received a Prolotherapy treatment while there and marveled over its effectiveness.

I have personally received immeasurable benefits from Prolotherapy. I had chronic lower back pain that was once severe but has virtually vanished with treatment of the more advanced form of Prolotherapy with platelets (PRP). Over the years, I have sent a number of coworkers, friends, and even strangers to be treated by Dr. Alderman. I have also copied excerpts from her articles and books, and handed them out to physically challenged people I have met. We are fortunate to live during a time when many miraculous medical remedies are being discovered and shared with the general public. Prolotherapy is one of them.

Legrand H. Clegg II
Former City Attorney for Compton, California

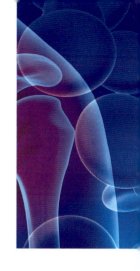

CHAPTER 6

Causes of Chronic Musculoskeletal Pain and Why Prolotherapy Works

As discussed in the previous chapter, injuries involving connective tissue are slow to heal because the blood supply to these structures is poor. This means that the growth and healing factors blood provides that help to regenerate injured tissue are in lesser supply. Also remember that after an injury, the stimulus to heal is reduced or gone after an initial healing period, usually four to six weeks. The result of incomplete healing is connective tissue weakness (also called "laxity"), which, if it continues, results in chronic musculoskeletal pain. In fact, connective tissue weakness is the most common cause of long-lasting musculoskeletal pain, and is exactly what Prolotherapy addresses.

CAUSES OF CONNECTIVE TISSUE WEAKNESS

Connective tissue weakness can result from an obvious accident or injury, such as a motor vehicle accident or sports injury. However, it can also, commonly, result from smaller, repetitive traumas that are not as obvious. A few examples of repetitive motions, which if done routinely may result in injury, are a mechanic turning a wrench, a delivery worker lifting boxes, a person texting on his/her cell phone, or an administrator or student typing at a computer. Many active individuals can experience these types of small ligament or tendon injuries without ever knowing what specifically caused them, resulting eventually in connective tissue weakness and pain.

Joint and connective tissue injuries are also common in athletes. Ideally, a player with a known ligament or tendon injury is put on the "injured list" and not allowed to play until it is believed that he/she is fully healed. However, as discussed earlier, even if someone is feeling better, most injuries do not result in 100 percent healing[1], leaving the area a little weaker and the player more susceptible to reinjury. Additionally, an athlete may not even notice small injuries and so continue to play with a weakened joint that has not yet gotten on his/her "radar." Indeed, small, repetitive injuries can accumulate in any joint until one day there is unrelenting pain (see Figure 6.1: Repetitive strain: an injury in slow motion).

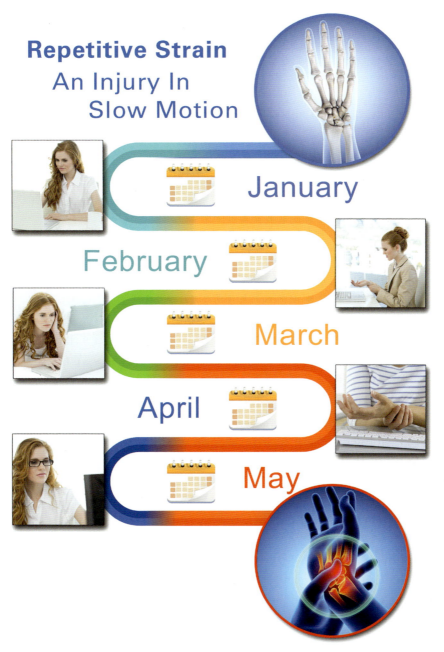

Figure 6.1: Repetitive strain: an injury in slow motion

TENDINOPATHY, TENDONITIS, AND TENDONOSIS

Tendinopathy (tendon + *pathy* from the Greek meaning "disease/disorder") is an umbrella term used
to describe any problem with a tendon. It used to be
that all injuries or pain in a tendon were referred to
as "tendonitis" (tendon + *itis* from the Greek meaning
"inflammation") because in the early stages of a tendon
injury, it is inflamed (trying to heal) and typically painful. If pain persists, it is sometimes called a *"chronic* tendonitis"; however, this terminology has turned out to
be inaccurate. Actual biopsies of tendons from patients
undergoing surgery for "chronic tendonitis" showed
that there was *no inflammation* present at all! In fact,
what was happening was degeneration of the tendon
fibers, with an absence of inflammatory cells.[2] The term
"tendonosis" is the more accurate term now used for
chronic tendon issues to emphasize that inflammation
is absent, and what is happening in those tissues is that
collagen breakdown is occurring faster than it is being
rebuilt; in other words, degeneration of the tissue is
occurring, resulting in connective tissue weakness.

THE CHALLENGE OF CONNECTIVE TISSUE HEALING
AND COLLAGEN REPAIR

An important element of connective tissue healing is
the rebuilding of collagen—a strong protein that is a
major component of ligament and tendon tissue. The
word *collagen* comes from the Greek *kola* for "glue," and
gennan for "to produce."[3] This strong, glue-like protein

is critical to healing an injured ligament or tendon. Various lifestyle factors can reduce or prevent collagen repair, such as poor nutrition, poor-quality sleep, smoking, and certain medications.

Certain nutrients and micro-nutrients are needed for proper collagen repair. For example, without vitamin C, the body cannot properly repair and rebuild collagen. Scurvy, a disease common among sailors in the eighteenth century, is an extreme example of vitamin C deficiency that prevents normal collagen repair, resulting in poor wound healing and joint pain, among other symptoms. The problem of scurvy was solved when a daily lemon, lime, or orange was added to the sailors' previously citrus-free diet. While this is a dramatic example of a severe nutritional deficiency, more subtle deficiencies may also exist in an individual that influence how his/her body repairs and makes collagen (for more detail, see Chapter 19: "Joint Pain: The Nutrition Connection").

Another factor affecting collagen repair is sleep. Sleep is important for repair and regeneration of normal, day-to-day small connective tissue injuries and joint wear and tear. This is because when we have quality sleep, our bodies make growth hormone, important for collagen and other tissue repair. A good night's sleep will generally repair these small, daily injuries. However, if sleep is disturbed or not adequate, even tiny injuries can accumulate, resulting in pain.[4]

Cigarette smoking also diminishes the body's ability to build and repair collagen. This is why smokers get facial wrinkles at a younger age than nonsmokers—collagen in the skin is not being adequately repaired—and also why smoking is not recommended before or right after surgical procedures when healing is important.[5] Ingredients in cigarettes, such as nicotine and other chemicals, prevent adequate collagen repair.[6] Even if the person quits smoking later, if he/she was smoking when the body was supposed to be healing, the damage has already been done.

Another possible reason for incomplete connective tissue healing is the use of anti-inflammatory medications[7], or other immune system lowering pain medications, at the time of the injury. Since inflammation is a necessary component of connective tissue healing, the use of anti-inflammatory medication for these types of injuries has been seriously questioned[8] (for more detail, see Chapter 11: "Pain Medication: A Double-Edged Sword").

INCOMPLETE CONNECTIVE TISSUE HEALING LEADS TO JOINT INSTABILITY

For the aforementioned reasons, joint connective tissue may not heal sufficiently after an injury, leaving the ligaments and tendons around the joint weaker. As you can imagine, this will logically result in the joint becoming less stable. If this instability does not resolve in a reasonable period of time, the body perceives this as a problem of survival. (For example, if you are running away from a wild animal, you need strong, and stable joints! Even a small amount of excess motion in a joint can trigger the body to try to resolve this problem.

The body responds to joint instability in three main ways. The first is that fluid is pulled into the joint or joint area. This frequently occurs in areas such as the knees, where cysts (fluid-filled sacks) or effusions (fluid in a joint) can occur in the body's attempt to stabilize the joint. Second, the muscles over the area will tighten, creating muscle spasm. This occurs especially where there are large muscle groups such as the back. And if muscle spasm continues for too long, the muscles may develop "trigger points"—areas of perpetual tightening. These trigger points can be felt as muscle knots, which are sore and tender to the touch, and can "trigger" pain. Thus the body's attempt to fix the initial problem (instability) can result in other problems: chronic joint swelling and/or muscular tightness and spasm!

JOINT INSTABILITY LEADS TO PAIN AND, ULTIMATELY, OSTEOARTHRITIS

If instability in a joint continues, the body initiates a third effort to stabilize it. Over many years, it will deposit calcium (bone spurs) in or on the joint. This is because calcium is hard, and likely to prevent the excess motion the body is perceiving. Calcium deposits in or on a joint is the definition of osteoarthritis (calcium deposits in or on a joint), also known as degenerative arthritis. Figure 6.2: The three ways the body responds to joint instability

THE THREE WAYS THE BODY ATTEMPTS TO STABILIZE AN UNSTABLE JOINT

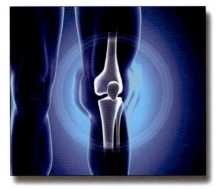

1 Fluid is pulled into the joint

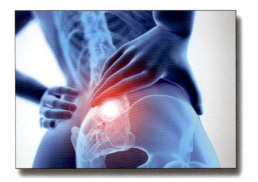

2 Muscles tighten/spasm around the joint

3 Calcium deposits into/onto the joint resulting in osteoarthritis

I	II	III	IV
Doubtful	**Mild**	**Moderate**	**Severe**

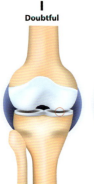 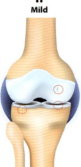 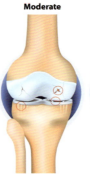

I	II	III	IV
Minimum disruption. There is already 10% cartilage loss.	Joint-space narrowing. The cartilage begins breaking down. Occurence of osteophytes.	Moderat joint-space reduction. Gaps in the cartilage can expand until they reach the bone.	Joint-space greatly reduced. 60% of the cartilage is already lost. Large osteophytes.

Figure 6.2: The three ways the body responds to joint instability

(see Figure 6.2: The three ways the body responds to joint instability).

Osteoarthritis (OA) is often diagnosed from an X-ray, which identifies the bony deposits. Many people have these types of calcium deposits on their X-ray images, without necessarily noticing any pain or symptoms. However, for others, OA progresses and may result in restricted movement and pain. You see, the calcium spurring creates an irregular stress and wear pattern on the joint surface (especially load bearing joints such as knees and hips), which can eventually break down protective cartilage. This uneven stress on the joint will then stimulate even more calcium spurring and OA because of Wolff's law (named after Dr. Julius Wolff), which states, "Bones respond to stress by making new bone."[9] Therefore, the presence of OA in a joint, over time, has a tendency to worsen the degeneration and OA in that joint.

As you can see, osteoarthritis is not just a disease of cartilage breakdown, as many people believe, but rather one of connective tissue instability.[10] And there is a direct relationship between connective tissue injury, joint instability, and the later development and progression of OA"[11] (see Figure 6.3: Ligament laxity and joint instability lead to osteoarthritis).

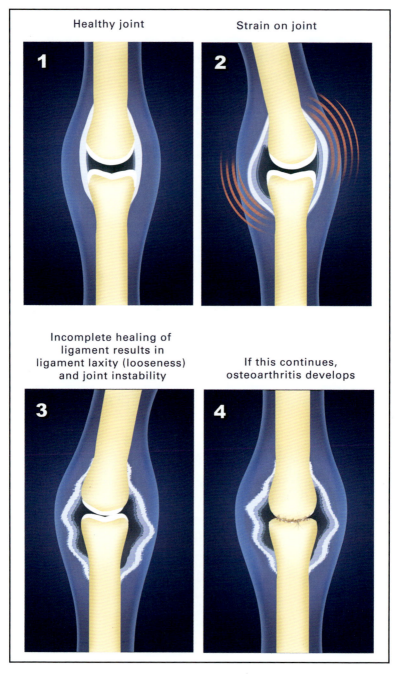

Figure 6.3: Ligament laxity and joint instability lead to osteoarthritis

Studies confirm this relationship. For instance, a very high percentage of female soccer players with knee ligament injuries were found to have knee OA 12 years later.[12] And there is an increased incidence of OA in individuals who have played certain sports, known to be hard on connective tissue, such as wrestlers, boxers, baseball pitchers, cyclists, football players, weightlifters, and others[13] (for more detail, see Chapter 13: "Prolotherapy Regenerative Medicine for Osteoarthritis").

THE IMPORTANCE OF JOINT STABILITY

Besides the aforementioned reasons why joint instability leads to osteoarthritis, other undesirable phenomena may occur when there is excess motion in a joint, such as bones hitting up and aggravating nearby nerves. Unstable low back joints may hit up against spinal or pelvic nerves and create pelvic, low back, or sciatica pain issues; or instability in a knee joint may result in excess movement of the bones, which start to irritate nearby nerves and create "shin splints." And if that were not bad enough, connective tissue weakness can also change an individual's biomechanics—forces and motion ("mechanics") in a living body ("bio"). An injured joint puts extra stress on other joints, which can then also overwork and weaken. For instance, someone with an injured knee will likely walk differently to decrease pain or discomfort. Over time, this may have an impact on other areas such as the foot, back, or hip. As the body compensates for the injury—taking stress off the injured joint by using other joints or body areas instead—the result can be a domino effect in which other joints then become overused, injured, and painful. Therefore, joint stability is not only important to prevent osteoarthritis but also to prevent other undesirable phenomena.[14]

BARRÉ-LIÉOU SYNDROME

A specific problem that may occur as a result of ligament instability in the neck is "Barré-Liéou syndrome," named after the doctors who first described it in 1928. This syndrome may occur after a neck whiplash injury or a long period of repetitive strain that slowly stretches out the neck ligaments. Over the years, there has been controversy about the existence of this syndrome, primarily because this type of ligament instability only shows up with motion and is not seen on magnetic

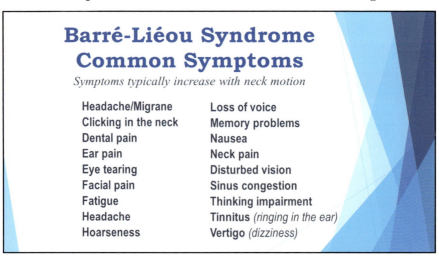

Figure 6.4: Barré-Liéou syndrome common symptoms

resonance imaging (MRI), where the patient is not moving. For that reason, it might not be suspected, so missed initially as a diagnosis. Increased scientific evidence has brought attention back to Barré-Liéou and its validity.[15] When ligaments holding neck bones (called "vertebrae") together become chronically over-stretched, there will be excess vertebrae motion. After a period of time, if the neck continues to experience this low level, but constant, slight excess motion every time the person moves his/her neck, nearby nerves become irritated, causing a wide range of symptoms, such as headache, allergy-type phenomena, ringing in the ears, dizziness, and head fogginess (see Figure 6.4: Barré-Liéou syndrome symptoms). Fortunately, Prolotherapy has been shown to improve neck ligament stability in the neck for not only average cases of whiplash or repetitive strain, but even this more complex syndrome[16] (see Figure 6.5: Neck ligament laxity and treatment).

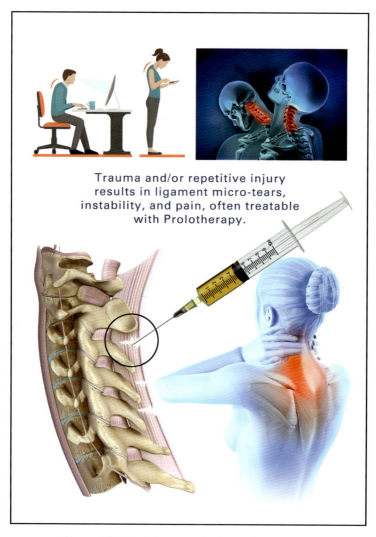

Figure 6.5: Neck ligament laxity and treatment

How Prolotherapy Regenerative Medicine Helps

Prolotherapy stimulates the repair of injured or weakened connective tissue, which increases joint stability.[17]

Prolotherapy for Hypermobility

The importance of stable and strong joints is further illustrated in a condition known as "hypermobility," where a person is born with connective tissue that is more elastic than the norm. This condition is both a blessing and a curse. Individuals are more flexible, which can help them to do certain movements more easily. However, it also increases the risk of overstretching, and injuring, these joints. Hypermobility has a spectrum and range of severities. At its very least, it is known as "benign congenital hypermobility," which can be mild, moderate, or severe. The person is very flexible, and may or may not have many problems, depending on the degree of flexibility and other lifestyle factors such as occupation, physical activity, or injuries. At its worst, the individual may have a severe type of hypermobility known as "Ehlers-Danlos syndrome." The joints of people with Ehlers-Danlos are so loose and unstable that they regularly dislocate, which can make for a painful, difficult existence. Often, multiple joint stabilization surgeries are needed over the course of their lifetimes for people with the most severe form of this syndrome. (See Figure 6.6: An example of joint hypermobility).

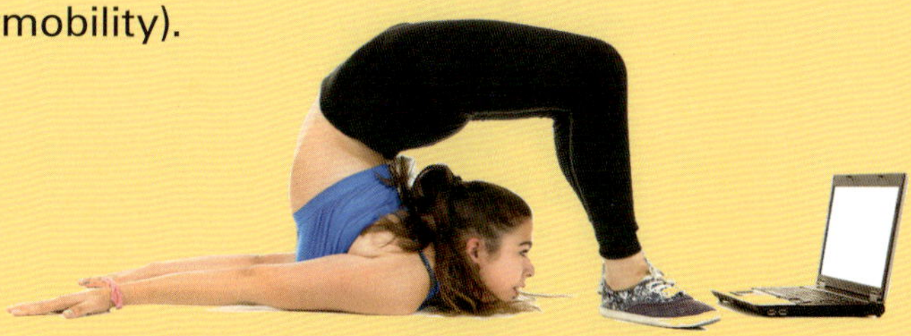

Figure 6.6: An example of joint hypermobility

Prolotherapy, fortunately, has the ability to strengthen connective tissue and joints in individuals with hypermobility, and has even helped those with Ehlers-Danlos. For more information, see the article in the *Journal of Prolotherapy* by Hauser and Phillips, "Treatment of Joint Hypermobility Syndrome, including Ehlers-Danlos Syndrome, with Hackett Hemwall Prolotherapy," available online at *http://journalofprolotherapy.com/treatment-of-joint-hypermobility-syndrome-including-ehlers-danlos-syndrome-with-hackett-hemwall-prolotherapy/.*

When ligaments and tendons are strong again, undesirable phenomena such as muscle spasm, fluid swelling, or aggravation of nearby nerves, triggered by the joint's instability, often resolve. Stress on other joints and body biomechanics also improves. Prolotherapy is also an excellent treatment for osteoarthritis (OA).[18] Prolotherapy treats the reason the arthritis developed (i.e., injured ligaments/tendons causing joint instability) as well as elevating growth-factor levels, helping the condition of cartilage (discussed further in Chapter 13: "Prolotherapy Regenerative Medicine for Osteoarthritis"). It is of course preferable to treat joint instability before OA develops. However, even if OA already exists, a remarkable thing has been observed after Prolotherapy: the pain often dramatically lessens or even goes away completely.[19] The reasons for this will be discussed in more detail in Chapter 13: "Prolotherapy Regenerative Medicine for Osteoarthritis."

In summary, the majority of chronic musculoskeletal pain comes from injured connective tissue that has not completely healed, resulting in joint instability, weakness, pain, and, eventually, osteoarthritis. Prolotherapy "wakes up" these incompletely healed and painful joint connective tissue areas, restarting repair even years after the initial injury—reducing or eliminating pain.

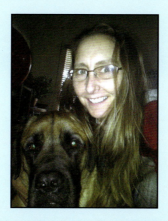

Executive, Nonprofit Organization

My pain started in 2013 after a severe auto accident that caused a whiplash injury in my upper neck. The pain, headaches, dizziness, and loss of concentration gained momentum in my life gradually, and although I would try to stay engaged in work and home life, it was becoming more difficult. The pain kept me in bed some days, and I was not able to keep work commitments. Simple things like conversing with family and friends were getting to be more difficult.

I saw a spine orthopedic doctor after the accident who treated me with physical therapy, chiropractic, and medications (muscle relaxers, anti-inflammatories) when needed, but when those didn't work, I received epidural injections for what I was told were cervical herniated discs. The decision to have an epidural was extreme for me; however, I was in pain and could see my symptoms were getting worse with more frequent headaches and dizziness, missing more work, and staying in bed longer. However, unfortunately, the epidurals did not bring me relief. At that point, the spine orthopedic doctor recommended I see a neurologist because I was complaining of dizziness. Upon my first visit, the neurologist requested an EEG and a CT scan, and then prescribed an antidepressant, but I wasn't depressed (yet). I was in pain! Once the tests were completed, I went back to the neurologist to consult about the results. He said they were negative, and there was nothing abnormal, and he prescribed an anti-seizure medication, Depakote, for migraine headaches. I didn't return to that doctor or fill the prescription.

I felt I was getting nowhere; my quality of life was no longer what I remembered. I was in bed daily, lying flat to relieve the pain in my head and to prevent the dizziness. Somedays, I couldn't drive myself, and now I was actually becoming depressed. I then heard about Prolotherapy and went for a consultation.

Dr. Alderman listened to me and understood what I was explaining when I told her what had happened to me. She showed me an illustration after my explanation of symptoms that depicted where/how/why this was happening. She explained about Barré-Liéou syndrome, where movement of the stretched ligaments causes pressure on the nerves going to the head, and that this problem does not show up on an MRI or CT because it happens with neck movement, and there is no neck movement during an MRI or CT. It made sense to me that the force of a whiplash could make the ligaments in my upper neck become stretched and weaker, and then normal movement could irritate surrounding nerves, which then could impact my head and focus, I knew at that point that I was going to be receiving the right treatment and embarked on a course of PRP Prolotherapy.

It was a long process, but a necessary process, and it worked! After three treatments, six weeks apart, I was 50 percent better and knew I was on the right track. After six treatments, I was 90 percent improved and back to my prior self. I am again doing the things I love and enjoy. Prolotherapy changed my life forever.

Elizabeth Clarke
Executive, Nonprofit Organization

CHAPTER

The Importance of a Correct Diagnosis

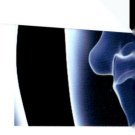

O btaining the correct diagnosis for a patient's pain is *extremely* important in determining the best treatment options. This cannot be stressed enough. Very often, patients come in telling me, "Doctor, I have a herniated disc. That's why I have this back pain," or, "My knee hurts because I have a torn meniscus." They identify the cause of their pain based on the results of an imaging study such as an MRI (magnetic resonance imaging) scan. As it turns out, and as discussed below, while an MRI does provide information, it doesn't tell the whole story.

MRIs Can Be Misleading in Diagnosing Musculoskeletal Pain

The simple truth is that abnormalities that show up in an MRI or X-ray could have occurred at some point in the past and may not be the source of a person's current pain. For example, let's say an MRI reveals a disc bulge. Sure, that bulge exists, but it is possible that the bulge already existed before the patient experienced any pain. The only way to know how long an abnormality has been present would be if the area had been scanned previously several times over the years, which is rare in a healthy person. In fact, a large number of studies have documented that individuals experiencing *no pain* can have abnormal MRI findings.[1] A well-known study published in the *New England Journal of Medicine* showed that out of 98 pain free people, 64 percent had abnormal back scans.[2] These were people with *no* pain! Many other studies have shown this same thing: abnormal findings exist in people with no pain. Shoulder rotator cuff tears and other shoulder abnormalities exist in MRIs for people with *no* pain or symptoms (medically referred to as "asymptomatic"),[3] including professional baseball pitchers.[4] Abnormal neck MRIs have also been found in asymptomatic individuals in multiple studies,[5] as well as abnormal knee MRIs in asymptomatic patients,[6] including in asymptomatic athletes.[7] Another study looked at the value of MRIs in the treatment of knee injuries and concluded, "Overall, magnetic resonance imaging [MRI} diagnoses added little guidance to patient management and at times provided spurious [false] information."[8] Therefore, one cannot assume when evaluating someone with musculoskeletal pain that an abnormality that appears on an MRI is automatically the cause of a person's pain. If every irregularity revealed in an MRI were the true cause of a person's pain, every surgery performed *because of* an MRI would result in a cure, but this is of course not the case.

On the other end of the spectrum, sometimes with musculoskeletal pain, X-rays or MRIs are negative or inconclusive and blood tests are normal. Yet the pain is real. There *is* a problem; it's just that the results, medical tests, and scans may not reflect a reason. Therefore, the physician has to go deeper into the history, or use other tools, such as diagnostic ultrasound, to arrive at a diagnosis. To determine the cause of a patient's pain accurately, it is very important to understand what happened *prior to* the problem starting, and other aspects of the pain pattern to determine a possible origin. An imaging study should only supplement—not replace—a diagnosis based on how the problem started, symptom progression, and pain pattern.

An Abnormal MRI Does Not Necessarily Mean Surgery Is Needed

As discussed above, abnormal MRIs in healthy individuals are common. Therefore, it should be obvious that an abnormal MRI does not necessarily mean surgery is needed. To further clarify this relationship, a study was done of elite overhead athletes—those who perform repetitive "overhead" activity, such as in tennis, swimming, baseball throwing, and above-shoulder, weight-training exercises. These are athletes who are more likely to suffer injuries to their shoulders because of continual and repetitive use. At the study's start, none of the athletes had any shoulder pain or problems, yet *40 percent* showed partial or full-thickness tears of the rotator cuff on their MRIs, and an additional 20 percent showed other shoulder abnormalities. The study then followed these athletes for five years. After five years, *none* of the athletes interviewed had any complaints and had not needed any evaluation, treatment or surgery for shoulder-related problems during the five previous years. The study's authors concluded, "MRIs alone should not be used as a basis for operative intervention." [9]

DIAGNOSTIC ULTRASOUND IN MUSCULOSKELETAL MEDICINE

You've likely heard of ultrasound being used to see the image of an unborn baby during pregnancy. Ultrasound uses sound waves to create this image, which it does in "greyscale" (black and white). These sound waves are too high to be heard by the human ear, and so are called "ultra" (ultra meaning "beyond") sound. In addition to its popular use in pregnancies, ultrasound has become a valuable tool in the diagnosis and treatment of musculoskeletal disorders,[10] and are fast becoming required training in some physician programs.[11] Ultrasound can be an invaluable tool in the diagnosis and treatment of musculoskeletal pain, especially in cases where an MRI was negative or inconclusive. It allows the physician to correlate the location of pain directly to an image—the patient says, "It hurts here," and the doctor can put the ultrasound probe there to see what is going on—providing additional information during a physical exam.

Advancements in technology have allowed for more portable machines as well as dramatically improved image quality (see Figure 7.1: High resolution, touch screen, portable ultrasound). Today's ultrasound images are exquisitely suited for musculoskeletal medicine, as they provide greater resolution of superficial muscles, ligaments, and tendons than any other diagnostic imaging method can, including MRI.[12] In fact, multiple studies have shown ultrasound diagnosis to be as accurate as MRI for many joint areas,[13] or, in some cases, better.[14]

Ultrasound diagnosis for musculoskeletal complaints has an advantage over MRI for several reasons. First, it can provide current, real-time, information about a patient's problem. It can be performed in an office setting where the doctor can immediately and precisely examine the site of injury or pain. Also, while MRI is done with the joint motionless, some connective tissue tears do not show up completely, or at all, unless the joint is moving.[15] Ultrasound is able to image joints "dynamically"—i.e., with movement—to see what happens to the tissue or joint. Ultrasound can also detect fluid in a joint and provide precise needle guidance in draining that fluid, or injection guidance for specific injury sites. Ultrasound can also offer a comparison between both sides of a patient—for instance, a patient's injured right knee and healthy left knee. Such differences are often very helpful in diagnosis, but seldom would a doctor order an MRI of the "good" side. Also of benefit is the ability to compare different ultrasound scans over a course of treatment in order to assess progress over time. And, finally, ultrasound can be performed on any patient, including one who has metal in a joint—something that is not always possible with MRI, since *magnetic* resonance imaging machines use magnets, and may not be safe for some patients.

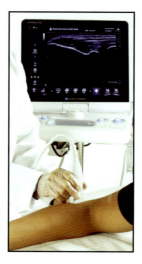

Figure 7.1: High resolution, touch screen, portable ultrasound machine
(photo courtesy of Konica Minolta, showing the Sonimage HS1 ultrasound system)

PATIENT EVALUATION

In addition to assessing general health status, it is important that the doctor take a complete history of the problem. The goal is to find out as much as possible about when and how the pain started, the pain location and pattern, what makes the pain better and what makes it worse, and what treatments or medications have been tried and if they helped or not. In

History and Advancements in Ultrasound Technology

In the late 1700s, an Italian scientist named Lazzaro Spallanzani observed that some animal species, such as bats, produce nonaudible sound in order to navigate. Because these sound waves were above the spectrum of sound that can be heard by the human ear, the term "ultra" sound was created. Over a century later, Canadian inventor Reginald A. Fessenden, saddened by the sinking of the *Titanic* in 1912, developed an instrument using ultrasound to detect icebergs up to two miles away. American inventors followed with a SONAR ("**SO**und **N**avigation **A**nd **R**anging") device, which used ultrasound successfully to detect enemy submarines during the two world wars. In 1942, neurologist Karl Dussik built an ultrasound apparatus designed to detect abnormalities in head and brain tissues, fluid, and blood flow. However, the use of ultrasound in medicine really started in 1958 when Dr. Ian Donald pioneered its use in obstetrics and gynecology to monitor pregnancies, where it has been used ever since.[16]

The first medical journal article about the use of ultrasound in examination of a joint was published in 1972 in the *British Journal of Radiology*.[17] Advancements over the last 20 years in image quality have allowed the use of ultrasound to see ligaments, tendons, nerves, and other musculoskeletal structures clearly. Ultrasound in musculoskeletal medicine in the United States has therefore grown rapidly over the last ten years to help in diagnosis, as well as needle guidance during procedures.

Color Sonoelastography

The most recent advancement in ultrasound technology is color "elastography"—also known as "sonoelastography." "Sono" is another term for ultrasound, and "elastography" describes the elasticity or density, measured as "hardness" or "softness," of tissue.[18] Ultrasound elastography has been used for many years to help doctors in diagnosing tumors since tumors are harder than the surrounding tissue. In the last several years, it has emerged as a useful tool in musculoskeletal medicine as another potential diagnostic tool to help detect early or small ligament, tendon, and muscle tears and weaknesses which would not otherwise be easily seen via either MRI or greyscale ultrasound. Color sonoelastography can also be used to help monitor improving tissue density over a course of treatment. There is a scale of tissue "softness" to "hardness" which shows up in colors ranging from red to blue. Tears show up as "softer" simply because the tissue is weaker and less dense than the surrounding stronger, "harder," healthy tissue (see Figure 7.2: Sonoelastogram showing a small muscle tear that did not show up in MRI or regular greyscale ultrasound).

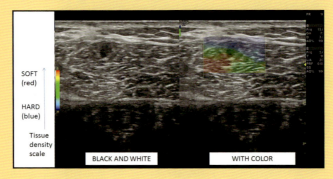

Figure 7.2: Sonoelastogram showing a small muscle tear that did not show up in MRI or regular greyscale ultrasound. [Note the muscle tear (red area) seen on the right (color) side. This is an image done on a 20-year-old runner who had persistent calf pain with activity. PRP Prolotherapy directed to the tear (red area) resolved this patient's pain.]

A large study done in 2015 evaluated 214 patients who had symptoms (including pain) of an injured tendon, but whose grayscale ultrasounds were negative or inconclusive. In 75 to 80 percent of these patients, a defect correlating to the patient's pain location was found on the color sonoelastogram. The authors concluded, "Sonoelastography can reveal tendon abnormalities of clinical relevance in a high percentage of cases, where the [black-and-white] ultrasound exam was negative, making the method a complementary tool to ultrasound evaluation."[19]

cases where there was an injury or accident, the doctor needs to understand the mechanics of that injury. Note that it is not unusual that pain can develop gradually, without any known prior injury or trauma, and this information is also important. An exam, and usually a diagnostic musculoskeletal ultrasound exam, is often conducted during the first consultation. The physician will also usually compare any available MRI scans or X-rays to the ultrasound findings done in the office.

Part of the diagnosis will be verifying the true origin of the problem. When someone feels pain in a particular location, the tendency is to think that the pain is coming from that location, but this is not always the case. Sometimes what is felt is in fact "referred" pain: pain that is actually coming from a different location from where it is felt. In these cases, the pain message travels along a "referral pathway." There are many kinds of referred pain: tooth pain that actually originates from an ear infection, for example, or a heart attack felt as left arm or jaw pain. These pain referral patterns have been mapped out for many joint areas, including the spine and hip (see Figure 7.3 Head and neck ligament referral patterns; and Figure 7.4: Low back and hip ligament referral patterns).

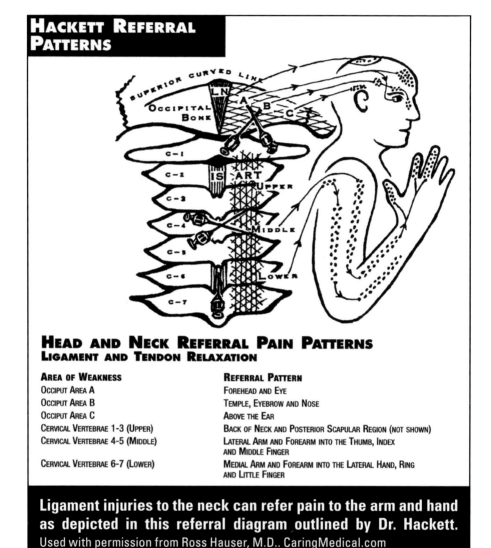

HACKETT REFERRAL PATTERNS

HEAD AND NECK REFERRAL PAIN PATTERNS
LIGAMENT AND TENDON RELAXATION

AREA OF WEAKNESS	REFERRAL PATTERN
OCCIPUT AREA A	FOREHEAD AND EYE
OCCIPUT AREA B	TEMPLE, EYEBROW AND NOSE
OCCIPUT AREA C	ABOVE THE EAR
CERVICAL VERTEBRAE 1-3 (UPPER)	BACK OF NECK AND POSTERIOR SCAPULAR REGION (NOT SHOWN)
CERVICAL VERTEBRAE 4-5 (MIDDLE)	LATERAL ARM AND FOREARM INTO THE THUMB, INDEX AND MIDDLE FINGER
CERVICAL VERTEBRAE 6-7 (LOWER)	MEDIAL ARM AND FOREARM INTO THE LATERAL HAND, RING AND LITTLE FINGER

Ligament injuries to the neck can refer pain to the arm and hand as depicted in this referral diagram outlined by Dr. Hackett.
Used with permission from Ross Hauser, M.D.. CaringMedical.com

Figure 7.3: Head and neck ligament referral patterns

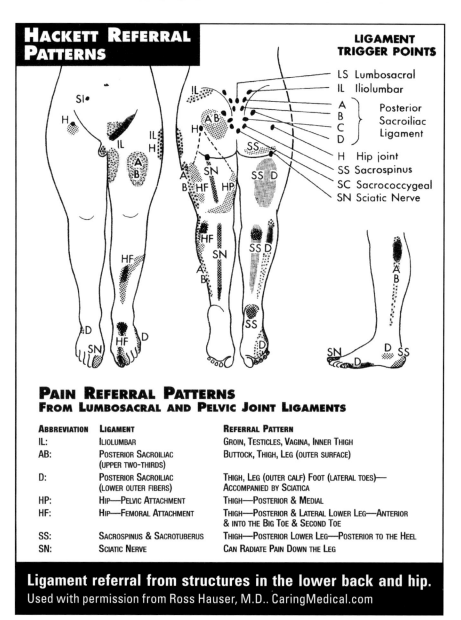

HACKETT REFERRAL PATTERNS

LIGAMENT TRIGGER POINTS

LS Lumbosacral
IL Iliolumbar
A ⎫
B ⎬ Posterior
C ⎬ Sacroiliac
D ⎭ Ligament
H Hip joint
SS Sacrospinus
SC Sacrococcygeal
SN Sciatic Nerve

PAIN REFERRAL PATTERNS
FROM LUMBOSACRAL AND PELVIC JOINT LIGAMENTS

ABBREVIATION	LIGAMENT	REFERRAL PATTERN
IL:	ILIOLUMBAR	GROIN, TESTICLES, VAGINA, INNER THIGH
AB:	POSTERIOR SACROILIAC (UPPER TWO-THIRDS)	BUTTOCK, THIGH, LEG (OUTER SURFACE)
D:	POSTERIOR SACROILIAC (LOWER OUTER FIBERS)	THIGH, LEG (OUTER CALF) FOOT (LATERAL TOES)— ACCOMPANIED BY SCIATICA
HP:	HIP—PELVIC ATTACHMENT	THIGH—POSTERIOR & MEDIAL
HF:	HIP—FEMORAL ATTACHMENT	THIGH—POSTERIOR & LATERAL LOWER LEG—ANTERIOR & INTO THE BIG TOE & SECOND TOE
SS:	SACROSPINUS & SACROTUBERUS	THIGH—POSTERIOR LOWER LEG—POSTERIOR TO THE HEEL
SN:	SCIATIC NERVE	CAN RADIATE PAIN DOWN THE LEG

Ligament referral from structures in the lower back and hip.
Used with permission from Ross Hauser, M.D.. CaringMedical.com

Figure 7.4: Low back and hip ligament referral patterns

As you can see from these charts, a ligament or tendon problem in the upper neck can refer pain into the head, causing headaches. Similarly, a low back connective tissue problem can send pain down the leg—a condition commonly referred to as "sciatica." This type of referral can also be seen in other joints—i.e., wrist pain can be actually coming from an injury in the elbow, or knee pain might be coming from a problem in the hip. To help in determining a pain's actual source, the doctor may test for a reaction known as the "jump sign." Typically, when the spot that is the *source* of the pain is pressed, the patient will automatically jump. Note, however, that sometimes these tender spots can be obscured by pain medication, or the individual has become very accustomed to her/her pain or has a high pain tolerance, so it isn't always clear-cut. However, referral patterns are considered during the exam, and all information put together by the physician to arrive at a conclusion.

ARRIVING AT A DIAGNOSIS AND TREATMENT PLAN

After the history, physical exam, diagnostic imaging, and evaluation for possible referral patterns have been taken into consideration, the doctor will arrive at a working diagnosis of what is likely causing the pain as well as if the problem is treatable. Again, it is *very, very, very* important (I cannot stress this enough) that all imaging be correlated to the patient's history, exam, and pain pattern, and not used as a diagnosis by itself. If the patient is a candidate for Prolotherapy treatment, the physician will recommend which formula would be most appropriate, including the treatment's injection sites and possible risks. After all of the doctor's conclusions have been discussed and all of the patient's questions have been asked and answered, if both doctor and patient wish to proceed, then the procedure is scheduled. In some cases, the first treatment is received the same day as the consultation.

The bottom line of all of this is best stated by Dr. James Cyriax (1904–1985), a British physician who designed a system of musculoskeletal diagnosis:

1. Every pain has a source;

2. Treatment must reach the source;

3. Treatment must benefit the source in order to relieve the pain; and

4. A specific [and correct] diagnosis leads to successful treatment.[20]

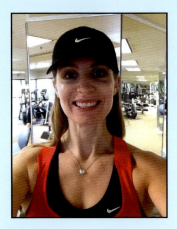

University Strength and Conditioning Coach

I have always been very physically active. I am now almost 40, and I have learned how important it is to take care of my body. My career as a strength and conditioning coach for a Division III athletics program and my work as a personal trainer require me to be in top physical shape at all times. My body is my moneymaker; exercise is my stress reliever, and I don't have time for injuries.

But life happens. When I was in my early 30s, my car was hit by a bus while in San Francisco, and I was left with injuries around the right shoulder and right side of my body that did not resolve and that none of the doctors I had seen could diagnose or knew how to treat. I went to numerous specialists to find a way to "fix" my issue. After six months of being in pain and not able to lift weights, I became depressed. To make the situation worse, I put on 40 pounds from my lack of exercise, stress, and depression.

I spoke to Dr. Alderman (one of my training clients) about my "issue," and her confident response was, "Let's shoot it." I, like many, had never heard of Prolotherapy before. I was a little skeptical that it could help, simply because I was running out of hope—although, scientifically, the treatment made sense to me. I read the first edition of Dr. Alderman's book so I could know what I was signing up for. I felt more comfortable about getting the treatment once I understood how it worked. Besides, at that point, I felt I had nothing to lose.

Dr. Alderman did four treatments of Dextrose Prolotherapy one month apart, and, much to my surprise, I was fixed! I was no longer in pain. I was then on a mission to get back to my workouts and was very motivated to lose the 40 pounds I had gained while injured. I took the weight off, returned to my pull-ups and lifting, and even got my six-pack back! I realized that prior to this injury, I had taken my physical ability for granted. However, now I had my life back and was determined to keep it.

Five years after that injury, which has never returned, I hurt my hip working out. I had excruciating pain that radiated from my groin down to the top of my thigh. I thought it would go away, so I ignored the pain for a good six months before I couldn't take it anymore. Finally, I saw Dr. Alderman, who did a diagnostic ultrasound and concluded I had a hip labral tear. Because of the type and location of this injury, this time she recommended PRP Prolotherapy. I noticed a huge difference after just one treatment; after three treatments six weeks apart, I was good to go. It's been over three years since the last treatment on my hip and over eight years since my last upper back/shoulder treatment, and I am going strong on both. Because of Prolotherapy, I was able to remain in my profession, got a job at a university as an assistant strength coach, and since then I was promoted to head strength coach at the university. I am still pain free.

I am grateful to have discovered Prolotherapy and am continuously telling people about it, especially my college athletes who deal with injuries often.

Jessica Balzano, BS, CSCS
University Strength and Conditioning Coach

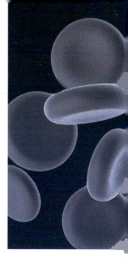

CHAPTER 8

Prolotherapy Regenerative Medicine Is Evidence Based

Prolotherapy Regenerative Medicine is evidence based. What this means is that it is based on the best available medical and research evidence, the doctor's clinical experience, and takes into account the patient's values and preferences. The purpose of this type of medicine is to get the best possible treatment outcomes along with patient satisfaction.

Prolotherapy is supported by multiple educational organizations and has its own peer-reviewed journal. Prolotherapy has also recognized by several premier medical facilities and academic institutions as an option in treating musculoskeletal pain, among these the Mayo Clinic. In April 2005, the *Mayo Clinic Health Letter* discussed Prolotherapy, stating, "In the case of chronic ligament or tendon pain that hasn't responded to more conservative treatments—such as prescribed exercise and physical therapy—prolotherapy may be helpful."[1] Then in March 2010, the same newsletter featured platelet rich-plasma, writing, "Mayo Clinic doctors are optimistic about platelet-rich plasma therapy."[2] On its website, the Mayo Clinic currently lists "Prolotherapy" and "Platelet-Rich Plasma Therapy" among the nonsurgical treatment options offered by its Physical Medicine and Rehabilitation Department, whose goal is to "use state of the art technology, to reduce pain and increase the activity of patients."[3] There is also a Center for Regenerative Medicine at the Mayo Clinic, which offers adult stem cell joint injections for certain musculoskeletal conditions.[4]

PUBLISHED SCIENTIFIC STUDIES AND RESEARCH

Since the 1930s, hundreds, if not thousands, of medical studies, reports, books, and papers have demonstrated the effectiveness of Prolotherapy for musculoskeletal complaints. In the appendix of this book, I have included a bibliography that lists some of these references. While this list is comprehensive, it by no means includes all studies, and there are new articles and research appearing constantly. To get an idea of these studies, following is a very abbreviated review, broken down by Prolotherapy formula.

TRADITIONAL DEXTROSE PROLOTHERAPY STUDIES

In 1983, a group of researchers showed a significant increase in the mass, thickness and strength of ligaments after treatment with Prolotherapy, confirmed microscopically.[5] A similar study showed increases in the number of cells, blood supply and new collagen after

Prolotherapy injections.[6] Similarly, biopsies of human tissue after a series of Dextrose Prolotherapy injections showed an increase in average fiber diameter from 0.55 to 0.88 micrometers.[7] That's a 60 percent boost!

Another study demonstrated that Prolotherapy injections raise growth factor levels and effectiveness.[8] Other studies have shown that patients receiving Dextrose Prolotherapy had improvement in low back pain,[9] knee osteoarthritis (OA),[10] knee instability,[11] thumb and finger OA,[12] temporomandibular joint (TMJ) dysfunction (jaw pain and instability),[13] painful rotator cuff tendinopathy,[14] knee anterior cruciate ligament (ACL) instability,[15] chronic groin pain,[16] cervical (neck) pain[17] and instability (whiplash),[18] sacroiliac (SI) joint pain (in which Prolotherapy was found to be superior to corticosteroids),[19] plantar fasciitis,[20] and lateral epicondylitis (tennis elbow),[21] among other conditions.

Long-term treatment results have also been tracked. Dr. George Hackett, one of Prolotherapy's pioneers, tracked 1,800 patients; he reported an 82 percent cure rate even 12 years after a patient's last Prolotherapy treatment.[22] Following in Dr. Hackett's footsteps in the 1950s, Dr. Gustav Hemwall ultimately treated over 10,000 patients, whose progress he studied over the years. In 1974, he presented his findings to the Prolotherapy Association. He reported that out of 1,827 patients he tracked who completed Prolotherapy treatments, 75.5 percent reported complete recovery and cure, 24.3 percent reported general improvement, and

Prolotherapy Studies and the
Problem with Saline "Placebo" Injections

A placebo is a medically ineffective treatment given to one group of patients during a study. This is done in a "blinded" fashion (the patient does not know whether he/she is receiving the active or inactive treatment). When there is an expectation that a treatment may work, some patients get better even if given the inactive treatment. In order to reach a valid conclusion about a particular treatment, there needs to be a "statistically significant" difference between the active and inactive groups. The classic placebo used in medical injection studies is saline (salt water). However, since saline can be used as an active Prolotherapy formula, calling a saline injection a "placebo" in the context of Prolotherapy could lead to inaccurate conclusions. In these types of studies, the outcome may be that both groups (one group receiving dextrose and/or platelet-rich plasma and the other group a saline "placebo") show improvement. Some study authors have erroneously concluded from such results that since both groups showed improvement that "Prolotherapy, or PRP, didn't work."

However, that's actually not a fair assessment; all those results convey is that there was "no statistical difference" between the results of the two groups. The fact is that both treatment and placebo groups received a legitimate form of Prolotherapy and—what do you know—both groups improved! In a study comparing saline and dextrose injections into the TMJ, both patient groups improved, which strongly suggests that both formulas were effective.[24] This is an important "FYI" point to keep in mind if you come across research studies designed in this fashion.

only 0.2 percent reported no improvement. The net result of Dr. Hemwall's study indicated that 99 percent of surveyed patients who completed treatment found some relief from their chronic pain.[23]

PLATELET–RICH PLASMA (PRP) PROLOTHERAPY STUDIES

Many excellent studies support the benefit of PRP Prolotherapy. The University of Alberta's Sports Medicine Clinic published results of its study using PRP for shoulder rotator cuff tendinopathy, which showed decreased pain, increased mobility, and documented tissue improvement (the MRI before and after showed structural change and a decrease in the size of rotator cuff tears).[25] Multiple studies confirm improvement when PRP is used for knee OA.[26] Other double-blind studies demonstrate PRP's effectiveness in disc disease,[27] patellar tendinopathy,[28] knee meniscal tears,[29] Achilles tendinopathy,[30] SI joint low back injections,[31] and lateral epicondylitis (tennis elbow),[32] as well as partial ulnar collateral ligament (UCL) elbow tears.[33] Comparison of PRP with corticosteroid injections showed PRP to be superior.[34] (for more detail, see Chapter 9: "Platelet-Rich Plasma (PRP) Prolotherapy").

BIOCELLULAR (STEM CELL–RICH) PROLOTHERAPY STUDIES

Biocellular Prolotherapy is a relatively new type of Prolotherapy. However, over the last ten years, multiple studies related to the use of adult stem cell sources for musculoskeletal complaints have been published. Both bone marrow–derived cells[35] as well as adipose-derived cells[36] have confirmed these injections to promote "significant improvements" in cartilage repair with less progression of cartilage disease.[37] Adipose-derived stem cell knee joint injections were given to 30 older patients (65 years plus); the patients showed "significant improvement" at a two-year follow-up in terms of "pain reduction, effective cartilage healing, and improved function." On arthroscopic examination, 87.5 percent of these patients also showed improved cartilage status.[38] Additional studies have shown successful outcomes using autologous adult stem cell injections into knees with partial tears of the ACL,[39] patellar tendonosis and tear,[40] large abdominal muscle tear, [41] and Achilles tendon tears[42] (for more detail, see Chapter 10: "Biocellular (Stem Cell–Rich) Prolotherapy").

PROLOTHERAPY HAS ITS OWN PEER-REVIEWED SCIENTIFIC JOURNAL

In addition to hundreds of articles and studies published in other peer-reviewed journals over the years, Prolotherapy has its own peer-reviewed scientific journal. The *Journal of Prolotherapy*, founded in 2009, publishes open-access, online, peer-reviewed scientific articles, studies, and research focused on Prolotherapy Regenerative Medicine with the stated purpose to "provide readers with new, cutting-edge information on Prolotherapy."[43] This also means that practitioners can share information via a collective knowledge base; in addition, the quality of research is improved and scholarly communities can form.[44] The editorial advisory board of the *Journal of Prolotherapy* includes Prolotherapy experts from around the world. In 2012, this board published a "consensus statement" regarding the use of Prolotherapy for musculoskeletal pain, detailing the theory, scientific evidence, and applications for all three types of Prolotherapy in the treatment of musculoskeletal pain.[45]

Of additional note is the monthly peer-reviewed scholarly publication *Physical Medicine and Rehabilitation Journal (PM&R)*, which is the official scientific journal of the American Academy of Physical Medicine and Rehabilitation. *PM&R* has published hundreds of articles on Prolotherapy and the use of regenerative injections for musculoskeletal pain. This is significant in that *PM&R* states one of its goals is to provide: "the timely delivery of clinically relevant and evidence-based research."[46]

PROLOTHERAPY ORGANIZATIONS AND UNIVERSITY AFFILIATIONS

There are several large educational nonprofit organizations dedicated to teaching and standardizing Prolotherapy protocols. Of particular note is the American Osteopathic Association of Prolotherapy Regenerative Medicine (AOAPRM), which is one of 24 specialty colleges affiliated with the American Osteopathic Association (AOA). This organization is "committed to the long-term education of Prolotherapy," offering training to physicians since 1938, including semiannual educational conferences.[47]

Prolotherapy is also taught as part of the curriculum of the University of Wisconsin School of Medicine and Public Health's Department of Family Medicine and Community Health medical residency program, which also sponsors a Prolotherapy education and research laboratory.[48] Research from this program has resulted in multiple publications that demonstrate Prolotherapy's value in primary care and musculoskeletal medicine.[49]

The American Association of Orthopaedic Medicine (AAOM), founded in 1983, offers information and educational programs in all three types of Prolotherapy Regenerative Medicine. In addition to hosting an annual scientific conference, AAOM also offers multiple hands-on injection workshops throughout the year in both the United States and other countries.[50]

The Hackett Hemwall Patterson Foundation, founded in 1969, offers classes, conferences, and clinical training in Prolotherapy; it also organizes educational trips during which medical professionals can provide Prolotherapy in underdeveloped countries through charity clinics.[51] In conjunction with the University of Wisconsin School of Medicine and Public Health, this foundation offers a comprehensive Prolotherapy course each year.

Another organization dedicated to training physicians and furthering the regenerative medicine field is The Orthobiologic Institute (TOBI), which holds an annual seminar "where global thought-leaders in ortho-biologics (use of the body's cells and blood to stimulate healing) convene to share cutting-edge research and advance regenerative medicine."[52] Although TOBI is a for-profit entity, it is associated with various charities and scholarship programs.

THE INSURANCE QUESTION AND THE "EXPERIMENTAL" LABEL

As you can see, Prolotherapy is supported by multiple professional organizations, universities and valid medical research, including quality peer-reviewed scientific studies and journals. Yet most insurance companies still consider it "experimental" and therefore typically won't cover it. This has been upsetting for some patients, especially when Prolotherapy has helped them avoid much more expensive surgeries that insurance *would* have covered. While the wheels of change in the medical world can be slow to turn, it is only a matter of time before this "experimental" label is removed.

The American Association of Orthopaedic Medicine (AAOM) openly disputes the categorization, insisting that Prolotherapy is *not* experimental. As the AAOM states on its website, most state boards of medicine determine their definitions of "experimental" based on two major factors. One, if a procedure is taught by postgraduate programs for the healing arts and, two, if it is supported by studies that meet certain criteria for research quality. If these things are present, then that procedure is considered to have graduated from the experimental stage. As discussed earlier, Prolotherapy is taught as an acceptable method of treatment by more than one approved postgraduate program for the healing arts, and there are many Prolotherapy studies that meet the specified research quality criteria.[53] It is true that Biocellular (Stem Cell–Rich) Prolotherapy may fall into the experimental category because it is still rather new and studies are still emerging. However, Dextrose Prolotherapy and PRP Prolotherapy certainly seem to fulfill the nonexperimental requirements.

However, there are some insurance companies that will cover these therapies. Unity Health medical insurance in Madison, Wisconsin, will cover some Prolotherapy treatments when performed by local doctors who have gone through the Hackett Hemwall Patterson Foundation training program. And in 2017, Arkansas passed a new law that grants state employees and teachers coverage for regenerative injection therapies for treatment of orthopedic conditions on their government health care plans. Arkansas is the first state to adopt a policy to include these emerging therapies in state employee health insurance, stating use of these effective regenerative therapies is expected to save the state *$100 million* as an alternative to more costly surgeries or drugs![54] This is promising indeed. I believe that in time, other states and/or insurance companies will follow, and that although this is a slow process, progress is being made.

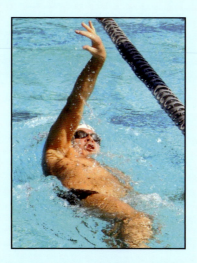

Family and Sports Medicine Physician

I am 62 years old. Over the course of the past several years, Dr. Alderman has treated my low back, hip, and shoulder. I initially injured my low back many years ago working as a lifeguard, then again 15 years later with another trauma. I also have a long history of shoulder issues; in fact, over the past 30 years, I have had a total of four surgeries on the left shoulder and two surgeries on the right. I tried multiple treatments for the pain: acupuncture, chiropractic manipulation, physical therapy, osteopathic manipulation, massage, and cortisone injections. None of these interventions helped much, or only temporarily, and I felt doomed to a life of coping with chronic pain. I reviewed my prior medical care and pain situation with my orthopedic colleagues. Their combined recommendation was to have multiple spine surgeries with fusion of the sacroiliac joint. During my career, I had seen more than enough failed back surgeries. I vowed I would not follow that path.

Through my years of practice as a family medicine/sports medicine physician and clinical instructor for medical residents, I would hear of multiple alternative medical therapies from my patients and students, including Prolotherapy.

I listened, but dismissed those treatments as "voodoo" medicine. Eventually, however, I became desperate to find an effective way to treat my increasing pain. I began an exhaustive review of the medical literature and found that the Prolotherapy literature indicated sound science—good evidence-based medicine with minimal risk. I looked for a physician who was not only experienced in Prolotherapy but also osteopathically trained and found Dr. Alderman. My first contact with Dr. Alderman's office was through her outstanding assistant, Michelle. Michelle thoroughly explained the procedure. I was anxious at the start of my first appointment, but not about the procedure itself. I was anxious that the treatment wouldn't be successful, as this was my last hope to prevent lifelong chronic pain.

This first consultation and Prolotherapy procedure lasted two hours. We decided to start with treatment on my low back, since this was the area bothering me the most. Walking out of the office after my first treatment, I felt 50 percent better. Four treatments later, my low back was pain free. With my back pain resolved, my activity level increased. I was once again distance running, swimming, and cycling. I hadn't been able to pursue these sports for the previous 15 years! Two years later, because of my now increased activity, I began experiencing right hip pain. The pain rapidly progressed to the point that I had to stop all physical activity. I had pain while walking, sitting, and working. An MRI scan showed right hip femoral acetabular impingement (commonly known as "FAI"), along with a hip labral tear and osteoarthritis. Again, I reviewed my case with my orthopedic colleagues. Their recommendation was a total hip replacement. Since I was determined to avoid this, I saw Dr. Alderman. We discussed my diagnosis and her experience in treating this problem with Platelet-Rich Plasma (PRP) or Biocellular (Stem Cell–Rich) Prolotherapy. She told me that hip issues can be challenging and often take more aggressive treatments, a larger number of treatments, require patience, and can have a lower success rate than other joint areas. However, because my hip range of motion was still good, and the other option offered to me (a replacement) had no guarantees either, I said, "Let's do it!" The PRP is a simple blood draw. The Biocellular using my own fat I was apprehensive about; however, turned out to be very tolerable. Initially, the results were unimpressive; then at about three months after the Biocellular procedure, my hip began to feel better. At six months after the procedure, I had no hip pain. I was back to swimming, running, and cycling pain free, and I became very active again. Two years later, I had a few twinges of pain again (not as bad as prior to the first treatment, however), so I repeated the Biocellular procedure, and a few months after that, I was pain free. It has been two years since that last treatment, and I continue to be free of hip pain.

After my hip pain was gone, I resumed activities that I had previously avoided, including joining a master's swim team. I was swimming and racing very intensely, and began to experience left shoulder pain and weakness. I had difficulty with my normal daily activities and then trouble sleeping because of shoulder pain. I couldn't perform a push-up or pull-up, and I certainly couldn't swim. So I received a PRP Prolotherapy treatment. Five weeks later, I was almost pain free. The subsequent ultrasound showed an impressive amount of healing. I chose to follow the PRP with a Biocellular treatment to ensure complete healing and because of the severity of my shoulder history. Six weeks after the Biocellular treatment, my shoulder was pain free and strong. It has been over a year since my last shoulder treatment, and I am still going strong.

In my 30-plus years' experience as a board certified family medicine and primary care sports medicine physician, I have never seen such profound tissue repair. Rotator cuff tears in 60-year-old males do not heal in five to six weeks, especially in a shoulder that has had four previous surgeries! However, ultrasound and physical exam follow-up confirmed essentially complete healing, and my pain is gone! Now my left (treated) shoulder, which used to be the "bad" shoulder, is better and stronger than my right one. I am now swimming three to four thousand yards a day, lifting weights, running, cycling, and surfing, totally pain free. I have evolved from describing Prolotherapy as "voodoo" medicine to being a strong advocate of the therapy. My wife and sister have both had chronic pain issues successfully treated with Prolotherapy, and I have referred multiple patients with amazing results.

Thank you for allowing me to tell the story of my journey. Hopefully, this will help other potential patients.

Terry Redding, M.D.
Family and Sports Physician

CHAPTER 9

Platelet-Rich Plasma (PRP) Prolotherapy

Many people have heard the term "platelet-rich plasma" in news stories in connection with athletic injuries, however do not realize that when platelet-rich plasma is injected into and around a joint, it is actually a type of Prolotherapy. In fact, platelet-rich plasma has been used as a formula in Prolotherapy since around 2005. Platelet-Rich Plasma (PRP) Prolotherapy has been shown to be effective not only for older injuries but also for recent ones,[1] making it ideal for athletic injuries. It has also successfully been used in the treatment of osteoarthritis (OA) and helpful for cartilage repair.[2] This chapter will discuss what PRP Prolotherapy is and how it works, its history, conditions it has been used for, and under what circumstances it may be the preferred Prolotherapy formula treatment choice.

PLATELET-RICH PLASMA BASICS

We will start with some very basic concepts. Our blood is composed of these basic elements: *red cells, white cells,* and *platelets,* all suspended within a liquid called *plasma.* Platelets are small, plate-shaped bodies (hence the term "platelets") that contain growth factors and other proteins that control natural wound healing.[3] Blood can be withdrawn from an individual, then placed in a machine that spins it (a "centrifuge"), and these blood components will separate from each other (see Figure 9.1: Composition of whole blood).

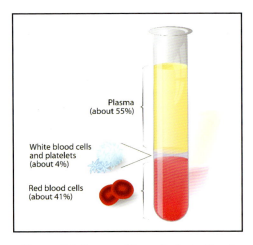

Figure 9.1: Composition of whole blood

The definition of PRP, as used in musculoskeletal medicine, is autologous blood (autologous: taken from the same person it is returned to, from the Greek *auto* for "self") in which platelets have been concentrated above their normal (baseline) levels.[4] By concentrating the blood in this way, the growth-factor rich platelet portion of the blood goes from *6 percent* to *94 percent,* increasing potential healing ability dramatically (see Figure 9.2: Composition of whole blood as compared to platelet-rich plasma).

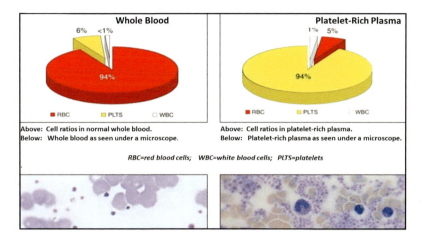

Figure 9.2: Composition of whole blood
compared to platelet-rich plasma

Adapted from Marx and Garg, *Dental and Craniofacial Applications of Platelet-Rich Plasma, 1st Edition,* January 2005. Courtesy of Quintessence Publishing Company.

PLATELET-RICH PLASMA IN MUSCULOSKELETAL MEDICINE

At the time of this writing, over 13,726 medical studies regarding platelet-rich plasma appear in the US National Library of Medicine's PubMed database,[5] and the term "platelet-rich plasma" appears in 1,340,000 references in Google Scholar,[6] with more being added every day. Platelet-rich plasma has been found to be effective for use in ligament and tendon injuries,[7] chronic tendinopathies,[8,] OA,[9] knee meniscal tears,[10] cartilage repair,[11] elbow pain[12] and other sports injuries,[13] patellar tendinopathy and muscle strain,[14] muscle tears,[15] jumper's knee,[16] Achilles tendinopathy,[17] plantar fasciitis,[18] temporomandibular joint (TMJ) disorders,[19] disc disease including cervical and lumbar disc herniations,[20]

History of Platelet-Rich Plasma

For many years, it had been observed that using platelet-rich plasma during a surgical procedure could improve how well a patient healed after surgery.[28] Orthopedic surgeons had been using PRP as early as the 1970s to assist in the healing of fractures and bone grafts with good results. However, preparing platelet-rich plasma required a large quantity of a patient's blood as well as big, expensive equipment; thus, the use of platelet-rich plasma was limited to hospitals.[29] By the 1990s, platelet-rich plasma machines were getting smaller and more portable. Multiple reports emerged showing dramatically improved healing when platelet-rich plasma was used during maxillofacial dentistry, periodontal surgery,[30] cosmetic surgery,[31] and skin grafting.[32]

These successes encouraged the use of platelet-rich plasma in sports medicine for connective tissue repair. In 2006, Mishra and Pavelko, associated with Stanford University, published the results of a study that used platelet-rich plasma injections for chronic tendon problems.[33] This study reported a 93 percent reduction in pain at two-year follow-up. Then, in 2008, just before the Super Bowl, Pittsburgh Steelers wide receiver Hines Ward received platelet-rich plasma injections for a knee injury. The Steelers went on to win Super Bowl XLIII, and Ward credited platelet-rich plasma with allowing him to get back in the game. Ward's success with platelet-rich plasma was publicized on national television,[34] making platelet-rich plasma more widely known. In 2010, the *Mayo Clinic Health Letter* discussed the use of platelet-rich plasma for enhanced healing of injured tendons.[35] Since then, not only has the use of platelet-rich plasma spread to the general public, but it has expanded to traditional orthopedic and sports medicine circles and continues to be used by many high-profile athletes.[36]

sacroiliac joint dysfunction,[21] hip pain[22] and other spine and low back pain[23] (even in older patients[24]), biceps and rotator cuff tears and tendinopathy,[25] and other musculoskeletal and orthopedic injuries.[26] Although discussion and some controversy exist in regards to which is the best concentration or type of PRP to use for various conditions,[27] there seems to be general agreement that platelet-rich plasma enhances musculoskeletal healing.

HOW PLATELET-RICH PLASMA ENHANCES HEALING

When platelets are injected at the site of an injury and then activated (turned "on," discussed later in this chapter), they release growth factors that signal for local adult stem cells (repair cells) to come to that injury site, which increases the rate of healing[37] (see Figure 9.3: Activated platelets signal for help from local adult stem cells in healthy tissue). This makes sense because the initial number of platelets at a wound site is directly related to how well and fast an injury heals.[38] And growth factors released by PRP have been shown to help increase blood supply and new blood vessel formation, a process called "angiogenesis" (*angio* for "blood vessel"; *genesis* for "new"),[39] important in tissue repair.[40]

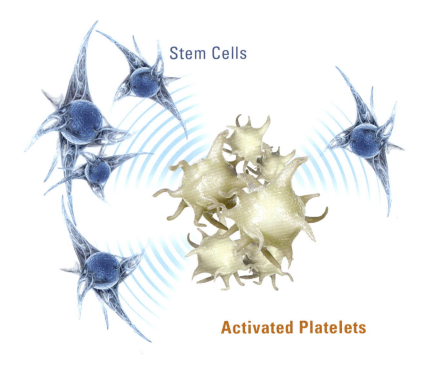

Stem Cells

Activated Platelets

Figure 9.3: Activated platelets signal for help from local adult stem (repair) cells in healthy tissue

NOT ALL PLATELET-RICH PLASMA IS EQUAL

As the use of platelet-rich plasma has grown, so has the demand for, and availability of, platelet-rich plasma–concentrating machines and methods; several manufacturers now make these systems. There are also doctors who "do it themselves" using a regular type of centrifuge rather than one of the systems developed for this purpose. The basic difference among all these various methods is 1) the amount of concentration of platelets (how many times a person's normal levels (called "baseline" levels) and 2) the presence and number of red or white blood cells.[41]

Platelet Concentration

There is debate in the medical community about what is the best platelet concentration or cell types for different conditions; however, most data supports a platelet concentration of four to six times a patient's normal level (baseline) for most musculoskeletal problems.[42] More specifically, since the average normal patient's platelet count is 250,0000 platelets per microliter, this means that the magic number is 1.0 million to 1.5 million platelets per microliter (4 to 6 times normal baseline). This concentration has shown better tissue regeneration when compared to lower platelet concentrations. It also seems that much higher concentrations could have an inhibitory effect,[43] which may decrease effectiveness[44]. Therefore, four to six times baseline has become the most commonly used concentration for platelet-rich plasma and this concentration range is known as "high-density."

Remember that platelets work by sending out biochemical messages so that nearby available stem cells will come and help repair injured areas. It has been found that when high-density PRP is used there is a stronger stem cell response when compared to whole blood or PRP with lower platelet concentrations (see Figure 9.4: Stem cell response related to platelet-rich plasma concentration).

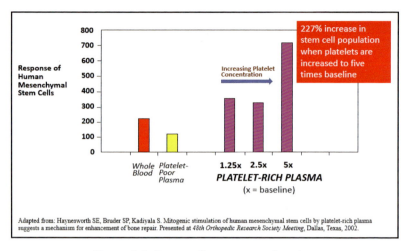

Figure 9.4: Stem cell response related to
platelet-rich plasma concentration.

Red and White Blood Cells

The other difference between PRP is the number of red and white cells. Keep in mind that most of the red cells are already removed in the making of platelet-rich plasma: whole blood is 94 percent red cells as compared to only 5 percent red cells in PRP (see Figure 9.2: Composition of whole blood compared to platelet-rich plasma). However, even though the remaining red cells are greatly diminished, it is believed that any red cells may still cause unnecessary aggravation after treatment. One issue has been that removing too many red cells may greatly reduce platelet levels since some platelets are within the red cell layer. Fortunately, recent developments in technology now permit the ability to remove most of the red cells while still maintaining high platelet counts. Another issue is that with Prolotherapy, we may prefer this additional red blood cell irritation to "wake up" certain tissue types that are not healing. Therefore, both formulas are used in Prolotherapy—the low red cell ("yellow") and the regular red cell ("red") —depending on the area treated, intended result, physician and/or patient choice and treatment plan.

Regarding white blood cells, some physicians argue that white cells may cause too much pain and should be reduced, especially in joints.[45] However, typically, white cells constitute only 1 percent of both whole blood and platelet-rich plasma, and therefore a *very* small percentage of the treatment formula (see Figure 9.2: Composition of whole blood as compared to platelet-rich plasma). Also, white cells are very difficult to remove without seriously sacrificing platelet numbers. [46] Most physicians also agree that white cells are important and improve wound healing; furthermore, white cells have antibacterial properties that are thought to potentially help reduce infection risk from, or after, the procedure (as long as done under appropriate sterile conditions of course.)[47] Therefore, it is generally agreed in the medical community that white cells are desirable and should remain in platelet-rich plasma formulas.[48]

How Platelet-Rich Plasma is Activated

In order to release growth factors, platelets must be activated. The activation process occurs in different ways. In a hospital setting, the surgeon activates platelet-rich plasma by mixing it with a commercially available protein called "thrombin." Thrombin thickens the PRP and causes a fast release of growth factors; this combination is then put on the desired tissue during surgery to help with healing. When PRP Prolotherapy is done in an office setting, some physicians add a very small amount of calcium chloride to the local anesthetic or to the platelet-rich plasma just prior to injection, which stimulates a slow release of platelet growth factors.[49] However, as it turns out, thrombin protein is also a natural component of connective tissue. That means that thrombin will naturally be released when the injection needle tip pierces the connective tissue that is being injected.[50] This is why Prolotherapy technique, which involves some needle peppering of the injection site, is important, especially if no other activating method is done. This needle irritation not only releases natural thrombin but also, as discussed earlier, "wakes up" nonhealing tissue so that platelets are directed where to start repair.

CORTISONE VERSUS PLATELET-RICH PLASMA

Cortisone injections are commonly recommended for the treatment of joint pain. However, the use of cortisone is controversial because it tends to break down, rather than repair, joints and connective tissue, especially if done repeatedly. Current evidence now supports platelet-rich plasma to be more effective than cortisone for treatment of joint and connective tissue issues,[51] especially long term. A well-designed, two-year, randomized, controlled, blind trial (meaning patients did not know which formula they were receiving), with a significant test group of 100 patients investigated cortisone versus platelet-rich plasma injections for elbow tendon problems. The researchers concluded that platelet-rich plasma reduced pain and increased function significantly, exceeding the effect of corticosteroid injection even after two years.[52] A similar study in 2017 agreed.[53] These two treatments were also compared for use in chronic, severe plantar fasciitis and concluded: "PRP was more effective and longer lasting than cortisone injection."[54] Platelet-rich plasma has also been found to be a "superior treatment option" versus cortisone for lumbar facet (low back joint) injections, with longer lasting effectiveness.[55]

PLATELET-RICH PLASMA FOR OSTEOARTHRITIS AND CARTILAGE PATHOLOGY

Multiple studies continue to emerge confirming the effectiveness of platelet-rich plasma for osteoarthritis (OA), Platelet-rich plasma also appears to have a protective effect on cartilage.[56] This is discussed in much more detail in Chapter 13: "Prolotherapy Regenerative Medicine for Osteoarthritis."

PLATELET-RICH PLASMA SAFETY CONCERNS/RISKS

Like Dextrose Prolotherapy, PRP Prolotherapy is low-risk and has few side effects. Concerns have been raised that the use of platelet growth factors can result in unwanted overgrowth of tissue; however, there have been no documented cases of hyperplasia (overgrowth), carcinogenesis (cancer), or tumor growth associated with the use of platelet-rich plasma that is autologous (taken from the same person it is given to).[57] Platelet-rich plasma growth factors do *not* enter the cells they are interacting with; rather, they act by binding to the outside of these cells.[58] This interaction causes normal healing but at a faster rate. Therefore, it has been concluded that platelet-rich plasma has no ability to induce tumor formation.[59] In addition, because the blood used in PRP Prolotherapy is taken from the same person it is given to, the risks of allergy or infectious disease are considered negligible.[60] As mentioned earlier, evidence also exists that platelet-rich plasma may have an anti-bacterial effect,[61] which also improves safety of the treatment when done under appropriate sterile conditions.

PRP PROLOTHERAPY VERSUS DEXTROSE PROLOTHERAPY

Both PRP and Dextrose Prolotherapy have been shown to stimulate natural healing.[62] Both can be effective, and both should be considered in the treatment plan for connective tissue repair. PRP Prolotherapy, however, may be deemed more appropriate in cases where the tissue or joint has become degenerated, there is osteoarthritis present or the problem is older and more chronic. When platelet-rich plasma is the formula used in Prolotherapy, it provides not only needed irritation (concentrated platelets are aggravating!) but also growth factors that provide a jump-start on healing. Using platelet-rich plasma is like adding fertilizer to newly planted seeds versus just planting the seeds; the condition of the "soil" can help to determine which formula is the best choice. Platelet-rich plasma may also be preferred over dextrose in cases of a tendon sheath or muscle injury; these areas are occasionally, but not typically, treated with dextrose.

Other factors to consider are that platelet-rich plasma is a more aggressive formula than dextrose; therefore, it can be more aggravating and uncomfortable for the patient afterward. The cost of PRP Prolotherapy is also higher than for Dextrose Prolotherapy because of the additional materials needed. Another difference is that PRP Prolotherapy seems to stimulate multiple healing episodes, sometimes creating more "ups and downs" in pain levels during the weeks following a treatment. With dextrose, on the other hand, there is usually only an initial period of discomfort, although there are variations from patient to patient. As a general rule, fewer treatments are needed with PRP than with dextrose. The bottom line is there are several factors to consider, and the determination of which type of Prolotherapy to use is made on an individual basis after careful evaluation and discussion between the doctor and the patient of all factors, including patient preference.

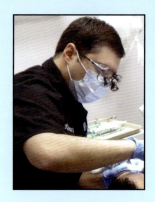

Dentist

In early 2013, I injured my wrist due to repetitive overuse at my busy dental office. This had happened before, but the first time it healed just fine. This last injury was different. No matter what I did, it wasn't getting better. I decided to try acupuncture with electrical stimulation, but it offered no relief. I tried applications of iontophoresis with dexamethasone (a steroid treatment like cortisone). I wore a wrist splint—I tried almost everything I could think of, and nothing was working.

I continued to have pain shooting up and down my hand every time I turned the knob to open a door, twisted the lid off a jar, or basically otherwise tried to use it. I was concerned that if I didn't receive proper treatment, it could eventually shorten my career. I decided that wasn't an option. I had heard about platelet-rich plasma (PRP) and regenerative medicine at a dental implant residency program; however, it wasn't until I heard about it again later from a medical colleague that I began to look into this emerging yet promising treatment option. Having a basic medical understanding about this particular type of treatment, I wanted to find someone who was skilled and specialized to perform it.

While I was researching PRP and Prolotherapy physicians, Dr. Donna Alderman's name kept coming up again and again, and I am glad it did. After the initial consult, she was optimistic that she could help me with PRP, sparing me from other therapies (and possible overtreatment). She was right! After only two PRP sessions, my wrist is now 99 percent better. I am able to work out again and do my normal daily activities, tending to my busy dental practice and all my patients while being virtually pain free. I *definitely* recommend PRP Prolotherapy to anyone who wants to handle their pain effectively without the burden, expense, and uncertainty of surgery. Yes, it is that good!

Ray Cros, D.M.D.
Family and Cosmetic Dentist

Using Your Own Tissues to Heal

To share the evolution of Prolotherapy into the use of autologous (one's own) adult stem cells as a treatment formula, I asked my colleague, Dr. Robert Alexander, to say a few words.

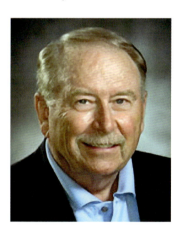

Robert W. Alexander, M.D., D.M.D., FICS

Dr. Robert Alexander is an internationally recognized aesthetic and reconstructive surgeon, author, teacher, and pioneer in the use of adipose stem/stromal cells in clinical practice, as well as a recognized leader for his accomplishments in *Biocellular Regenerative Medicine*® Dr. Alexander's contributions in the areas of aesthetic surgery, chronic wound therapy, and regenerative medicine and surgery is respected worldwide.

From the beginning of the use of Prolotherapy in the 1930s, practitioners have realized great success with stimulated healing within damaged ligaments, tendons, and joint structures. The last ten years has seen many advances in the field, especially involving the use of autologous (one's own) tissue. The value of using a patient's own cells and tissue to help in repair has long been proven in general and orthopedic medicine and surgery. For example, for decades, we've used adipose (fat) tissue for contouring issues and structural grafting for aesthetic purposes in reconstructive surgeries. Liposuction, which was introduced to the United States from Europe in the late 1970s, originally required the use of a large pump to remove fat. However, in the mid-1980s, aesthetic and reconstructive surgeons developed a gentle method for more effective fat removal (called "harvesting"), which used small blunt-tipped instruments (called "cannulas") rather than large pumps. That refinement offered both more predictable outcomes and much improved cellular survival.

Then in the 1990s, surgeons began combining platelet concentrates (platelet-rich plasma) with the adipose used for surgical reconstruction since the platelet-rich plasma both greatly aids healing and repair, and maximizes safety and efficacy. This combination resulted in enhanced wound site healing. Today, the relocation of undesired fat deposits to areas needing additional volume and structure, such as the breasts, buttocks, and face, has become the most requested elective aesthetic surgical procedure in the world.

In the late 1990s, researchers at UCLA and the University of Pittsburgh School of Medicine conducted in-depth studies of adipose with the goal of better understanding the character of the cells within it. Their findings demonstrated that adipose tissue holds vast numbers of "adult" stem-type cells. These cells are contained within the fat cellular tissue (called "stroma"). Subsequent research showed adipose to contain more than 2,000 times as many of these adult stem-type cells as compared to bone marrow; in addition, adipose can retain its regenerative capabilities in an older population much better than bone marrow does. Adipose has also been found to possess remarkable capabilities of becoming different types of connective tissue cells—cartilage, muscle, ligament, tendon, etc.—depending on the microenvironment in which it is placed, as well as possessing positive anti-inflammatory and healing properties that promote repair and regeneration.

Clinicians in orthopedic surgery and medicine were also encouraged to use this combination of platelet concentrates plus adipose tissue as an optimal cell source for replacement cells within musculoskeletal applications. Successes in such applications brought about a paradigm shift (a new model of how to do things) in orthopedic surgery and medicine, both as a minimally invasive alternative to surgery and as an adjunct (an additional step) done with surgery to improve post-surgical outcomes. Understanding that this adipose/platelet-rich plasma combination is a very potent stimulus to blood flow within wound sites, many practitioners started to apply this potential, with great success, in chronic wounds such as pressure sores, diabetic ulcers, burn ulcers, and blast, avulsion, and crush injuries. Many clinical papers and studies available in the medical literature confirm the safety and efficacy of these treatments.

All of these early steps led advanced Prolotherapy practitioners, starting about ten years ago, to begin to use this combination of stem/stromal cells in what is now known as Biocellular Prolotherapy or Biocellular Regenerative Medicine® for many conditions, including arthritis and degenerative joints; ligament, tendon, and muscle injuries; and other musculoskeletal pain. These applications are greatly aided by use of musculoskeletal ultrasound, which enables the practitioner to both accurately diagnose the condition and identify the optimal site of injection. It goes without saying that the more accurate the treatment is, the better its outcome will be. In the following chapter, Dr. Alderman explains the basics of this therapy, and how it is used in Prolotherapy to heal injured connective tissue and joints, helping to reduce or eliminate pain. Literally, thousands of successful Biocellular Prolotherapy treatments have been performed since 2009, with both remarkable results and a remarkable safety track record.

Biocellular (Stem Cell–Rich) Prolotherapy

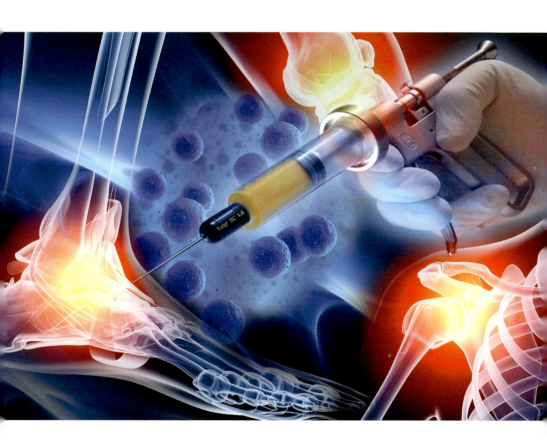

Biocellular (Stem Cell–Rich) Prolotherapy is the most advanced and aggressive form of Prolotherapy. It is used either when other forms of Prolotherapy have stopped working, or as a first procedure when a condition is severe. This type of Prolotherapy is called "Stem Cell-Rich" because tissue used is rich in stem cells, specifically "adult" stem cells. Because tissue used is taken from our own body, it is called "autologous" (auto meaning "self"). The two main tissue sources used in this type of Prolotherapy are either fat (medical term "adipose") or bone marrow, and the term "Biocellular" is an umbrella term that covers either tissue source. Like other forms of Prolotherapy, both chronic or acute problems can be treated. Biocellular Prolotherapy is especially well suited for sports injuries because of its tendency to encourage repair using new, normal tissue rather than weaker scar tissue.[1]

To be clear, adult stem cells are *not* embryonic or fetal stem cells. Adult stem cells exist within our own adult bodies; embryonic or fetal stem cells are those that exist in an unborn baby. While there seems to be immense potential with fetal and embryonic stem cells, there are also unanswered questions regarding safety; therefore, in the United States, use of fetal or embryonic stem cells is restricted. Fortunately, there is a lot of regenerative potential within the existing adult stem cells we all have within our own bodies.

BIOCELLULAR BASICS:
THE AUTOLOGOUS ADULT STEM CELL

All the tissues in the body are made up of cells. Any particular kind of cell—such as skin cells, muscle cells, ligament or cartilage cells—are referred to as being "specialized" because they have already developed into an established, distinct type of cell. However, we also have cells in our bodies that are *partially* specialized; that is, they have developed to a certain point only, and then stop there, waiting until they are needed for repair, at which point they have the ability to "stem" into the specific kind of cell needed. These partially specialized cells within our own bodies are called "adult" stem cells, and it is believed that their primary role is to maintain and repair the tissue in which they are found. [2]

The adult stem cell that interests the prolotherapist is the mesenchymal stem cell ("MSC"). This is the cell type from which the musculoskeletal system develops. The MSC is partially specialized to the point where it can become ligament, tendon, cartilage, muscle, fat, or bone, but it does not commit to a specific cell type until the need arises. For this reason, MSCs are called "multi-potential" or "multipotent," since there are multiple potential directions these cells can develop. The process of becoming more specialized into a needed cell type is called "differentiation" (from Latin for "to develop into"). Therefore, the term used to describe what an MSC goes through when it matures is "multipotent differentiation." Because MSCs have the ability to stem into needed cell types, they can greatly help healing when concentrated around an injured area. In addition to this, it is believed that MSCs simply improve the tissue microenvironment to make it more favorable towards healing because they release growth factors and cytokines (proteins that help with healing)[3] (see Figure 10.1: The mesenchymal stem cell).

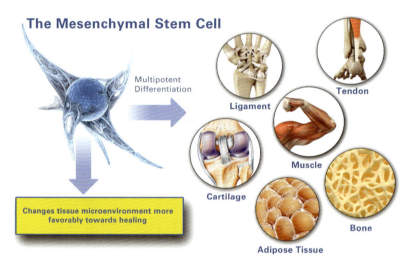

Figure 10.1: The mesenchymal stem cell

As mentioned earlier, the two biggest storage locations for MSCs in the body are fat (medical term: adipose) and bone marrow. Bone marrow had been used as an MSC source for many years, yet it was known that other tissues also contain MSCs. So in the late 1990s researchers began investigating other potential tissues for these cells and discovered that adipose had nearly identical regenerative abilities as did bone marrow.[4] In fact, as mentioned by Dr. Alexander in his introduction to this chapter, adipose was also found to contain up to 2,000 times as many MSCs as bone marrow.[5] There also exists strong evidence that, as a person ages, the regenerative power of MSCs is better maintained in adipose than it is in bone marrow.[6] These facts make adipose a more ideal regenerative stem cell source, especially for older patients. Adipose is also easier to obtain, and its extraction is better tolerated by patients, with less risk, than is bone marrow extraction. All the same, depending on the circumstances, bone marrow may be preferred, so both stem cell sources are used in Biocellular Prolotherapy.

MESENCHYMAL STEM CELLS: ADULT STEM CELLS FOR CONNECTIVE TISSUE HEALING

Mesenchymal stem cells (MSCs) are essential to tissue regeneration and wound healing.[7] Multiple studies have confirmed that MSCs help in healing of musculoskeletal tissue, specifically: ligament,[8] tendon,[9] cartilage,[10] disc,[11] and muscle.[12] An interesting observation about MSCs is that the amount and potency of these cells in patients with degenerative joints are often severely low.[13] Therefore, it is logical that using MSCs in the treatment of degenerative conditions would be beneficial.[14] Indeed, in degenerative diseases such as osteoarthritis (OA), regenerative therapies using MSCs have been shown to be quite effective.[15]

ADIPOSE AS AN
ADULT MESENCHYMAL STEM CELL SOURCE

Adipose as a stem cell source has been well recognized for many years, with studies and papers appearing regularly in the medical literature. There is even an organization dedicated to the use of adipose for regenerative purposes, the *International Federation for Adipose Therapeutics and Science ("IFATS")* which has been holding annual international scientific conferences since 2001. Scientists, engineers, and physicians from all over the world meet at these conferences every year to present and discuss the latest research, clinical uses, and controversies.[16]

Adipose as a stem cell source for repair within one's body is logical because it is the one of the most abundant cell types, found near or in almost every organ. Adipose itself is a very complex tissue (see Figure 10.2: The structure of adipose). There are several different cell types within it, and there is regular discussion about which cell type does what. Some researchers claim it is not actually the MSCs but another cell type in the adipose that are the true stem cells. These other cells surround blood vessels, and for that reason are called "pericytes" (*peri* meaning "around" and *cyte* meaning "hollow vessel").[17] Since it is not known exactly which cells are the most regenerative, and since in adipose these cells exist in such high numbers, isolation of specific cells is usually not necessary or even desirable[18] In Biocellular Prolotherapy, we do not typically extract or isolate the MSC, but rather use the entire "smorgasbord" of cells (called "stroma"), letting the body take what it needs. This is why the term "stem/stromal" cell is sometimes used.

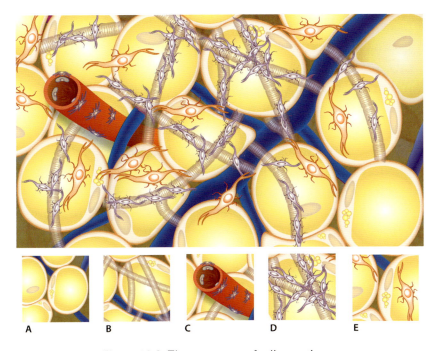

Figure 10.2: The structure of adipose tissue

[Note there are several different cell types, as explained in this key:

A. Adipose cells

B. Fluid and tissue outside of the cells, called "Extracellular Matrix"

C. Pericytes (surround blood vessels; important in new blood vessel formation)

D. Mesenchymal Stem Cells (MSCs) (the little guys)

E. Pre-Adipose cells]

Adipose and Platelet-Rich Plasma: Better Together

Studies have shown that using platelet-rich plasma and adipose tissue together "significantly improves" regeneration versus using adipose cells alone.[19] When adipose is used as the stem cell source, platelet-rich plasma is thus typically used at the same time since this combination has been shown to work synergistically (enhancing results) in multiple studies.[20] In one study, using adipose-derived cells with platelet-rich plasma, versus platelet-rich plasma alone on Achilles tendon injuries showed tendon strength for the adipose/platelet-rich plasma group to be greater, with a statistically higher production of collagen and growth factors.[21] Therefore, typically, adipose and platelet-rich plasma are done together during a Biocellular procedure.

The Phenomena of "Cellular Depletion" and the Extra Benefit of Biocellular Prolotherapy

When an area of the body has been repeatedly injured over a long period, a phenomenon called "cellular depletion" occurs. This means that in that depleted area, many of the adult stem cells present at birth that would normally be used for repair have already been used up, thus reducing the capacity for healing there. If local repair cells have been depleted, less aggressive forms of Prolotherapy may only go so far. Remember from the previous chapter that platelet-rich plasma works by sending biochemical signals for stem cells to come in to help repair an injury site. This signal is *local* (think of Bluetooth, which is a short-range signal), which means there must be stem cells within a certain distance of the platelets' signal in order for the signal to be effective. When there is cellular depletion, very few stem cells are close enough to "hear" the platelets' cry for help. (see Figure 10.3: What happens when there is cellular depletion). Such is the beauty of Biocellular Prolotherapy, since the treatment itself provides healthy adult stem cell sources directly to the depleted injury site.

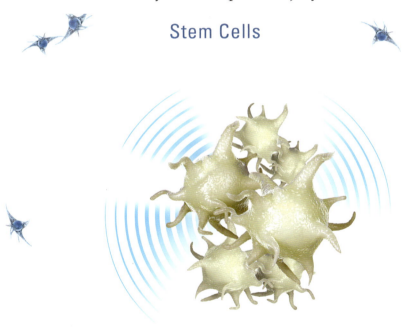

Figure 10.3: What happens when there is cellular depletion. Activated platelets signal for help, however few or no adult stem (repair) cells are within range to respond.

Biocellular Formula and Procedure Terminology

Multiple names exist to describe stem cell sources; therefore, the term "Biocellular" was created as an umbrella term to include any form of Prolotherapy involving the use of adult stem cell sources. This term may also contain the modifier *adipose-derived* or *bone marrow-derived* to clarify which stem cell source is being used. There are other various terms used by medical professionals and in the medical literature to describe terms relevant to Biocellular procedures. It is helpful to understand these terms should you have an interest in doing more research on your own in this area.

Terms relevant to Biocellular Prolotherapy:

- **ADIPOSE** is the medical term for fat.

- **ADSC** is the abbreviation sometimes used for "adipose–derived stem/stromal cell" tissue sources.

- **ADSC/PRP** is the abbreviation sometimes used for the combination of adipose-derived stem cell tissue sources and platelet-rich plasma.

- **ASPIRATE** refers to the cells or fluid removed from a person during a medical procedure known as ASPIRATION (aspiration is a medical term meaning "to draw up" or "to remove something from an area of the body").

- **AUTOLOGOUS** means "one's own." A patient's own fat and bone marrow are autologous tissues used in Prolotherapy treatment.

- **BONE MARROW ASPIRATE CONCENTRATE** (abbreviated "BMAC") consists of cells that have been removed (aspirated) from bone marrow and then concentrated.

- **LIPOASPIRATE** (*lipo* means "fat" + "aspirate") is what is taken during the adipose aspiration procedure. Therefore, "Lipoaspirate Prolotherapy" is a term sometimes used to describe Biocellular Prolotherapy using adipose.

- **STEM/STROMAL CELL** is sometimes used to describe the lipoaspirate. This is because the lipoaspirate is a combination of stem cells and the tissue "stroma." (Stroma is the tissue and liquid within which the cells exist.)

- **STEM CELL–RICH** is the most recent term, indicating the formula being used is the patient's own tissue (adipose or bone marrow), and that this tissue is naturally high (rich) in stem cells.

- Terminology used in the medical literature for lipoaspirate is **TISSUE-STROMAL VASCULAR FRACTION** (abbreviated "t-SVF"), so named since the cells are unprocessed "tissue" stroma and contain blood vessels (vascular). If this same tissue is digested with an enzyme to isolate the mesenchymal stem cells, it is then called **CELLULAR-STROMAL VASCULAR FRACTION** (abbreviated "c-SVF").

Biocellular Prolotherapy for Osteoarthritis (OA)

Osteoarthritis can be inflammatory, destructive, and progressive. Adult stem cells have been shown to both control inflammation and improve blood flow in joints, thereby slowing OA's progression.[22] Studies in animal OA models consistently demonstrate that adult stem cells prevent both the destruction of cartilage and further OA bone spurring, as well as improve existing ligament and meniscal damage.[23] An advantage of adult stem cells is that they seem to have the ability to "home in on"—to perceive and travel to—injured tissue; once there, they secrete growth factors and other elements that both help stop destructive inflammation and contribute to tissue repair.[24] This is in contrast to conventional treatments such as medication, physical therapy, hyaluronic acid, and cortisone injections; although these traditional remedies can relieve pain, they neither stop the progression of joint degeneration nor offer any regenerative capacity.[25] Both types of stem cell sources, bone marrow and adipose, are used in the treatment of OA.

The Choice of Biocellular Formula: Adipose versus Bone Marrow

The choice of which stem cell source to use in Biocellular Prolotherapy depends on several factors, including the condition being treated, the age of the patient, the physician's background and training, and the patient's preference.

While adipose and bone marrow formulas have demonstrated similar treatment capabilities, there does appear to be functional differences between them. Some animal and laboratory studies indicate that bone marrow may be preferred and more efficient for osteochondral (bone and cartilage) regeneration.[26] However, adipose has shown an excellent ability to stimulate cartilage regeneration,[27] and there are many studies that indicate similar chondrogenic (ability to make cartilage) potential between bone marrow–derived and adipose-derived MSCs.[28] In a recent case report, a patient received surgery for a cartilage defect, which is the traditional treatment. This particular patient had a condition called osteochondritis dissecans (a joint condition in which bone underneath the cartilage of a joint dies due to lack of blood flow; the bone can break lose and cause pain), which can be serious. However, that surgery failed. The patient then received an injection of autologous adipose-derived MSCs into the area. The result was structural and functional improvement, as well as reduction of pain levels.[29]

In multiple studies, both adipose and bone marrow stem cells have shown the ability to change the microenvironment more favorably toward healing and to decrease "bad" inflammation while promoting "good" inflammation and blood supply, helping to *reduce pain* and *stimulate repair*. However adipose is considered by some researchers to be better in this ability.[30] There are also several advantages that adipose has over bone marrow for ligament, tendon, and muscle repair,[31] especially in certain joints. For these reasons, adipose is becoming the preferred choice for connective tissue injury.

The Advantage of Adipose-Derived Biocellular Prolotherapy for Knee Osteoarthritis: The Fat Pad

Adipose-derived Biocellular Prolotherapy can also be an excellent treatment for knee OA because of its ability to replenish a structure in the knee called the "infra-patellar fat pad" [32] (*infra* meaning "under" and *patella* for the kneecap, so named because this fat pad sits directly under the kneecap). The fat pad is believed to be an important reservoir of regenerative cells,[33] including potent mesenchymal stem cells that have the ability to become cartilage. [34] A healthy fat pad has been found to help in the prevention or progression of OA.[35] In fact, a simple fat transfer (taking fat from another place in the body and injecting it into the knee joint) has been shown to help knee osteoarthritis pain in a recent study. The authors believed that this not only improved cushioning provided by the fat pad, but supplied stem cells to replenish that important tissue. [36]

As a person ages or experiences trauma, and there is wear and tear, the fat pad may lose volume, along with the stem cells within it becoming depleted (used up) or injured.[37] Age-related, fat-pad depletion has been associated with anterior knee pain and the development of OA,[38] and there is a strong correlation between the size and condition of a patient's fat pad and the severity of his or her pain and OA progression.[39] Also interesting is that removal of the fat pad during surgery has been associated with increased pain,[40] so, clearly, this structure is important in the health of the knee. With the adipose-derived Biocellular procedure, good fat taken from elsewhere in the body is transferred to a depleted fat pad. It is logical that this has the potential to restore this regenerative reservoir of cells and to improve the healing environment. The many cases of adipose-derived Biocellular Prolotherapy that have been completed since 2011 show just that: not only pain reduction and improved function but also objective ultrasound evidence demonstrating infrapatellar fat-pad improvement after treatment (see Figure 10.4: Ultrasound appearance of fat pad before and after adipose-derived Biocellular (Stem Cell–Rich) Prolotherapy). For all these reasons, adipose (fat) as a stem cell source appears to be a more logical choice to treat knee OA.

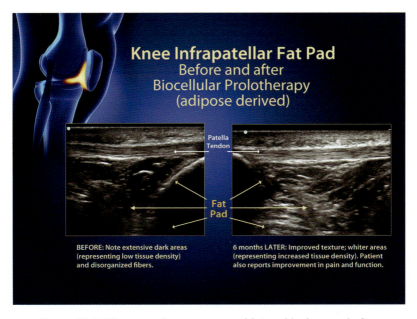

Figure 10.4: Ultrasound appearance of fat pad before and after adipose-derived Biocellular (Stem Cell–Rich) Prolotherapy

Biocellular Safety Concerns/Risks

As with any medical procedure, Biocellular Prolotherapy involves some risk, although when done by a properly trained professional, the risk is low. There is the risk of bruising and very mild discomfort at the extraction site; this typically lasts for a few days up to perhaps a few weeks, but rarely longer. There is also the risk of infection at the extraction site, but this is extremely rare. An additional risk when extracting adipose could be minimal skin surface irregularity or dimpling at the fat extraction site, but since the amount of fat needed is so small, this is also extremely rare, especially when done by an experienced physician. With bone marrow extraction, there is the risk that the extraction site may remain sore for a period of time; however, this is also rare.

There is also the question of safety which arises whenever cells capable of growth are introduced into a person. However, taking a person's own stem cell–rich tissues and then giving them back to that same person has been shown to be very safe. One study monitored 1,873 patients for 21 years who had been treated with bone marrow cells between 1990 to 2006. During that monitoring period, the researchers found "no increased cancer risk" either at the treatment site or elsewhere.[41] Another study followed 91 patients for over two years who had been treated for various orthopedic conditions with adipose-derived cells mixed with platelet-rich plasma and found no tumor formation at any site treated (a total of 100 joints).[42] Both bone marrow and adipose stem cells have also been used to repair injured cardiac muscle. As of 2014, more than 700 heart disease patients worldwide have received adult stem cell–based therapies with no indication of tumor growth ever reported.[43] In 2016, the *Journal of Orthopaedic Surgery and Research* concluded that the "use of MSCs in the clinical setting can be considered safe, since no major adverse events related to the treatment nor to the cell harvest have been reported," and that regardless of cell source or method, studies showed a high success.[44]

A few other procedure-related risks involving the extraction and injection of cells during this type of procedure exist in theory. This includes the theoretical risk for a blood clot; however, at the time of this writing, there have been *zero* such events reported with the use of the microcannula harvesting system (a gentle method used in extracting adipose). Nonetheless, all potential risks should be discussed prior to treatment with the physician performing the procedure.

FOOD AND DRUG ADMINISTRATION GUIDELINES

The Food and Drug Administration (FDA) is the government agency responsible for protecting the public health by assuring the safety and security of foods and cosmetics, human and veterinary drugs, biological products, and medical devices. Although the FDA does not regulate the practice of medicine, guidelines regarding the use of adult stem cells were established in 1997 and continue to be discussed and updated. [45] These guidelines conclude that using cells removed from a patient and returned to that same person (autologous) during the same procedure poses no greater risk of disease transmission than the procedure itself does, and so this practice is thus permitted. Procedures in Biocellular Prolotherapy follow these guidelines, which are continually discussed and redefined so as to keep pace with the rapidly growing field of regenerative technologies.

WHEN TO USE BIOCELLULAR (STEM CELL-RICH) PROLOTHERAPY: TREATMENT ALGORITHM

Biocellular Prolotherapy may be the preferable treatment for chronic or degenerative conditions where cellular depletion is suspected and a more aggressive approach is needed or preferred.[46] In many cases, prior to doing Biocellular treatment, the doctor will recommend one or two dextrose and/or platelet-rich plasma treatments to prime the area and see how much improvement can be obtained, and then advance to Biocellular if needed. The decision of which formula to use must be evaluated on a case-by-case basis, considering the problem to be addressed, the particular injury site, and the person's medical history—in addition to the individual's age and health status. Only after a thorough evaluation by a physician trained in these techniques, and an extensive discussion of a patient's needs and expectations, can the best decision be made to determine the optimal course of treatment. To get an idea of how a treatment plan is mapped out, see Figure 10.5: Typical Prolotherapy treatment algorithm (an "algorithm" is commonly used in medicine as a tool in problem-solving and creating a treatment plan).

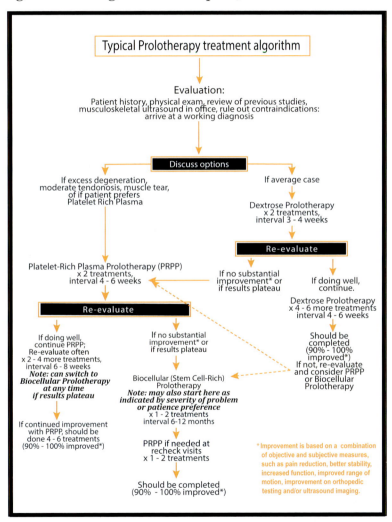

Figure 10.5: Typical Prolotherapy treatment algorithm

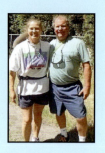

Businessman

A few years ago, I saw a respected surgeon in San Francisco for pain in my right knee and was told it was time for a knee replacement. As I was leaving the surgeon's office, one of his medical assistants pulled me aside and said I might want to have a consultation with a doctor in Alameda who was doing amazing things with Prolotherapy. At the time, I couldn't make it up a staircase without pulling myself up using the railing. Long story short, Dr. Alderman examined my knee and treated it with Biocellular (Stem Cell–Rich) Prolotherapy, and my wife and I now hike in the hills four to five miles, multiple times a week. It has been over two years since my treatment, and I continue to be active and pain free.

I describe the treatment to friends as being *"Star Trek*–like," as you could see the numerous tears of tendons, cartilage, and ligaments with ultrasound imaging, and then later, sometimes only weeks after the treatment, the ultrasound showed where these tears were filling in or had healed. Having seen a colleague recently go through a knee replacement, I know I was fortunate to have been given a better option.

Glenn H. Spoerl
Businessman

CHAPTER 11

Pain Medication: A Double-Edged Sword

In June 2016, Prince, a legendary artist in the music world, was found dead from an accidental overdose of opioid pain medication. The singer had been suffering for years with hip and knee pain, a result of jumping up and down in high heels while performing, and had been secretly taking pain medication to cope.[1] What began as a temporary solution for pain turned into dependence—and ultimately loss of life. Of course, pain medication is at times needed, especially on a short-term basis. However, the rapid increase in abuse of opioid medications has recently come into question. In 2016, the *New England Journal of Medicine* reported on an opioid crisis, with deaths from prescription-opioid overdoses now the leading cause of accidental death in the United States.[2] Another class of medications, nonsteroidal anti-inflammatory drugs (known by the abbreviation "NSAID"), have also come into question for long-term use, especially with musculoskeletal pain. Evidence suggests that both opioids and NSAIDs may have a negative impact on healing as well as potentially serious side effects.[3]

BOTH OPIOIDS AND NSAIDS
CAN NEGATIVELY IMPACT HEALING

The term *narcotic* is an older name for a class of medications now called "opioid analgesics." This class includes morphine, codeine, OxyContin, Percocet, Vicodin, and fentanyl, among others. For more than 100 years, opioids have been observed to negatively affect the immune system.[4] This is demonstrated in laboratory studies that show the long-term use of opioid medications can increase the size and spread of cancer cells.[5] Opioid medications may also prevent the body's ability to fight off infection.[6] This is supported by observations that patients abusing opioids have a higher level of infections than nonabusers.[7]

Clearly, opioids have the ability to negatively affect healing and should be used only when absolutely necessary—and then for only a brief period. Patients taking opioid analgesic medications during Prolotherapy treatment are advised to restrict usage to the minimum needed to alleviate pain. In some cases, a short course of opioids will be prescribed for post-treatment pain after Prolotherapy, but, again, with the recommendation to only take if needed and for the shortest time period possible.

Like the opioid medications, NSAIDs have been questioned for their impact on the immune system. With more than 70 million prescriptions written each year, NSAIDs are among the most commonly prescribed drugs in the United States. However, since NSAIDs are also available without a prescription, use is esti-mated at more than 30 billion doses per year![8] In one study, a common NSAID, ibuprofen, was found to have a negative effect on wound healing, resulting in both decreased numbers of fibroblasts (collagen-forming cells) and delayed formation of new skin and blood vessels.[9] Another study found that among patients admitted to hospitals for certain infections, those who had been taking NSAIDs prior to admission had longer hospital stays than those who had not.[10]

NSAID History and Types

NSAIDs are widely used to treat pain and musculo-skeletal injuries[11] (see the common NSAID medications listed in the sidebar). Aspirin is the original NSAID, first developed in 1853 and later refined by the Bayer company in 1899.[12] While there are positive health ben-efits of using aspirin in low doses, it has been linked to excessive bleeding, ringing in the ears, or stomach issues, especially when used in larger doses.[13] In the 1950s and 1960s, research to find a safer anti-inflam-matory medication resulted in the discovery of the first "non-aspirin" anti-inflammatories: indomethacin (brand name Indocin), approved by the US Food and Drug Administration (FDA) in 1965, and ibuprofen (brand names Motrin and Advil), first available in the United States in 1974. This first group of NSAIDs work by blocking not only inflammation but also have the side effect of blocking an enzyme responsible for pro-tecting the stomach lining. This means the stomach

List of Common NSAID Medications

CURRENTLY AVAILABLE

Aspirin (Bayer)

Celecoxib (Celebrex)

Diclofenac (Voltaren, Cataflam)

Etodolac (Lodine)

Fenoprofen (Nalfon)

Flurbiprofen (Ocufen)

Ibuprofen (Advil, Actiprofen, Motrin IB)

Indomethacin (Indocin)

Ketoprofen (Orudis)

Ketorolac (Toradol)

Meloxicam (Mobic)

Naproxen (Aleve)

Norboletone (Relafen)

Oxaprozin (Daypro)

Piroxicam (Feldene)

Salsalate (Disalcid)

Sulindac (Clinoril)

Tolmetin (Tolectin)

CURRENTLY IN CLINICAL TRIALS

Tanezumab

Fulranumab

Fasinumab

RECALLED OR NOT AVAILABLE

Lumiracoxib (Prexige)

Meclofenamate (Meclomen)

Rofecoxib (Vioxx)

Valdecoxib (Bextra)

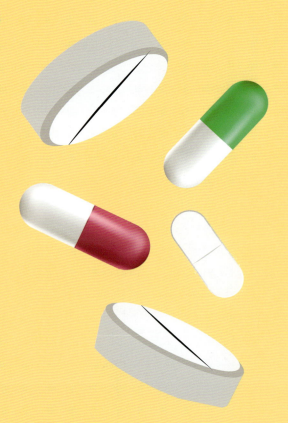

lining may lose valuable protection, resulting in ulcers and other stomach issues, for individuals who take them. This discovery inspired the development and release in the 1990s of a newer class of NSAIDs that were able to block the inflammatory enzymes without a negative effect on the stomach. Unfortunately, these newer NSAIDs—celecoxib (Celebrex), rofecoxib (Vioxx), meloxicam (Mobic), and valdecoxib (Bextra)—were found to increase the risk of heart attacks and strokes, leading to the recalls of Vioxx in 2004[14] and Bextra in 2005.[15] Since then, the link between all types of NSAIDs and heart problems has been well established.[16]

In the 2000s, there was testing done for a new class of NSAIDS that target nerve growth factor—a protein that works by reducing pain signals being sent to the brain. Early clinical trials showed good results in lowering patients' pain and inflammation. Unfortunately, reports of rapid cartilage loss and joint destruction—severe enough in some to require joint replacement—prompted the FDA to place a hold on all clinical trials in 2010. Although the FDA later lifted this hold in 2013 and allowed new trials, the long-term efficacy and safety profile of these medications are yet to be established.[17]

THE IMPORTANCE OF INFLAMMATION DURING ACTIVE HEALING AND WHY NSAIDs ARE CONTROVERSIAL FOR MUSCULOSKELETAL INJURIES

NSAIDs are commonly prescribed for pain related to muscle or tendon injuries, ligament sprains, low back pain, and osteoarthritis (OA). However, not all in the medical field are in agreement regarding this use of NSAIDs for musculoskeletal pain.[18] While there are studies that support the use of NSAIDs for musculoskeletal injuries, these studies look at short-term symptom relief and benefit, not long-term outcomes or recurrence rates. Remember from Chapter 5: "Prolotherapy Basics" that inflammation is a necessary part of healing, especially with connective tissue injuries. Blocking inflammation decreases blood flow, which may ultimately result in incomplete healing.[19] And remember from previous chapters, that even under the best of circumstances, connective tissue repair may be as little as 50 to 60 percent of preinjury strength.[20] NSAIDs may lessen this already slow, imperfect process even more.

Many health-care professionals have also begun to question, and to encourage their colleagues to question, the effects of anti-inflammatory medications on the *quality* of the tendon, ligament, bone, or muscle repaired while a patient was using NSAIDs for pain.[21] Taking an NSAID may not be a big issue if there is no active healing going on at the time. However, if there was recently a joint or musculoskeletal injury, then reducing inflammation may be counterproductive to healing.[22] Some studies even suggest that long-term use of NSAIDs may actually increase the degeneration of articular cartilage[23] (discussed in more detail later in this chapter). Because of the potential risks and controversy surrounding the use of NSAIDs for musculoskeletal pain—in addition to the potential adverse effects on the stomach, kidneys, and heart, as well as on bone health in general—a 2017 report questioned the high levels of NSAIDs prescribed to military personnel for musculoskeletal injuries.[24] Sports medicine physicians are also realizing the potentially detrimental effects of NSAIDs. Authors in the *Annals of Physical and Rehabilitation Medicine* wrote, "We do not recommend [NSAID] use for muscle injuries, bone fractures (also stress fractures), or chronic tendinopathy. In all cases, if chosen, NSAID treatments should always be kept as short as possible and should take into account the specific type of injury [and] the level of dysfunction and pain."[25]

NSAIDs MAY REDUCE MUSCLE, BONE, AND LIGAMENT HEALING

Muscle Healing

In general, muscles heal quickly because of their excellent blood supply (remember they are reddish in color for a reason!). While there are some who believe NSAIDs may actually help muscles in the early phase of healing,[26] other researchers have found NSAIDs may cause negative effects in the later phases of muscle healing[27] with subsequent loss of muscle function.[28] Therefore, NSAIDs are generally *not* recommended for use in muscle injuries.[29] A Scandinavian sports medicine journal reports, "It appears that a potential beneficial effect of NSAIDs in the early phase after injury is not maintained in the long term. . . . At the cellular level, evidence exists for a negative influence of NSAIDs on the muscle stem cell population."[30] In a study of athletes with acute (recent, sudden appearance with rapid worsening) hamstring injuries, one group was given NSAIDs while another was given a placebo. When the treatment period was over, the researchers noted that those who had been taking the NSAID were in more pain than those who had taken the placebo—inferring that better overall healing had occurred *without* medication. They concluded that using NSAIDs for muscular injuries was not recommended.[31]

Bone Healing

NSAIDs have also been linked to poor bone and fracture healing.[32] The authors of an article appearing in the *Journal of the American Academy of Orthopaedic Surgeons*, state, "When fracture healing or spine fusion is desired, nonsteroidal anti-inflammatory drugs should be avoided."[33] Indeed, several studies over the years have shown disturbances in bone healing and immune system functioning, decrease in bone mineral density,[34] failure to heal/delayed healing, [35] and even bone loss,[36] in many patients taking NSAIDs.[37] One study examined 288 patients who underwent spinal fusion (an operation where two bones in the spine are fused together), and determined that those patients who took NSAIDs immediately following surgery were *five times* more likely to experience "fusion non-union"—meaning the bones didn't grow together as expected—than those patients who'd taken a placebo.[38] Thus NSAIDs are not recommended when bone healing is important.

Ligament Healing

Several studies done with athletes have shown NSAIDs to have a negative effect on ligament healing. It was found that athletes who took NSAIDs after an ankle ligament sprain often return to their sport sooner than those who did not, probably related to reduced pain. However, those taking NSAIDs may have poorer ligament healing and increased joint instability later.[39] And in animal studies, animals taking NSAIDs showed a decrease of ligament strength (32 percent loss) versus animals who did not take this medication.[40] Other findings were that NSAIDs taken after a shoulder dislocation were detrimental to ligament healing and stability, and should be avoided or limited.[41] Fortunately, many doctors no longer recommend NSAIDs for ligament injuries.[42]

NSAIDs May Cause Cartilage Damage and Progression of Osteoarthritis

NSAIDs are often prescribed as a treatment for osteoarthritis (OA), but, unfortunately, these medications may do more harm than good—in some cases, significantly more harm. Specifically, some NSAIDs have been found to inhibit the production of a protein needed for cartilage formation, especially when taken in higher doses.[43] A study in the well-respected journal *The Lancet* noted a "highly significant association" between NSAID use and hip joint destruction.[44] Other studies have shown more rapid and severe progression of OA in patients taking NSAIDs than in those not taking them.[45] And a large double-blind study evaluated the progression of OA in 812 patients taking either the NSAID *indomethacin* or a placebo. After one year, the study concluded that there was a statistically significant increase in the rate of joint deterioration and reduction of joint space in those patients taking the NSAID versus the ones that were just taking the placebo.[46] So while taking an NSAID may help with the pain of osteoarthritis, it may actually worsen the condition for which it is being taken.

NSAIDs May Worsen Tendinopathy

Remember from Chapter 6 (Section entitled: Tendinopathy, Tendonitis, and Tendonosis) that tendinopathy is a term used to describe any pain or dysfunction in a tendon, commonly thought of as *"tendonitis."* Also recall from Chapter 6 that tendons previously labelled as "chronic tendonitis" are actually often nonhealing, *non-inflamed* tendon tissue where collagen is, in fact, actually degenerating—a chronic condition called *"tendonosis."*[47]

Given that revelation, consider the effect that an anti-inflammatory with the potential to delay healing would have on non-inflamed, already degenerating tissue; such would, at the very least, be ineffective and counterproductive. In fact, NSAIDs may actually accelerate the develop of tendonosis by turning a tendonitis, an inflamed tendon that is trying to heal, into one that is not (tendonosis). Indeed, studies have confirmed that NSAIDs can hamper the healing of tendons, especially immediately after an injury. One study showed that taking such medication in the first week after rotator cuff tendon surgery significantly decreased healing.[48] There is also evidence that NSAIDs decrease the body's ability to make collagen within the tendon itself,[49] significantly decreasing tendon strength, along with diameter (thickness).[50] Using NSAIDs for tendinopathies is summed up in this editorial statement from the *Clinical Journal of Sport Medicine*: "From our understanding of the etiology and development of this condition [tendinopathy], we believe that there is no scientific basis to manage chronic tendinopathy with NSAIDs."[51]

NSAIDs Have Side Effects

As if all of the aforementioned weren't enough, anti-inflammatory medications have negative side effects on other parts of the body. Using NSAIDs can raise blood pressure.[52] They can also increase dehydration, and they have been implicated in case reports of kidney failure in both runners[53] and military personnel.[54] The *New England Journal of Medicine*, evaluating NSAID use in the general population, concluded that long-term use increases the risk of kidney failure.[55]

Unfortunately, the list goes on. Complications related to gastrointestinal (stomach, intestine) side effects from using NSAIDs are responsible for approximately 100,000 hospital admissions—and 16,500 deaths—in the United States each year.[56] And these figures don't even include deaths possibly related to cardiovascular side effects,

FDA Warnings on NSAID Use

Following numerous adverse events from the use of NSAIDs, in 2005, the FDA issued a warning regarding the risks of taking these medications.[59] Then in 2015, the FDA strengthened its warning,[60] writing that "nonsteroidal anti-inflammatory drugs (NSAIDs) can increase the chance of a heart attack or stroke [in patients with or without risk factors for heart disease], either of which can lead to death. Those serious side effects can occur as early as the first few weeks of using an NSAID, and the risk might rise the longer people take NSAIDs. (Although aspirin is also technically an NSAID, this revised warning doesn't apply to aspirin.)"[61] In 2016, the FDA also required that NSAID labels be updated to warn that use of NSAIDs has been associated with "increase[d] cardiovascular thrombotic risk [stroke]" which were "observed most consistently at higher NSAID doses," along with "increased risk of heart failure," and "an approximate two-fold increase in hospitalizations for heart failure" in NSAID-treated patients compared to placebo-treated patients."[62] The FDA also recommends that prescriptions be the lowest effective NSAID dose for the shortest duration possible that would still facilitate the ideal treatment goal. Other medical associations support this recommendation, including the American College of Cardiology/American Heart Association,[63] the American College of Rheumatology,[64] the National Kidney Foundation,[65] and the Alliance for Rational Use of NSAIDs.[66]

which are now thought to exist with every NSAID (see page 148: "FDA Warnings on NSAID Use). The awareness of this side effect began in 2004 during a study of the NSAID *Vioxx*. During that study, done to see how effective it was for pain, participants taking it were having heart attacks and strokes, in fact twice as many heart attacks and strokes as those not taking the drug![57] Although the reasons for these cardiovascular complications aren't completely clear, it's believed that, in addition to inhibiting the enzyme that causes inflammation, these types of NSAIDs may also inhibit an enzyme that protects the heart, thus increasing the likelihood of heart attacks and blood clots.[58] Therefore, it is clear that NSAIDs are not a long–term solution for pain. If needed, these should be taken for the briefest period possible, and at the lowest effective dose.

NSAID Use during Prolotherapy Treatment

What we are trying to do with Prolotherapy treatment is increase good inflammation, necessary for healing in the musculoskeletal system.[67] Without inflammation, there will be an insufficient healing response. Because of this, and because of the potential for NSAIDs to negatively impact healing and immune function—let alone all the other potential side effects—Prolotherapy patients are instructed to avoid anti-inflammatory medications during their treatment course, especially immediately preceding and following treatment. In some circumstances, a patient wishing to receive

Prolotherapy treatment might need to take NSAIDs for another condition. It is believed that the degree of NSAID negative effects on healing are related to the specific NSAID used, when it was started, and the duration of therapy.[68] While not ideal, a good Prolotherapy treatment outcome may still be possible even if a person needs to take NSAIDs (especially with the more advanced Prolotherapy formulas), depending on timing and amount taken. However, all medications being taken, or questions regarding usage, should, of course, be discussed with the treating physician prior to beginning a course of Prolotherapy treatment.

Prior NSAID Use and Pain Perception after Prolotherapy Treatment

An interesting phenomenon I have observed in patients who have been in the habit of regularly taking NSAIDs for pain prior to starting Prolotherapy is that it may take longer for that patient to notice improvement from treatment. This is because NSAIDs, especially if taken on a regular basis prior to treatment, have been masking a person's true level of pain (called "baseline" pain). When NSAIDs are stopped prior to treatment, then you will feel your original pain at its true level (not masked), as well as possibly additional pains in your body that have been covered up and that you might not have even known about. The body has become accustomed to having NSAIDs covering up these pains, and then when you stop taking them, followed by a

Prolotherapy treatment, you can experience what I call the "double whammy" effect: expected after-treatment pain on top of a higher baseline pain level. Therefore, it may take longer for you to perceive improvement from Prolotherapy treatment. The important thing is to realize this can happen and to hang in there. Usually, things will normalize after the second treatment. What really matters is the fact that, instead of just *masking* pain that had no end in sight, after healing starts to take place and the *cause* of the pain improves, so will the pain.

An example of this is a patient I saw years ago. She had been taking 2,400 mg of ibuprofen a day—a huge amount—for years prior to treatment. Just before beginning Prolotherapy, she went "cold turkey" off the medication. After a few treatments, she told me she still didn't notice any difference—that she was in the same amount of pain. I then asked her how much ibuprofen she was taking now. She replied "none," and I was able to point out the difference: she had the same level of pain, but *without* the medication. That is improvement! She then realized how much better she had become, how much stronger she felt, and how much more she was able to do. Therefore, it is important to understand this phenomena and how prior use of NSAIDs (or other medication) prior to treatment may affect the treatment course.

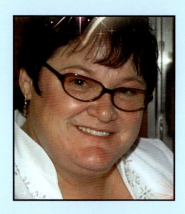

Flight Systems Design Engineer

In August 2013, at 52 years old, I reached behind my chair to pick up my cell phone and suddenly felt extreme pain in my shoulder—so strong I couldn't move my arm. For years, I had experienced episodes of shoulder pain, but those always resolved; however, this time felt different. I went to urgent care that night and was given an injection to relax the muscles. The next day, I went to my primary care physician, who gave me a cortisone injection and prescribed pain medication, along with a referral to an orthopedic surgeon. This surgeon took a brief glance at me and dismissively remarked, "It's just a touch of bursitis, dear." He didn't examine me or try to get me to lift my arm...nothing—not even an X-ray! I was in the most pain I have ever felt in my life. In the past, I have had torn ligaments, broken bones. I've given birth, but nothing compared to the pain I felt in my shoulder. Add to that the fact that I'd lost all the use of my arm since it had now become frozen. The surgeon gave me another cortisone injection and some pain pills, and he sent me home with instructions to try an ice bag.

I had a follow-up appointment with this surgeon a few weeks later. I was still in a great amount of pain despite the anti-inflammatory medication I'd been prescribed. I couldn't lie down to sleep. I had to sleep sitting up in a chair, but even then, I couldn't find a comfortable position. I couldn't even pull up my underwear. So for the follow-up appointment, I brought my daughter with me, and she demanded I receive some kind of imaging. The surgeon then ordered an MRI, which revealed a labral tear, SLAP type (stands for "superior labral tear from anterior to posterior"), along with some arthritis and bursitis. I was told these results didn't mean anything, but because I couldn't move my arm, the doctor sent me to physical therapy, which did not help. I was off work for over two months seeing doctors and trying to get functional. During that time, I tried another orthopedic doctor in my network who looked at the MRI and agreed it was just "a touch of bursitis." Over the course of the next two years, I had 23 visits to doctors, and I received multiple injections of cortisone or painkillers. I was also prescribed medications such as morphine, Norco, oxycodone, tramadol, trazodone, and Vicodin, as well as lidocaine patches, muscle relaxants such as Robaxin and Soma, and NSAIDS (nonsteroidal anti-inflammatory drugs) such as Mobic and others. Nothing worked very well. I continued to be in tremendous pain and had to continue to sleep sitting up. Eventually, I suffered a mild heart attack from taking so many NSAIDs. This is when I knew I had to do something else; otherwise, what I was doing was going to kill me.

I saw a third orthopedic surgeon who said the cortisone shots had actually made my shoulder worse and that surgery might help, though at that point, the odds weren't good. Fortunately, I had heard about Prolotherapy from a coworker and decided to try it before surgery. I saw Dr. Alderman in July 2016, almost three years after my injury. She did a diagnostic ultrasound that imaged my shoulder not only at rest but also when moving, and saw a rotator cuff tear that increased with motion. Because of the severity of the problem, Dr. Alderman recommended Biocellular (Stem Cell–Rich)

Prolotherapy. She took cells from my own fat and platelets from my blood, and used the ultrasound to find the tear in my shoulder and injected the cells and platelets into it. That injection hurt all the way to my elbow, but it was well worth it. I was amazed when within a week I stopped needing pain medication. A follow-up ultrasound three months later showed dramatic improvement. The pain started to resolve, and I am now able to sleep lying down, lift my arm, and use it again. Nine months have passed since my Biocellular treatment and still no shoulder pain! I am so amazed, after suffering through all that pain, all that time, and all those drugs, that my shoulder is better after just one Biocellular Prolotherapy treatment. Most importantly, my shoulder is now not just masked with pain medication, but *healed*, and I have my life back.

Barbara Smith
Flight Systems Design Engineer

CHAPTER 12

Prolotherapy Regenerative Medicine for Tendinopathy, Ligament Sprains, Muscle and Meniscal Tears

endon and ligament injuries represent almost half of the 32 million musculoskeletal injuries reported every year in the United States.[1] These injuries have long been a challenge for classic orthopedic medicine because of their poor response to traditional treatment.[2] Meniscal tears are also common, and challenging to treat, with the traditional approach being the surgical removal of the injured tissue. However, because there is a high risk for the development of osteoarthritis (OA) after even a minor surgical procedure, many physicians have moved toward surgical repair rather than removal of meniscal tears, but there are limitations here as well.[3] Fortunately, Prolotherapy offers a nonsurgical low risk, high reward, treatment option. Both acute and chronic problems can also be treated.

TENDINOPATHY

As discussed previously, tendinopathy is an umbrella term for any tendon problem. Remember from previous chapters that a tendon injury may start out as a "tendonitis" (an inflamed tendon), but if it becomes chronic, inflammation is usually no longer present. For that reason, it is not called a "chronic tendonitis" but rather a "tendonosis," a nonhealing, non-inflamed degenerative tendon condition.[4] With Prolotherapy, what we are really trying to do is turn a nonhealing, degenerative tendon back into a tendonitis, on purpose, in order to stimulate repair and healing.[5] All three of the Prolotherapy formulas have successfully been used to help with healing tendinopathies. Injecting even a low concentration of the traditional Prolotherapy formula, dextrose, into a tendon will stimulate natural growth-factor elevation within minutes to hours.[6] Multiple studies for multiple joint areas have also shown the effectiveness of Dextrose Prolotherapy.[7]

As mentioned previously, both Platelet-Rich Plasma (PRP) and Biocellular (Stem Cell–Rich) Prolotherapy formulas have been found to be safe and effective treatments tendinopathies. PRP has been shown to improve quality of tendon repair and reduce pain for many tendon areas, including wrist, rotator cuff (shoulder), knee patella tendon,[8] plantar fasciitis,[9] and other tendinopathies.[10] Biocellular formulas have been used for multiple tendon areas as well, including chronic patellar tendinopathy.[11] When PRP and Biocellular formulas were directly compared to each other, both were found to be beneficial, however the Biocellular formula obtained "faster results," making it particularly suitable for patients who need to return to physical activities sooner.[12]

Of note is a case series (more than one patient case report) describing the use of Biocellular Prolotherapy for severe achilles tendonosis and a large achilles tendon tears. Improvement was seen as soon as 3 to 4 weeks after treatment, and at 12 weeks after treatment, all patients returned to full activity without pain or dysfunction. Ultrasound images before and after treatment are noteworthy for dramatic healing of this large tendon tear (see Figure 12.1: Ultrasound of an Achilles tendon tear before and after Biocellular (Stem Cell–Rich) treatment). During follow-up at three to four years after the procedures, all patients were still symptom-free, with no recurrence of any problems or pain.[13]

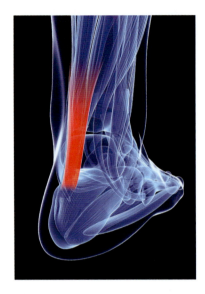

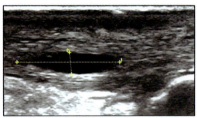

BEFORE TREATMENT: Large tear (black measured area) and tendonosis present

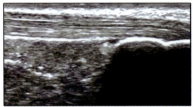

AFTER TREATMENT: Tendon has normal appearance with complete resolution of tear and tendonosis (images taken at one year follow up)

Adapted from Tate-Oliver K, Alexander RW. Combination of autologous adipose-derived tissue stromal vascular fraction plus high-density platelet rich plasma or bone marrow concentrates in Achilles tendon tear. *Journal of Prolotherapy*. 2013; 5: e895-912, used with permission.

Figure 12.1: Ultrasound of an Achilles tendon tear
before and after Biocellular (Stem Cell–Rich) treatment

LIGAMENT SPRAINS

Ligament tissue is meant to be strong in order to hold bones together and provide stability for the joint. These ligaments are supposed to have a little "give," but are not designed to be overly flexible. They can be over-stretched, either suddenly, or gradually, resulting in a "sprain." Sprains are common, and can be acute (sudden, short-lived) or chronic (ongoing, recurrent). There are also degrees of sprain, all the way from mild to severe.

All three Prolotherapy formulas have shown a high success rate with ankle ligament injuries and pain,[14] even when the ankle sprain is old.[15] Dextrose and PRP Prolotherapy have also been used successfully with many other joint ligament injuries,[16] including knee ACL (anterior cruciate ligament) tears.[17] Autologous bone marrow has been found to accelerate ligament healing in animal studies, where dissection and thorough investigation of tissue quality can be verified.[18]

The system used by many doctors to determine the severity of a sprain ranges from Grade I (over-stretching) to partial tear (Grade II), and then complete tear (Grade III) (see Figure 12.2: How sprains are graded as to severity). If a ligament has a severe, complete tear (Grade III), surgery is often recommended, especially in cases where the injury is new and the demand on the joint is high, as in an active person or athlete. Fortunately, most sprains are Grade I or II and can be treated with Prolotherapy. And even in some cases of Grade III sprains, where surgery is not recommended (discussed next), Prolotherapy has been successful.[19]

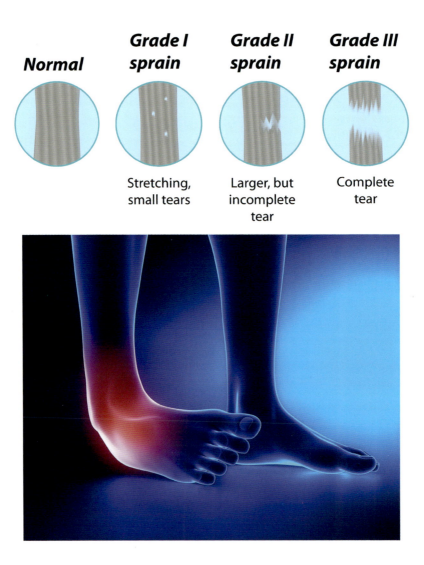

Figure 12.2: How sprains are graded as to severity

When it comes to complete ligament tears (Grade III), there is some controversy over whether surgery should always be done, especially when injuries are older, or the individual is not very active. Although surgery for severe ligament injuries does appear to decrease the re-injury rate, it increases the risk for the subsequent development of osteoarthritis.[20] Balancing the advantages and disadvantages of surgical and nonsurgical treatment for ankle sprains specifically, authors in the *Archives of Orthopedic and Trauma Surgery* concluded that the majority of all ankle sprains could be managed without surgery.[21]

MUSCLE TEARS

Muscles have a very good blood supply, and so generally heal quickly without any intervention. However, if a muscle tear is large enough, it may not heal well, or heal with scar tissue formation. Since scar tissue is weaker tissue than normal tissue, this is not ideal. Platelet-rich plasma has been used for acute muscle injuries because of its ability to accelerate repair[22] and potentially prevent scar tissue formation. Biocellular (Stem Cell–Rich) Prolotherapy has also successfully been used to stimulate faster and better repair, without scar tissue. A case report showed complete healing, without scar tissue formation, when an athlete was treated with Biocellular (adipose-derived) two weeks after sustaining a large, painful abdominal muscle tear which was not resolving on its own. One month later, the patient was pain free; ultrasound imaging showing complete healing without scar tissue, confirmed up to the final three-year follow-up[23] (see Figure 12.3: Ultrasound of an abdominal muscle tear before and after adipose-derived Biocellular (Stem Cell–Rich) treatment).

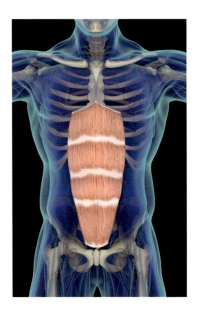

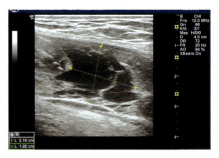

BEFORE TREATMENT: Large tear present (black measured area)

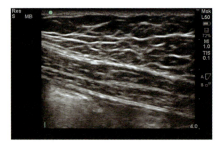

ONE MONTH AFTER TREATMENT: Tear healed without scar tissue formation

Adapted from Alexander RW. Biocellular regenerative medicine: Use of adipose-derived stem/stromal cells and its native bioactive matrix. *Physical Medicine & Rehabilitation Clinics of North America*. 2016; 27(4): 871-891, used with permission

Figure 12.3: Ultrasound of an abdominal muscle tear before and after adipose-derived Biocellular (Stem Cell-Rich) treatment.

MENISCAL TEARS

The meniscus is a C-shaped piece of cartilage that provides cushioning in the knee. The word "meniscus" comes from Latin for "crescent moon," which is what the meniscus looks like. The plural of meniscus is "menisci" (see Figure 12.4: The menisci).

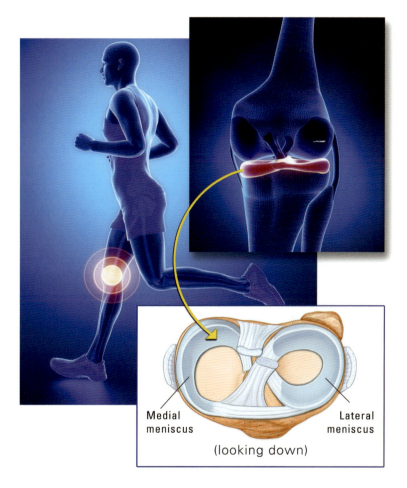

Figure 12.4: The menisci

As you can see from this drawing, there is a "medial" (towards the middle of the body) meniscus and a "lateral" (towards the outside of the body) meniscus.

The presence of healthy menisci is important for proper functioning of the knee.

Meniscal tears are frequent injuries seen by orthopedic medicine physicians. Traditional treatment has focused primarily on surgical repair or removal of all or part of the meniscus. Unfortunately, surgery may not always be successful, for a couple of reasons. First, meniscal tissue is very limited in its ability to heal because most of it (the inner two-thirds, which is also where most tears occur[24]) has *zero* blood supply.[25] Secondly, a meniscal tear may not be the cause of a person's pain. Most people do not realize that the inner two-thirds of the meniscus, in addition to having no blood supply, has *zero* nerve fibers, so a meniscus tear there does not actually cause pain. This makes perfect sense when, as discussed in Chapter 7, a high number of abnormal MRI findings, such as meniscal tears, exist in people without any pain[26]; in fact, meniscal tears even exist on MRIs of pain free, high functioning professional athletes.[27] So the presence of a meniscal tear on MRI may not necessarily explain what is causing a person's pain, and so surgery on that tear may not resolve the problem.

What is more likely causing pain in these situations? To answer this, I will explain a little more about how the meniscus helps to provide stability in the knee. A common place for knee pain is the inner side of the knee, called the medial knee. This is where the medial meniscus connects to the medial collateral ligament (abbreviated "MCL"). In a healthy knee, the medial meniscus and the MCL are firmly attached to each other in order to provide knee stability (see Figure 12.5: Medial meniscus/medial collateral ligament interface normal anatomy).

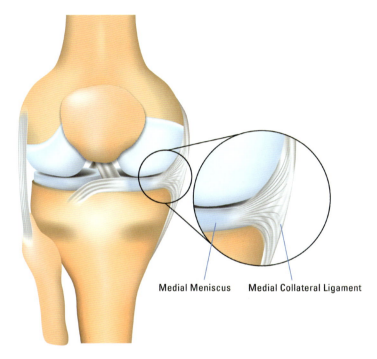

Medial Meniscus   Medial Collateral Ligament

Figure 12.5 Medial meniscus/medial collateral ligament interface, normal anatomy. As can be seen, the medial collateral ligament is firmly attached to the medial meniscus in order to provide stability in a healthy knee. Disruption of this interface connection can result in instability and pain.

Because these two tissues are connected, whenever there is an injury to any part of the medial meniscus, there will almost always be corresponding microtears and injury to the MCL. This causes a disruption at the interface, eventually resulting in ligament laxity, instability and pain. An MRI is done, which will show the medial meniscus tear, but not usually the corresponding ligament laxity and microtears. Therefore, meniscus surgery can fail because the ligament injury, which may actually be causing the pain, is never addressed. And remember, as discussed previously, that even with minimal surgery, there is an increased risk for the early onset or acceleration of osteoarthritis (OA).[28] Therefore, unless there is a clear-cut surgical need, an alternative nonsurgical approach is desirable.

All three Prolotherapy formulas have been used successfully to stimulate the repair of meniscal tears, in addition to being able to directly treat ligament injury and laxity. Dextrose and platelet-rich plasma injections have been shown to be effective in many studies,[29] improving pain as well as halting the progression of meniscal damage, as documented by MRI.[30] Biocellular (Stem Cell–Rich) treatment also has the therapeutic potential to directly and indirectly contribute to meniscal healing.[31] In a case report, a patient with an MRI-documented meniscal tear and a two-year history of knee pain received one adipose-derived Biocellular treatment. Three months later, a repeat MRI showed almost complete disappearance of the meniscal tear, along with significant pain reduction.[32] Other research papers agree that the Biocellular therapy has much potential in meniscal treatment, especially the adipose-derived sources.[33]

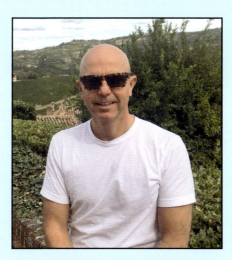

Investment Banker

I was diagnosed with a rotator cuff tear in March 2016. I could hardly use my arm, was unable to lift anything above my head, or reach behind to grab anything—not even a napkin. I was unable to really lift or carry anything or move anything with any weight to it. I just watched, feeling helpless, as my physique diminished. I was in a low level of constant nagging pain, often waking up from pain multiple times per night. The whole thing was very frustrating, affecting my mood and ultimately my ability to do the things I enjoy most: fishing and weight training. I saw my doctor, who sent me for rehab physical therapy, but, unfortunately, that didn't work. I was then told that the only solution was to surgically repair the 6.5mm tear in my rotator cuff. By then it was mid-October 2016. Feeling totally hopeless, I scheduled the surgery. However, several friends and my wife urged me to give regenerative injections a chance. That is when I contacted Dr. Alderman, who started with a PRP treatment to prime the area and then advanced to Biocellular Prolotherapy with adipose. Three months later, my pain was essentially gone, and my range of motion was back to normal. I had lost muscular strength from inactivity, so the next step was to begin an exercise program under the guidance of my trainer, Adam. He brought me along beautifully, slowly building strength and careful not to allow me to overdo it. Six months after my treatment, an ultrasound scan showed full healing of the rotator cuff tear with dramatic tissue quality improvement. Best of all, by then I was back to full function. I am able to work out and go fishing, as well as lift or carry objects—all activities I was not able to do before. I want to point out the importance of sticking with the treatment, as results take time. Shortly after the first injection, I still wanted to give up and get the surgery. I am so glad I hung in there and did not do the surgery, which I believe would have been a mistake for me. I am getting stronger and stronger every day—I'm fully functional. I'm back to lifting weights, pull-ups, and push-ups, following the program designed for me. I'm excited to get back to training and achieving fitness goals again.

Tim Woodall
Investment Banker

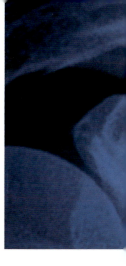

CHAPTER 13

Prolotherapy Regenerative Medicine for Osteoarthritis

"Arthritis" is a diagnosis frequently given to a patient as the reason for his or her joint pain. The word itself comes from *arthr*, meaning "joint," and *itis*, meaning "inflammation." There are several different types of arthritis, the most common being osteoarthritis (abbreviated "OA")[1] (*osteo* for "bone"). OA is also known as "degenerative joint disease" or "wear-and-tear" arthritis. OA is diagnosed when bony spurs, calcium deposits, and/or cartilage breakdown appear in an X-ray or other imaging of a joint.

Typical medical recommendations for OA are pain medication or NSAIDs (nonsteroidal anti-inflammatory drugs), which offer short-term relief but, as discussed earlier, may have unwanted side effects. Cortisone injections are also often recommended, which may sometimes help temporarily; however, they can have adverse effects on joints and joint tissue. Hyaluronic acid (a jelly-like substance that provides padding) may help, but only temporarily. More hands-on approaches such as physical therapy or osteopathic or chiropractic treatments may help, but not in every case. And, of course, there is surgery, which may not be clear-cut as to need, has additional risk, and may fail. Clearly, there is a need for a safe and effective nonsurgical treatment for OA. Fortunately, we have Prolotherapy Regenerative Therapies. To understand how Prolotherapy helps with OA, it is important to understand how and why OA develops.

JOINT INSTABILITY: A COMMON CAUSE OF OSTEOARTHRITIS

As discussed in Chapter 5, unresolved ligament injury results in ligament looseness (laxity) and joint instability, which then ultimately leads to abnormal loading of that joint, uneven wear and tear, and, eventually, OA.[2] This is seen in athletes who suffer ligament or tendon injuries, then later are seen to have OA.[3] In fact, insufficient healing and weakness of ligament or tendon connective tissue supporting a joint is believed to be one of the most important factors in the later development of OA.[4] Therefore, OA is, in most cases, a result of the problem—connective tissue weakness—rather than the cause.

LIGAMENT INJURY PRECEDES OSTEOARTHRITIS

As early as 1972, researchers noticed this relationship between ligament injury, joint instability, and the later development of OA.[5] A very large, well-done study investigated this relationship by seeing what happens to a particular joint in the hand over time. Patients were seen for 25 years, interviewed as to pain or issues, examined for stability, and received regular hand X-rays to see the condition of that joint. At the beginning of the study, these joints were stable, and there was no OA seen in the joint. What was noted, over the years, is that the first thing that occurred was ligament weakness, followed by joint instability—long *before* any signs of OA in X-rays.[6] In 2006, a similar study was done, using MRI, with the same conclusion, that ligament injury occurred *before* any OA or cartilage defects developed. This resulted in the conclusion that ligament and tendon injuries "have a central role" in the development of osteoarthritis, a conclusion now shared by many other researchers.[7] It also appears that the more severe the ligament injury is, the more severe the progression of OA.[8]

SURGERY FOR OSTEOARTHRITIS

If OA gets severe enough, it may eventually affect joint structure and function—causing both restriction in range of motion and continual pain. In those very severe cases, surgery may be needed. This is especially true with hips, which are by far the least forgiving joint when it comes to OA. However, as noted previously, abnormalities such as OA exist on imaging studies in pain free individuals.[9] Or, if pain is present, it may be the result of the connective tissue injury that caused the OA, rather than the OA itself. Although the following has been said, it bears repeating: *the presence of OA alone does not necessarily indicate that a surgical procedure is called for.*

In May 2016, *Orthopedics Today* reported on a study in which nearly 40 percent of 272 patients "reported persistent knee pain" one year after total knee replacement surgery.[10] But in a way, this makes perfect sense: since knee replacements do not treat connective tissue injury, pain and instability coming from these tissues remain, even after knee replacement.[11] In other words, although a symptom (the OA) had been addressed by having the knee replaced, in those cases where the pain was coming from connective tissue weakness/instability, the problem remained. Fortunately, surgeons themselves are starting to question whether surgery is always the best answer.[12] The current recommendation by the *American Academy of Orthopedic Surgeons* is that knee replacement be reserved for only the most severe cases and then only after nonsurgical management has failed.[13]

A less invasive type of surgical procedure, arthroscopy, has also been widely used to treat OA of the knee for many years. Surgical procedures were done to "clean out" the joint using this method. However, scientific evidence to support this as an effective treatment has been lacking. A very famous study done and published in the New England Journal of Medicine in 2002 asked the question whether surgical intervention for knee OA ("cleaning up" the joint) was worthwhile. The study involved three groups. One group of patients received an actual arthroscopic "cleanup" procedure; the second group received a slightly more aggressive "cleanup" and clipping procedure; the third group received only a "placebo" procedure that involved going through the motions of being taken to the operating room, an incision made, etc., but without the actual procedure being done. This was a double-blind study, which meant that neither the patients nor the doctors doing follow-up knew which patients had received the actual, versus the placebo, procedures. After two years, the study concluded that outcomes with the actual procedures were no better than those with the placebo, and at some points during follow-up, results were worse in the actual treatment group.[14] A repeat of this study published similar results in 2008.[15] And a 2013 study evaluating arthroscopic surgery for degenerative meniscal tears produced similar results: showing no advantage of surgery for these conditions.

In other words, a large number of people have undergone surgical procedures for OA based on an X-ray or MRI that didn't necessarily provide the benefit that was needed. And if this weren't bad enough, remember that *any* surgery to a joint can be aggravating, potentially promoting, or even accelerating, OA! Patients receiving even minimally invasive knee arthroscopy were found to have three times the risk that future knee replacement would be needed.[16] And those receiving a larger surgery involving the meniscus had a 10 to 18 times likelihood that OA would develop.[17] Therefore, in 2017, the American Academy of Orthopaedic Surgeons published a strong recommendation *against* the use of arthroscopy in nearly all patients with degenerative knee disease.

Fortunately, Prolotherapy has been shown to be effective in stimulating connective tissue repair, stabilizing the joint, and preventing further OA. However, if the "horse is already out of the barn," and OA has already progressed to the point where it is part of the reason for the pain, Prolotherapy has also been shown to be effective in stimulating cartilage regeneration, discussed further in the study summaries that follow.

PUBLISHED SCIENTIFIC STUDIES AND RESEARCH

Traditional Dextrose Prolotherapy Studies

Multiple investigations[18] have demonstrated that Dextrose Prolotherapy effectively reduces OA pain[19] and stimulates cartilage regeneration.[20] Improvement in cartilage has been verified both with X-ray[21] and tissue biopsies before, and after a Prolotherapy treatment course.[22] Patients receiving Dextrose Prolotherapy have also been found to be better when compared to patients receiving traditional arthritis treatments when evaluated six months later.[23]

Platelet-Rich Plasma (PRP) Prolotherapy Studies

PRP for OA has been extensively studied, especially for knee OA, and conclusions are that it may indeed be an effective option.[24,] An analysis of 1,543 patients who received platelet-rich plasma injections concluded that PRP improves function and pain in patients with knee joint cartilage degeneration more effectively than hyaluronic acid (a popular traditional treatment).[25] Another analysis of 1,423 patients showed that PRP was more effective for knee OA than not only hyaluronic acid, but also more effective than ozone or corticosteroids (other popular treatments).[26] Multiple studies demonstrate a reduction in knee pain[27] after as little as three PRP treatments, with a 2017 study showing pain reduction after just one treatment.[28]

Although the knee joint has been the most studied, other joints have been found to receive benefit from PRP treatment. When used in the ankle, it was found to improve pain, cartilage[29] and potentially prevent the need for surgery.[30] PRP injections into the hip have been shown to improve function and quality of life.[31] And for the temporomandibular joint (TMJ), PRP showed pain reduction and increased mouth opening at one-year follow-up.[32]

Some of these PRP studies have concluded that only those patients with early arthritis and lower degrees of degeneration had good benefits from platelet-rich plasma injections;[33] however, that conclusion does not tell the whole story. Obviously, the more advanced a patient's condition, the more treatment is needed, but studies by their very nature have to give every patient identical treatment, and they tend to be limited to just a small number of treatments, usually just one or two. However, it has been found that a series of platelet-rich plasma injections given over time give better results than a single treatment for OA.[34] Also, protocols in these types of studies do not typically include injections of joint connective tissue; rather, they are usually just an injection into the joint. In real clinical practice, Prolotherapy treatment plans (number of treatments, intervals, aggressiveness) are customized for the specific condition of the patient[35] and usually include injections into the connective tissue attachments around the joint. The good news is that many patients with more advanced arthritis and greater degrees of degeneration have benefited when given more aggressive PRP Prolotherapy treatments targeted to, and customized for, the severity of the condition for that specific patient.

Biocellular (Stem Cell–Rich) Prolotherapy Studies

Studies using both bone marrow[36] and adipose[37] have confirmed that such treatments can stimulate cartilage repair while also slowing the progression of OA and cartilage disease. Even with more advanced OA, Biocellular treatments have been shown to be successful. In a study of severe knee OA treated with adipose, 100 percent of patients showed significantly improved joint function and increased cartilage thickness (verified by MRI), eight months after treatment. In addition, zero side effects or complications were noted.[38] Another report showed MRI-documented improvement in joint space and cartilage six months after an adipose-derived injection.[39]

As you may recall from Chapter 10, adipose-derived Biocellular Prolotherapy lends itself very well to treatment of the knee because of the fat pad located there. In fact, just transferring fat into the fat pad has been found to be an effective treatment for knee OA.[40] You may also recall that adipose has been found to retain its regenerative abilities better than bone marrow as an individual ages.[41] A study of patients 65 years old or older with knee OA showed adipose-derived cells were found to be very effective in cartilage healing, reduction of pain, and improved function, with 87.5 percent of these patients showing improved cartilage status on arthroscopic examination.[42] Increased cartilage thickness after knee treatment with adipose was verified by MRI in other studies,[43] and a review of 11 additional adipose studies concluded it was safe and effective.[44]

Bone marrow studies also show good results. One hundred and two patients treated with bone marrow for symptomatic shoulder joint OA and/or rotator cuff tears showed "substantial symptomatic and functional improvement" as soon as one month after treatment, which was sustained until the final follow-up exam two years later.[45] Bone marrow also has been shown effective in other joints. [46]

MICROFRACTURE VERSUS BIOCELLULAR PROLOTHERAPY FOR CARTILAGE REPAIR

A surgical treatment used for OA since the 1970s is "microfracture," a technique that irritates the bone surface to try to stimulate cartilage to grow. However, microfracture has mixed, often unsatisfactory, long-term results.[47] Articular cartilage (the smooth, white tissue that covers the ends of bones, allowing the joint to move smoothly) has a very limited ability to repair itself—or to be repaired with surgical interventions—because of its lack of blood supply. A 2013 study compared two groups of patients over the age of 50 with ankle cartilage lesions. One group received only microfracture; the other group received microfracture along with an injection of bone marrow–derived cells. The study concluded that there was "significantly greater improvement" in the group that also received the bone marrow injection.[48]

OSTEOARTHRITIS APPEARANCE ON IMAGING STUDIES AFTER PROLOTHERAPY

It is important to understand that while visual improvement in the quality of the fat pad, as well as the tendons and ligaments that were treated can usually be observed via ultrasound over a period of months, the many bony deposits on an osteoarthritic joint surface may not appear to change much. Over a longer period of time, increased joint space may be noticed on imaging studies; however, in most joints with OA there is such a large number of bony spurs and calcium deposits that being able to perceive small, slow improvement of the bony surface is difficult. It is important to understand, however, that positive changes may be occurring nonetheless. This is made clear by an interesting case report. There, a large, isolated calcium spur is clearly seen on a shoulder X-ray within a rotator cuff tendon. Three platelet-rich plasma treatments were given to this patient's rotator cuff tendon, and a year later another X-ray was done, showing that the large calcium spur was now gone! [49] (See Figure 13.1: Calcium spur in a tendon before and after platelet-rich plasma).

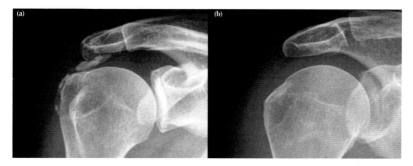

Figure 13.1: Shoulder X-rays showing: (a) large calcium deposit in a tendon, and (b) one year after platelet-rich plasma injections showing calcium deposit gone. (Used with permission, from Seijas R, Ares O, Alvarez P, Cusco X, Garcia-Balletbo, Cugat R. Platelet-rich plasma for calcific tendinitis of the shoulder: a case report. *Journal of Orthopedic Surgery.* 2012; 20 (1): 125-130.)

This is significant in that it demonstrates the potential of regenerative treatments such as platelet-rich plasma to improve calcified areas. Since it was just one isolated calcium spur, the improvement can be easily seen. In areas with a large number of calcifications, it is logical to assume that there are small improvements that, while not easily seen, are nonetheless occurring. Remember that even a small difference in a body can result in a big change in outcome; for instance, a bullet could miss a vital structure in the body by a few millimeters, and the patient could live or die. So even small changes in the surface of an osteoarthritic joint may result in a huge clinical benefit, even if the image of the joint surface itself does not seem to change.

How Prolotherapy Regenerative Medicine Helps Osteoarthritis

Prolotherapy treats one of the most common causes of OA—connective tissue injury/laxity and joint instability—by promoting strengthening and repair of those tissues, stabilizing the joint and potentially preventing further OA. There is also evidence that all three formulas used in Prolotherapy treatment can stimulate the regeneration of cartilage,[50] especially the more advanced formulas. In brief, in a high percentage of patients with OA treated with Prolotherapy, the result is that the joint and surrounding connective tissue becomes stronger, function improves, and pain diminishes or resolves.

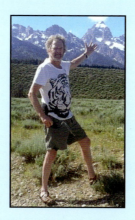

Medical Doctor/Author

Years ago, I noticed pain in my knee, but it went away, and I was good for many years. Then one day, at age 71, I developed severe left knee pain with osteoarthritis that limited my activity; for example, I couldn't walk for more than 15 minutes. I hadn't changed my activity; it just gradually came on. Pain was always present with movement. Sometimes, it was even present at rest, and occasionally it woke me from sleep.

I went to Dr. Alderman for Prolotherapy on the recommendation of one of my patients. Over the next seven months, I had four PRP Prolotherapy treatments, followed by Biocellular (Stem Cell–Rich) Prolotherapy treatment. After the first PRP treatment, I experienced the expected post-treatment pain for about a week. After that, treatments were only moderately painful for a day or two.

My knee gradually got better, and I began to exercise more normally, until I was walking an hour and a half four times a week. After the PRP treatments, I had an 80 percent reduction in pain. After the Biocellular treatment, I was 95 percent pain free. At the time of this writing, it is a year after finishing my treatments, and I am still 95 percent pain free.

I now hike regularly and no longer take NSAIDs or any other medication for my knee.

I have been asked by physician colleagues of mine if the results of the treatment were possibly the product of placebo or other psychological effects. Dr. Alderman and her staff were very cordial and supportive, which certainly helped. However, the swelling and tenderness resolved, and my experience was more analogous to the way someone would feel if taking antibiotics for an infection or after a successful surgery. It was a remarkable experience—a happy one.

Arthur D. Colman, M.D.
Medical Doctor/Author

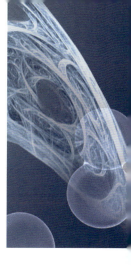

CHAPTER 14

Prolotherapy Regenerative Medicine for Low Back Pain and Sciatica

L ow back pain is a very common problem that affects at least 80 percent of all individuals at some point in their lifetime. It is also a frequent reason for physician visits,[1] and causes more disability worldwide than any other condition.[2] Indeed, low back pain is the leading cause of work absence in much of the world.[3] A large majority of these individuals recover within a few months; however, some will have recurring episodes[4] or may even develop chronic—perhaps even constant—low back pain.[5] In the United States, it is estimated that more than five million people are *disabled*—not just troubled—by low back pain, half of whom are permanently disabled.[6] Despite advanced medical technology, the number of patients suffering from low back pain continues to increase.[7]

COMMON CAUSES OF LOW BACK PAIN

Low back pain can be acute (meaning it comes on suddenly and lasts for only a short time) or chronic (meaning it tends to come on slower and lasts longer than three months). It can appear after a sudden trauma or injury, but also may seem to appear suddenly after an innocent cough or small movement. In those cases, it had been accumulating over time—that last small motion was simply "the straw that broke the camel's back," as it were. Engaging in a variety of sports activities—gymnastics, football, weight lifting, rowing, golf, dance, tennis, baseball, basketball, and cycling—increases the odds of having low back pain,[8] as do increased age, previous episodes of low back pain, hard physical labor, and poor posture, especially with certain activities— such as lifting or carrying heavy loads. Other contributing factors include mental stress, osteoporosis,[9] joint hypermobility,[10] or, surprisingly, physical *inactivity*.[11]

There are various causes of low back pain. Most (estimated at 90 percent) low back pain is caused by ligament sprains, muscle pulls, or disc herniations resulting from either overuse or straining, spraining, lifting, or bending.[12] This is known as "mechanical low back pain." In many cases, the back pain is localized to the back itself; in other cases, the pain may travel into the buttocks or legs as well. Other reasons for low back pain—usually more chronic—include osteoarthritis (OA; inflammation caused by calcium spurs in the joint), central canal stenosis (where the spinal canal has become narrowed because of arthritis or other degenerative changes), facet joint dysfunction (when the joints that connect the vertebrae—the facets—don't function properly, often because the ligaments connecting them have been injured), and spondylolisthesis (slippage of one vertebra over another, which can be congenital or a result of trauma). Another, often overlooked, cause of low back pain is the sacroiliac (SI) joint,[13] responsible for causing at least a third of cases of low back pain in one large study.[14]

In Chapter 7: "The Importance of a Correct Diagnosis," I discussed how MRIs can be misleading in diagnosing musculoskeletal pain. This is especially true for low back pain. To convey why, let's start with a thumbnail history of back pain diagnosis. In 1905, the *Boston Medical and Surgical Journal* (later renamed the *New England Journal of Medicine*), published a paper that proposed SI joint dysfunction and ligament laxity as being the main generators of low back pain.[15] For the next 30 years, the medical community largely agreed. Then in 1934, the research of William Mixter and Joseph Barr became popular.[16] They focused attention on the intervertebral disc: a circular, collagen-type tissue that sits between the bones (vertebrae) in the spine. From that time forward, attention to "disc disease" overshadowed that given to the SI joint and ligaments. Then the 1970s saw the introduction of CT scanners (computed tomography, a very sophisticated type of three-dimensional X-ray), and the 1980s heralded the MRI—and both have been used readily ever since. It so happens that intervertebral discs are easily seen with both types of scans, which inspired further attention to the disc as being the *cause* of low back pain.

Understandably, patients—and their doctors—are eager to find the cause of their pain; an abnormality on an MRI provides a seemingly obvious "reason." But, as a well-respected textbook of orthopedic medicine states, "The results of radiographic examinations should never be given to the patient as a diagnosis."[17] Medical studies have documented over and over again that what the scan shows may *not* be the reason for the person's pain. In fact, although a diagnosis of disc herniation is frequently given as the cause of pain, it has been widely reported that *only 4 percent of low back pain is due to a herniated disc.*[18] Ligament injury is in fact a more common cause of low back pain,[19] because ligament laxity in the spinal ligaments always precedes disc herniations.[20]

The trouble is, ligament injury is difficult to prove with an MRI or CT scan unless the injury is significant, which is usually not the case. And, as discussed earlier, MRI scans require that the patient remain still. However, small ligament or tendon abnormalities may not show up on imaging until the joint is moving, so an MRI may not identify the problem.

This isn't to discount those who suffer from true intervertebral disc problems, nor to say that MRI and CT scans are useless. It is simply to say that radiographic findings should not automatically be accepted as the cause of pain until other sources have been proven unlikely.[21]

We will discuss disc disease and concerns at length in the next chapter. For now, let's continue with other common causes of low back pain.

SURGERY FOR LOW BACK PAIN

During recent years, the general public has accepted the idea that a herniated disc requires surgery, especially if the pain has not resolved after a few weeks and there is an abnormal MRI or CT. However common, this opinion has not been supported by evidence in long-term studies which show, instead, that equally good or better results are obtained after conservative nonsurgical treatment. This will be discussed in much more detail in the next chapter. Suffice it for now to say most doctors recommend that conservative treatments should be undertaken first[22], and that a large percentage of the time, disc herniations seen on MRI scans resolve on their own without surgery.[23]

THE SACROILIAC JOINT

The sacrum is a triangular shaped bone that sits at the bottom of the spine. On each side of the sacrum is another bone called the "iliac bone." The joint between each side of the sacrum and the iliac bone is therefore called a "sacroiliac" joint (abbreviated "SI"), and all these bones together form the "pelvis." The pelvis is held together by a large number of ligaments—and where there are ligaments, the possibility of injury and pain exists. In fact, as early as 1905, the SI joint was identified as a significant source of low back and posterior pelvic pain[24] (see Figure 14.1: The sacroiliac and pelvic ligaments can be a source of pain).

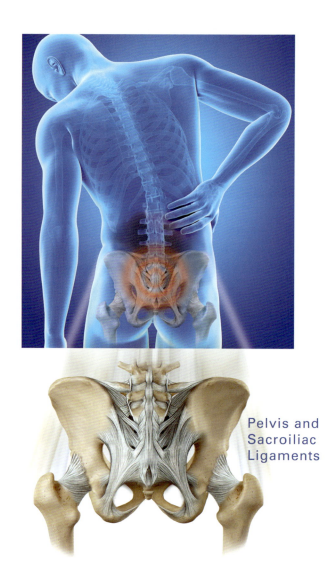

Pelvis and
Sacroiliac
Ligaments

Figure 14.1: The sacroiliac and pelvic ligaments,
a potential source of pain

In the last several years, there has been renewed interest in the SI joint as an underappreciated cause of low back pain in patients of all ages.[25] Multiple studies and investigations have also discovered that SI ligament or joint injuries may also "refer" pain into the buttocks, thigh, hip, groin, leg, ankle, and even the foot[26] (remember from earlier that "referred" pain is pain that is felt at a distance from where it is coming from—for instance, when a person is having a heart attack, he or she may feel pain in the left arm, which is being "referred" there from the heart). Such injuries can also imitate sciatica[27] (sharp buttocks and leg pain), discussed in the next section. The ability of the body to refer pain from the SI joint and other ligaments in the low back was previously discussed in "Chapter 7: The Importance of a Correct Diagnosis," however bears repeating here (see Figure 14.2: Low back and hip ligament referral patterns).

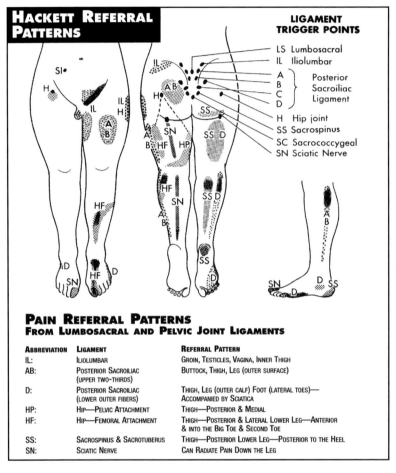

HACKETT REFERRAL PATTERNS

LIGAMENT TRIGGER POINTS

LS Lumbosacral
IL Iliolumbar
A
B — Posterior Sacroiliac Ligament
C
D
H Hip joint
SS Sacrospinus
SC Sacrococcygeal
SN Sciatic Nerve

PAIN REFERRAL PATTERNS
FROM LUMBOSACRAL AND PELVIC JOINT LIGAMENTS

ABBREVIATION	LIGAMENT	REFERRAL PATTERN
IL:	ILIOLUMBAR	GROIN, TESTICLES, VAGINA, INNER THIGH
AB:	POSTERIOR SACROILIAC (UPPER TWO-THIRDS)	BUTTOCK, THIGH, LEG (OUTER SURFACE)
D:	POSTERIOR SACROILIAC (LOWER OUTER FIBERS)	THIGH, LEG (OUTER CALF) FOOT (LATERAL TOES)— ACCOMPANIED BY SCIATICA
HP:	HIP—PELVIC ATTACHMENT	THIGH—POSTERIOR & MEDIAL
HF:	HIP—FEMORAL ATTACHMENT	THIGH—POSTERIOR & LATERAL LOWER LEG—ANTERIOR & INTO THE BIG TOE & SECOND TOE
SS:	SACROSPINUS & SACROTUBERUS	THIGH—POSTERIOR LOWER LEG—POSTERIOR TO THE HEEL
SN:	SCIATIC NERVE	CAN RADIATE PAIN DOWN THE LEG

Figure 14.2: Low back and hip ligament referral patterns

COMMON CAUSES OF SCIATICA

The term *sciatica* is often used to describe any type of pain that follows the course of the sciatic nerve that runs from the buttocks down the back of the leg. Although the term "sciatica" is descriptive of where the pain is located, it is a general term that does not necessarily convey the cause of the problem. There can be several reasons for sciatica. As mentioned earlier, a common cause of sciatica is "SI joint dysfunction" or "SI joint instability." There are several ways instability there can cause sciatica. If ligament laxity develops there, muscles around it spasm in an attempt to stabilize it, and this spasm then puts pressure on nearby nerves running down the leg. Or the excess motion of the sacrum may eventually directly aggravate nearby nerves. Another cause of sciatica is "Piriformis Syndrome," which can exist all by itself or in combination with SI joint instability. This is not hard to understand when you review the anatomy and how close the SI joint is to the piriformis muscle (see Figure 14.3: Relationship of sacroiliac joint to piriformis muscle and sciatic nerve).

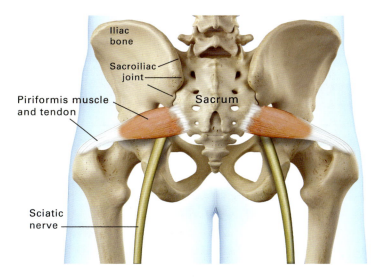

Figure 14.3: Relationship of sacroiliac joint
to piriformis muscle and sciatic nerve.

If any of these pelvic ligaments are sprained, this swelling will also put pressure on nearby nerves that travel down the leg. Just as a sprained ankle swells after an injury, sprained connective tissue in the pelvis will swell when injured, putting pressure on the sciatic—or other low back nerve roots—causing "sciatica." This is especially true when the piriformis muscle and tendons are irritated, because this large muscle runs directly over the large sciatic nerve. (see Figure 14.4: Piriformis syndrome).

PIRIFORMIS SYNDROME

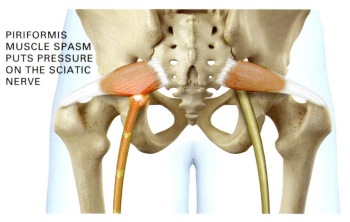

PIRIFORMIS
MUSCLE SPASM
PUTS PRESSURE
ON THE SCIATIC
NERVE

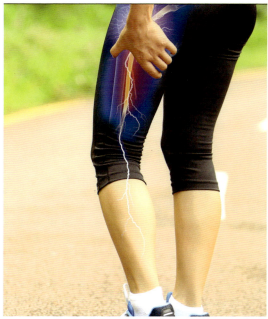

Figure 14.4: Piriformis syndrome

These are very common causes of sciatica. In fact, a large study of 1,293 patients who were followed over a 12-year period of time concluded that SI joint syndromes (and posterior joint syndromes) are the *most common* referred-pain syndromes, occurring twice as frequently as nerve root compression caused by a herniated disc or stenosis, and they often mimic those symptoms[28]

Fortunately, Prolotherapy can help. A 1964 study by Dr. John Merriman compared Dextrose Prolotherapy treatment to lumbar fusion surgery as a treatment for sciatic pain. His conclusion was that 80 to 90 percent of more than 15,000 patients experienced relief from sciatica with Prolotherapy, with far fewer side effects than those patients who had undergone a fusion operation.[29] Other investigations have also confirmed the efficacy of Prolotherapy to resolve sciatica-like symptoms.[30]

SACROILIAC JOINT VERSUS TRUE RADICULAR (SPINAL NERVE–GENERATED) PAIN

A (thankfully) much less common source of sciatica results from true nerve root compression—when something is actually structurally pressing against a nerve. Remember, a nerve can experience pressure from a swollen ligament or a spasmed muscle pushing against it, as in Piriformis Syndrome, and this type of nerve compression will get better once the ligament, tendon, or muscle weakness and injury is addressed and resolved. You see, the nerve doesn't know what's pressing on it and will respond way whether it's a temporary pressure because of swelling nearby or an actual true nerve root being compressed. True radicular pain, however, is structural in nature and can be caused by stenosis (narrowing of the spinal canal), or a true, active herniated disc or fragment that is pressing on a nerve. Because SI joint pain can imitate the pain that's generated by true nerve compression, it is important for the doctor to determine the actual cause of the pain. To confuse the issue further, both types of pain can coexist in the same person. It is estimated that 33.5 percent of patients with low back pain have both.[31] But there are certain differences between these two types of pain.

Pain coming from the SI joint is usually deep, achy, and ill defined, and will often feel tender in response to light pressure. There may be muscle weakness from inactivity, but rarely muscle loss (atrophy). There are also a few simple tests to determine if the origin of pain is likely coming from the SI joint. A basic test was proposed in 1960 by Dr. John Mennell: if the patient, when asked where the pain is, "points over one or the other sacroiliac joints, then the cause of the pain probably lies within that [SI] joint."[32] Almost 40 years later, Dr. Joseph Fortin published the "Fortin Finger Test" in the *American Journal of Orthopedics*. This study involved pushing on the SI joint line to see if it caused any discomfort or pain. If so, a local anesthetic was injected into the SI joint to see if there was any temporary reduction in pain, and if so, chances were that at least some of the problem lay within that SI joint. [33] Fortunately, multiple studies have shown the efficacy of Prolotherapy for SI joint pain.[34]

Lumbosacral Transitional Vertebrae/Bertolotti's Syndrome

Lumbosacral transitional vertebrae (LSTV), also known as Bertolotti's Syndrome, is a common congenital (at birth) abnormality, with a prevalence of as much as 30 percent in the general population, affecting males more than females.[35] It was first described in 1917 by Mario Bertolotti, who noticed that one or both sides of the lowest vertebrae was enlarged in some patients with low back pain, especially in younger ones.[36] While many individuals with these enlarged vertebrae are pain free, there does appear to be a higher incidence of low back pain in individuals with this condition.[37]

There are several different types of LSTV, depending on the amount of enlargement of the vertebrae, whether it is moving freely or fused to the sacrum, or whether it is on one or both sides of the pelvis. The part of the vertebra that is enlarged is the part of the bone on the side, called the "transverse process" (transverse is from Latin for "laying across"; process comes from French for "a journey"). In Figure 14.4, you can see the way this bone looks normally, and how it might vary depending on the specific type of LSTV that is present (see Figure 14.4: Lumbosacral transitional vertebrae types).

The presence of LSTV may affect movement in the region and could lead to irregular lumbar and SI joint motion, with eventual pain and dysfunction. It has been found that because LSTV results in less motion at the L5-S1 level, there is excess motion at the level above it (L4-5), which increases the likelihood of degenerative changes and disc breakdown there.[38] A study of 300 patients with low back pain showed that 37 percent had LSTV;[39] another study of 500 patients with low back pain showed that 28.5 percent had not only LSTV but also SI joint dysfunction.[40]

Lumbosacral Transitional Vertabrae

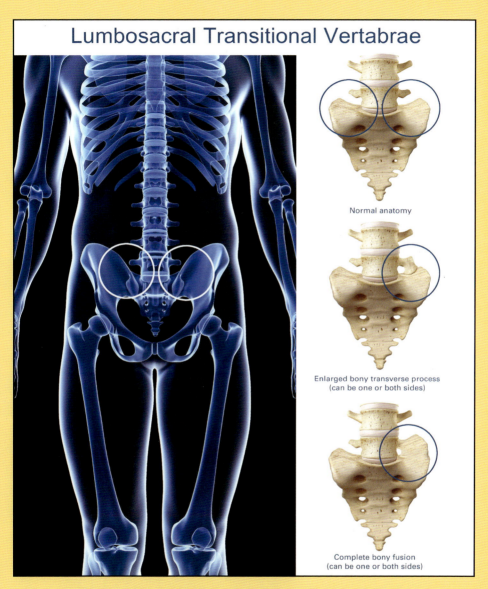

Normal anatomy

Enlarged bony transverse process
(can be one or both sides)

Complete bony fusion
(can be one or both sides)

Figure 14.5: Lumbosacral transitional vertebrae (LSTV) types

Radicular (true spinal nerve compression origin) pain, on the other hand, typically involves sharp pain, which can feel "electric." The patient can have numbness, tingling, burning, or coolness—and sometimes worse pain in the leg than in the back. There may also be actual muscle loss (atrophy) in the leg, in addition to weakness.

As you might imagine, a proper diagnosis for the cause of sciatica calls for both a comprehensive analysis of a patient's history as well as a thorough physical exam. As long as there are no neurological warning signs, such as loss of bowel or bladder function, profound muscle atrophy, loss of tendon reflexes, unrelenting sharp leg pain inhibiting the ability to walk, or other alarming signs, the doctor may determine that a trial treatment with Prolotherapy is reasonable based on the origin of the problem most likely being primarily musculoskeletal rather than coming from true nerve root compression. However, treatments and progress should be monitored closely to ensure improvement. In a very small number of cases, surgery may be needed to relieve pressure on the nerve if symptoms do not improve with conservative treatment.

How Prolotherapy Regenerative Medicine Helps Low Back Pain

Traditional Dextrose Prolotherapy stabilizes low back, sacroiliac and pelvic ligaments and has been used successfully for these problems for many years.[41]

Platelet-rich plasma (PRP) has been found effective for SI joint dysfunction, demonstrating in one study continued pain reduction and functional improvement up to the last patient follow-up four years after the treatment.[42] PRP has also been successfully used for lumbar facet joint (the joints between the vertebrae),[43] as well as muscular-based low back pain.[44] PRP has also been compared to a traditional treatment—cortisone—and found to be superior.[45] Biocellular formulas, although newer, have also shown success when used for these conditions.[46]

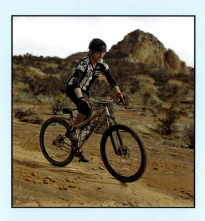

Graphic Designer/Wanderer

My entire adult life has been spent enduring some form of constant back pain, at times debilitating. At age 20, I learned I had been born with a congenital fusion of a lumbar vertebrae (Lumbosacral Transitional Vertebrae, or "LSTV"). My issue was specifically at L5/SI, where my L5 and the sacrum were fused together on the right side, preventing either from moving normally. This in and of itself isn't always a root cause of back pain. Many people have this same condition and live long pain free lives, unaware of their congenital fusion. But in my particular case, the congenital fusion, combined with an undersized disc, and my very active lifestyle was the perfect storm. I have not been kind to my body over the years. I have broken over 30 bones and damaged a variety of soft tissue from a long history of sports-related injuries: skateboarding, inline skating, mountain biking, motorcycle racing—the list goes on. But I was managing my back pain reasonably well until my early 40s, when things deteriorated quickly. I was not able to sit or stand for any length of time, which affected my ability to work. I was also unable to sleep more than a few hours per night; I often went several consecutive nights without sleep because of pain. My typical heavy, burning type backaches started shifting, replaced by sharp, piercing stabs that caused tingling and numbness down my left leg. It came to a head when, while riding my mountain bike with friends,

I experienced what I can only describe as the sensation of "Velcro tearing," along with the worst pain of my life.

After that event, I spent months researching both surgical and nonsurgical options—research I was forced to conduct from bed, as I was no longer able to function. A walk around the block left me unable to move for hours. Opening the refrigerator door meant risking a pain so severe I would drop to my knees. I was immobile, unable to function on even a basic level. As my pain worsened, and I saw my life slip away, I became more and more desperate for relief. So after even more sleepless nights, I boarded a plane for Germany and underwent artificial disc replacement at L4/L5, which had been diagnosed as damaged and the likely source of my pain.

The recovery from that surgery was long, painful, and frightening. Days, weeks, and months passed, and my recovery crawled along at a glacial pace. I was able to walk, but my gait was awkward, and my hips and spine felt like two separate entities trying to connect. Something just didn't feel right, so a year after surgery, I contacted Dr. Alderman for an evaluation. An ultrasound of my sacroiliac joint revealed chronic and severe ligament damage and tearing, which was causing pelvic instability. I decided to try Biocellular (Stem Cell–Rich) Prolotherapy.

Within days of the first treatment, I felt a small improvement. As the weeks went by, improvement increased and then snowballed, and became better and better. Eager to take advantage of the healing process, I returned for another treatment six months later, and, again, my strength, flexibility, and overall body movement and function continued to improve. The ultrasound images of my sacroiliac joints "before" and "after" Biocellular Prolotherapy were dramatic. What was once "desiccated chewing gum" in my SI ligaments was now dense tissue, and my pelvis and hips could now maintain their position after being adjusted by a chiropractor, whereas before they would slip out of place once I stood up from the chiropractor's table.

I went on to have a third Biocellular treatment, mainly for good measure, but also to treat my entire lumbar facet joints. It's been three years since my disc replacement surgery and one year since my last Biocellular treatment. Three years ago, I was confined to bed, struggling to simply take a shower. Today, I can spend five hours in the saddle, riding my mountain bike over jarring, rocky terrain. I can sit at a dinner table and enjoy a feast with friends without mind-numbing pain ruining a pleasant evening. I'm also engaged in a regular and highly intensive calisthenics program where I target parts of my body with body weight exercises that I thought impossible even a year ago. The proof, as they say, is in the pudding. At 47, I'm getting stronger each day and regaining my life back one pedal stroke at a time. This is thanks in large part to Biocellular Prolotherapy, which has rebuilt tissue in my back that once seemed beyond repair.

Ian Gillies
Graphic Designer/Wanderer

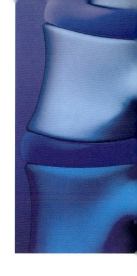

CHAPTER 15

Prolotherapy Regenerative Medicine for Disc Disease

Τhe diagnosis of "disc disease," "bulging disc" or "disc herniation" is so common that it deserves its own chapter. As you may recall from Chapter 6, it is believed that ligament weakness exists *before* a disc herniates. It is important to understand what a disc is, the natural course of disc disease, how ligament weakness/laxity fits in, and how Prolotherapy can help.

DISC DISEASE BASICS

The disc is a circular, collagen-type tissue, which acts like a cushion and shock absorber between the bones (vertebrae) in the spine. The center of the disc is a jellylike, watery material called the "nucleus pulposus" (Latin for "center pulp"). The disc does not have a direct blood supply of its own, and therefore has limited healing ability. The outer portion of the disc is called the "annulus fibrosus" or simply "annulus" (Latin for "fibrous ring"); it is composed of strong, ligament-like tissue, with nerve fibers only on its outermost edges. Because the disc sits between the vertebrae, it is called an "intervertebral" disc (see Figure 15.1: The intervertebral disc).

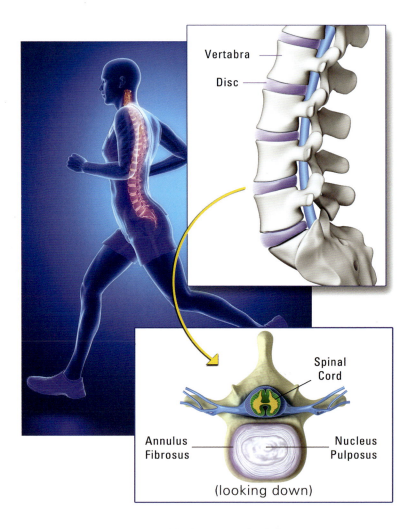

Figure 15.1 The intervertebral disc

DISC DEGENERATION

Like other parts of the body, discs experience "wear and tear" as we age. The center of the disc (the nucleus pulposus), which is 85 percent water in a young person, tends to become dehydrated over time, and may only be 65 percent water in an older person.[1] Factors that lead to disc degeneration are lifting heavy objects, excessive bending, and sitting for long periods of time, all of which can put extra strain on the discs, leading to flattening and dehydration. This usually occurs over many years with small injuries that slowly accumulate. Since discs lack direct blood supply, they cannot easily regenerate and repair themselves; once flattened, they remain so. However, the presence of disc degeneration does not necessarily mean pain, or a problem exists. In fact, disc degeneration is an MRI finding for many individuals who have *no pain* at all.[2] This should not be a surprise since, as discussed earlier, abnormal findings on MRI exist in pain free individuals. Disc degeneration is, in fact, so common that it is considered part of the normal aging process.[3]

LIGAMENT LAXITY HAPPENS BEFORE DISC BULGE, HERNIATION OR RUPTURE

Disc degeneration, bulge, and *herniation* (sometimes called a *ruptured* or *slipped disc)* describe the increasing stages of disc disease (see Figure 15.2: The stages of disc disease).

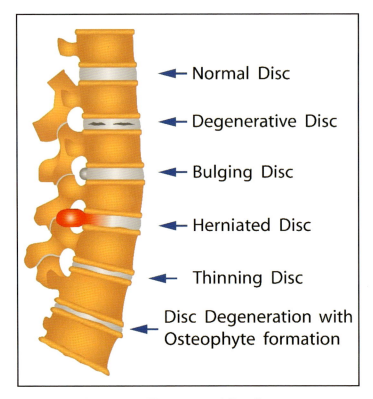

Figure 15.2: The stages of disc disease

It is important to understand that for a disc to bulge or herniate, there must first be ligament weakness allowing it to do so.[4] Ligaments surround the disc and are designed to hold it securely in place. In a younger person, these ligaments fit snugly around the vertebrae and disc between them. But as a disc loses moisture and flattens over time, or as there are traumas or micro-traumas, the ligaments stretch and become lax. Imagine if you lost six inches around your waist, but didn't tighten your belt! (see Figure 15.3: What happens to the ligaments when the disc flattens).

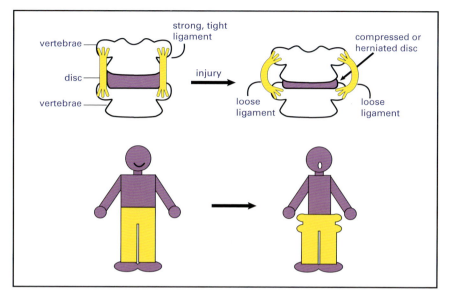

Figure 15.3: What happens to the ligaments when the disc flattens

Since the disc has no blood supply and cannot regenerate, a flattened disc means there is no longer a snug fit between the disc and the ligaments—in the same way that you'd be swimming in your old bigger pants after losing weight. The extra space around the disc allows excess disc and ligament motion—joint instability—leading to a disc *bulge,* and then, eventually, to the next stage: *disc herniation.*

Once a herniation occurs, the outside edges of the disc may become cracked or torn,[5] allowing the fluid in the disc's center (the nucleus pulposus) to leak through these cracks, causing irritation. As you can imagine, this leakage also decreases disc height, resulting in further instability and a *thinning disc*, which in turn means more laxity of the surrounding ligaments. Over time, and in a further effort to stabilize the continuing instability, the body starts to put hard calcium deposits ("osteophytes," also called "bone spurs") in that joint to stop the excess motion, and the final stage of disc disease occurs: osteoarthritis. After the first disc herniation, other discs are more likely to be affected and eventually bulge and herniate. Simply put, the ligament holds the disc in place, so if the ligament weakens, the disc can herniate through it. Increased pressure on the disc (high demand activities), together with increased ligament laxity, is the perfect recipe for further disc herniation.[6] If instability continues long enough, the result will be degenerative osteoarthritis.

Natural Course of a Disc Herniation

When a disc first herniates, it can be painful enough to knock a person flat, so to speak, and the effects can last for several days. But this injury can heal; in a few days, or maybe a few weeks, the protruding disc segment slowly reduces in size.[7] In fact, most disc herniations resolve within two to six weeks, restoring the patient back to 90 percent of normal activity within one month, even without treatment.[8]

However, it has been estimated that 10 percent of people who suffer a disc herniation continue to have pain; usually this involves chronic muscle pain, spasm, and stiffness (a sign of ligament laxity and a weak joint, see Figure 6.2, in Chapter 6: The three ways the body responds to joint instability). These symptoms may persist long after the disc herniation has reduced in size and is no longer causing a problem because the ligament laxity and weakness is still present (see Figure 15.4: Natural course of a disc herniation).

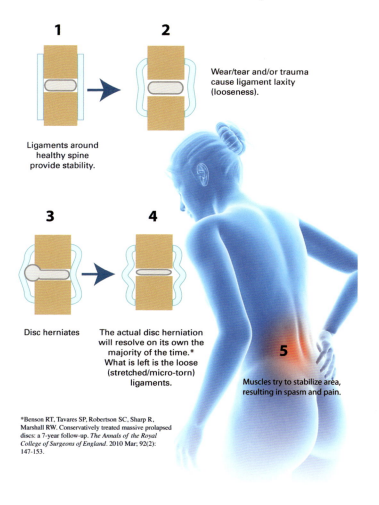

1

Ligaments around healthy spine provide stability.

2

Wear/tear and/or trauma cause ligament laxity (looseness).

3

Disc herniates

4

The actual disc herniation will resolve on its own the majority of the time.* What is left is the loose (stretched/micro-torn) ligaments.

5

Muscles try to stabilize area, resulting in spasm and pain.

*Benson RT, Tavares SP, Robertson SC, Sharp R, Marshall RW. Conservatively treated massive prolapsed discs: a 7-year follow-up. *The Annals of the Royal College of Surgeons of England*. 2010 Mar; 92(2): 147-153.

Figure 15.4: Natural course of a disc herniation

While someone can suffer a disc herniation because of sudden or severe trauma, such as lifting something heavy, as mentioned earlier, many herniations occur over time due to repetitive trauma—some large, some small, which accumulate. There may not even be a history of back pain, but then one day a minor event, even just a cough or sneeze, is enough to trigger herniation.[9]

I have had numerous patients tell me a similar story: "I was just lifting a plate out of the sink," "I just sneezed," or "I was just getting out of a car" when suddenly severe back pain brings them to their knees. While the innocent activity seems to be the cause, it was just the proverbial straw that broke the camel's back. Over the years damage to the area has been adding up, until a person is, in a sense, sitting at the edge of a cliff, so it may not take much of a push to fall off. Most people don't notice the slow process of disc degeneration and ligament weakening, and so may not even know there is a problem—that is, until the camel's back breaks.

Most Disc Herniations Resolve without Surgery

As discussed in the previous chapter, most disc herniations resolve without surgery. Two studies found *no difference* between the final results of surgical and non-surgical therapy after 7 and 20 years of observation.[10] Another study found a 92 percent return-to-work rate in a group treated conservatively without surgery, even though 60 percent of those individuals initially had muscle weakness and 26 percent showed disc rupture on the CT scan.[11] A more recent analysis of multiple studies compared changes in MRI scans over a period of a year for patients with low back pain and sciatica. This review reported that up to 93 percent of herniations reduced or disappeared in size without surgery, and up to 91 percent of nerve root compressions (where the nerve is being pressed by the herniated disc) also reduced or disappeared without surgery.[12]

This explains why surgeries for disc herniations based only on an MRI may fail. The MRI may show an old remnant (small remaining piece) of a previous disc herniation that resolved on its own long before, and is not actually responsible for the patient's *current* pain. Therefore, surgery addressed to that area may fail to resolve the problem. A review of 1,108 patients who, based on their MRI results, received disc surgery, found that one year later *more than 50 percent* of these patients were still experiencing pain.[13] Put simply, the presence of even large herniations or disc ruptures should not be taken as an absolute reason for surgery.[14] While there can be emergent needs that call for surgery—such as trauma resulting in back fracture, or sudden loss of bladder or bowel function—only a very small percentage of disc herniations truly require surgery.[15] Most practitioners agree that conservative non-surgical approaches should be recommended first.[16]

PLATELET-RICH PLASMA FOR DISC HERNIATIONS

Platelet-rich plasma injections are a safe and effective treatment for disc herniations. Patients with MRI proven disc herniations, who also had neck or low back pain, were treated with platelet-rich plasma injections in and around the joints and ligaments of the spine where the herniation was. Not only were the injections themselves safe with no complications, but eight years after these injections, 87 percent of these patients continued to have improvement. The authors concluded that in comparison to spinal surgery, with its higher risk and complication rate, platelet-rich plasma was an effective option and a much safer alternative.[17] This study also confirms that treatment to the spine area around the disc is an effective treatment for disc herniation.

Another approach is the direct injection of platelet-rich plasma (PRP) into the disc. This would be done in those less common cases of low back pain where there is a high certainty that pain is being generated from the disc itself ("discogenic" pain).[18] Results have been encouraging,[19] however studies are still ongoing.[20] Small investigations into the use of bone marrow concentrate[21] or adipose-derived mesenchymal stem cells[22] injected directly into the disc have also been promising, although additional studies are still needed and ongoing.[23]

How Prolotherapy Regenerative Medicine Helps Disc Disease

There are two very important points to remember about disc disease: 1) disc herniation is almost *always* a result of ligament weakness/laxity and 2) the majority of disc herniations resolve on their own without surgery. When pain continues, it is usually because the reason for the herniation—weakness of the ligaments supporting the disc—has not resolved or been addressed. The pain also comes from muscular spasm, which is how the body tries to stabilize the weakness. This muscle spasm can last long after the disc has healed. Prolotherapy helps these issues by stimulating repair and strengthening of weakened ligaments around the disc and in the region, making the joints stronger, and reducing or eliminating pain.

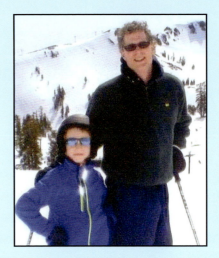

Fashion Designer

I have a very active lifestyle. Roughly, 14 years ago, at age 43, a neck injury from competitive tennis and other stressors put me in the worst pain of my life. I visited four of the top neurosurgeons and orthopedists in the San Francisco Bay Area for their opinions on treatment. Based on a truly ugly MRI showing disc disease, I was told that my condition would require a double fusion of my cervical spine with a plate installed. This seemed like a no-go, as all I could imagine was living the balance of my life in crippling pain.

The last doctor I saw offered yet another extensive surgical solution. Then he mentioned Prolotherapy, literally, as I was walking out his office door. I had heard a Prolotherapy success story from a friend who had been suffering from a condition similar to mine, so I reached out to him to get Dr. Alderman's contact information.

Dr. Alderman and Prolotherapy treatments—both Dextrose and PRP—became my medical miracle. By the time I'd had three treatments, I was feeling better. After my sixth treatment, my pain had been reduced by 80 percent, and I was able to return to my normal life. While there's no telling how my highly active and busy life would have been affected if I had not found Prolotherapy, I think it's fair to say that a surgery of the kind I was headed for would have been a terrible mistake. It's also fair to say that I couldn't have gone on much longer in the condition I was in, so something had to change.

Since those days, I have become even more active and have had periodic treatments when I felt I'd re-injured myself. That said, if I do have a flare-up, it never approaches the level of pain I had before I met Dr. Alderman. In that state of severe pain, I never imagined that feeling this good again would be possible. I couldn't be more grateful.

As a result, I have sent many family members and friends for Prolotherapy, including my wife, and all have experienced successful results. Anyone looking at a potential surgery involving the musculoskeletal system would do well to consider Prolotherapy as a possible alternative before going forward.

Henry Jacobson
Fashion Designer

CHAPTER 16

Prolotherapy Regenerative Medicine for Sports Injuries: Returning the Athlete Safely to His/Her Sport

An important goal in sports medicine is returning the athlete safely back to his/her sport.[1] This goal is made more difficult because of the number of both acute and chronic connective tissue injuries in sports, and, as has been discussed earlier, the challenges with connective tissue healing. Even if an injury improves, there is a high risk that healing may be incomplete, leaving the athlete with decreased strength and increased likelihood of repetitive injury.[2] If acute injuries remain unresolved, these can become chronic and more difficult to treat.[3] Athletes also experience a high incidence of muscle injuries, with the potential for scar tissue formation or weakness if not quickly resolved. Treatment of these acute muscle injuries with Platelet-Rich Plasma (PRP) Prolotherapy has been gaining popularity with a growing body of evidence supporting its use.[4]

Standard Treatments for Sports Injuries

Typical treatments for sports injuries include nonsteroidal anti-inflammatory drugs (NSAIDs) and corticosteroids, but, as discussed in Chapter 11: "Pain Medication: A Double-Edged Sword," these have been shown to be detrimental to tissue healing[5] and can promote cartilage loss,[6] which ultimately leads to both chronic pain and deterioration of sports performance—not attractive options. The good news is that patients treated for sports injuries with Prolotherapy Regenerative Medicine have achieved the exact opposite outcomes: decreased pain and increased sports performance and function.[7]

Prolotherapy Regenerative Therapies for Sports Injuries

Traditional Dextrose Prolotherapy

Traditional Dextrose Prolotherapy has been used for decades in the treatment of sports injuries. Ross Hauser's book *Prolo Your Sports Injuries Away!* published in 2002, explains at length the many ways Prolotherapy can treat sports injuries. Multiple studies have demonstrated the benefit of Dextrose Prolotherapy treatment for sports injuries. One such study concerned chronic groin pain that had "prevented full sports participation" for an average of 16 months in a group of 24 elite rugby and soccer athletes for whom conservative treatment for groin pain had failed. After an average of less than three monthly Dextrose Prolotherapy treatments, 22 athletes returned to playing at their previous level, and 20 of them were pain free.[8] Other studies have confirmed Prolotherapy's effectiveness for rotator cuff lesions,[9] Achilles tendinopathy,[10] osteitis pubis,[11] coccydynia,[12] and golfer's elbow,[13] as well as other sports injuries.[14]

Platelet-Rich Plasma (PRP) Prolotherapy

Many people have heard about platelet-rich plasma being used for sports injuries but do not know that Prolotherapy practitioners have been using PRP as a formula long before its use was widely known. Initially when it broke upon the sports medicine scene in the early 2000s, not much was understood about it, and the World Anti-Doping Agency (WADA) put it on their "prohibited" list. Fortunately, in 2013, it was removed from that list, and WADA declared that despite the presence of some growth factors, "current studies on PRP do not demonstrate any potential for performance enhancement beyond a potential therapeutic effect."[15] While there is still controversy regarding the best PRP type or method, it is now widely accepted in the sports medicine and orthopedic medicine communities,[16] as well as in professional sports.[17]

Just as with Dextrose Prolotherapy, multiple studies have demonstrated the benefit of PRP treatment for sports injuries, including a study that showed successful repair of ulnar collateral ligament tears (an important ligament in the elbow and commonly injured in throwing athletes such as baseball pitchers). That study concluded, "PRP injections may be particularly beneficial in young athletes who have sustained acute damage to an isolated part of the ligament and in athletes unwilling or unable to undergo the extended rehabilitation required after surgical reconstruction of the ligament."[18] Athletes suffering from high ankle sprains have also been shown to benefit from PRP injections, with a shorter "return to play" and less long-term residual pain.[19]

Muscle injuries, also common in athletes, have demonstrated the remarkable ability to recover faster when PRP was used almost immediately after injury. Ultrasound-guided PRP injections were given to athletes suffering with moderately severe muscle tears. All patients had *complete healing* of the muscular lesion and returned to complete muscular function and sports activity, with complete resolution of pain.[20] Another study showed that even a single ultrasound-guided platelet-rich plasma injection was an effective, long-term treatment for nonresponsive, chronic, distal biceps tendinopathy.[21] Another treatment area where PRP was found successful are jumper's knee (patellar tendinopathy).[22] Hines Ward (Pittsburgh Steelers wide receiver who received PRP just before Super bowl XLIII) isn't the only big name to boost PRP's reputation; a number of celebrity athletes recovered sooner than expected from injuries treated with platelet-rich plasma injections, including golfer Tiger Woods, tennis player Rafael Nadal, soccer player Cristiano Ronaldo, basketballers Kobe Bryant and Steph Curry, and baseball players Joey Votto and Alex Rodriguez.[23]

Biocellular (Stem Cell–Rich) Prolotherapy

Starting around the year 2000, many professional athletes received Biocellular procedures, both instead of surgery and to accelerate recovery after surgery—among them high-profile US National Football League (NFL) players, many of whom publicly credit these treatments as helping them extend their careers.[24] A 2014 report in *Sports Illustrated* reported that the NFL considers stem cell–based treatments to be medical—not performance enhancing—and has permitted such treatments as long as they don't include any banned substance (such as human growth hormone).[25]

An interesting case report describes a baseball athlete who underwent knee reconstruction surgery. After the surgery, he continued to have pain and was unable to play, run or jump because of a large tendon tear in his patella tendon. He received Biocellular Prolotherapy using adipose, bone marrow, along with PRP, and was able to return to play, essentially pain free, six weeks later. Ultrasound imaging also showed dramatic improvement in the tendon.[26]

Even when surgery is needed, Biocellular sources used during that surgery may be helpful in speeding recovery and preventing recurrences. A study compared shoulder surgery with and without bone marrow applied during the surgery. The results showed significantly better outcomes, with reduced re-injuries, in the group receiving the bone marrow, as long as ten years after the procedure.[27]

Finally, remember from Chapter 12: "Prolotherapy Regenerative Medicine for Tendinopathy, Ligament Sprains, Muscle, and Meniscal Tears" that when regenerative injections are done soon after an injury, faster, better healing is possible. There is also evidence that healing may occur without weaker scar tissue, and rather with new, normal, strong tissue, preventing recurrences.

THE FUTURE OF PROLOTHERAPY REGENERATIVE THERAPIES IN SPORTS MEDICINE

As Albert Einstein said, "The world as we have created it is a process of our thinking. It cannot be changed without changing our thinking." Older thinking about the best ways to treat sports injuries is slowly giving way to newer fundamentals of regenerative medicine. Sports medicine professionals and the athletic community are beginning to embrace regenerative therapies that enhance tissue and joint repair while also avoiding the risks of surgery. Although there are still controversies about protocols, every year, more studies offer information that help to clarify the fine points of these regenerative therapies, and more and more athletes—professional and recreational—are discovering Prolotherapy Regenerative Medicine.

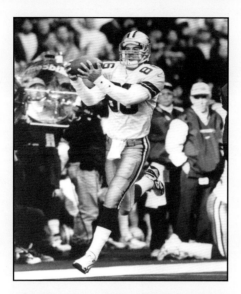

Professional Football Player

I played quarterback/receiver at University of Washington from 1990 to 1994 and tight end for the Dallas Cowboys from 1995 to 1999 and the New England Patriots in 2000. I had a chronic case of turf toe for about six years. It is a really painful injury, and it contributed to pain in my back, knees, and hips due to my trying to compensate for this. I could only wear certain shoes; it bothered me to walk and also while I slept. I had tried all the traditional treatments, including ice, electrical stimulation, orthotics, cortisone injections, and then the alternative treatments, including chiropractic, acupuncture, acupressure, and a variety of supplements, all with little or no success. I constantly had to take anti-inflammatory medication to play because the pain affected my performance.

My chiropractor suggested I try Prolotherapy. I went through six treatments and noticed a significant improvement in my condition. It is by far the best my toe has felt in years, and I only wish I had known about Prolotherapy while I was still playing football.

Eric Bjornson
Former Tight End, Dallas Cowboys

CHAPTER 17

Frequently Asked Questions

What areas of the body can be treated?

Almost any painful joint area can be treated if that area is deemed to have an appropriate problem after an evaluation. This includes pain in the knee, shoulder, neck, back, elbow, wrist, fingers/toes, hip, ankle, and foot. In addition, painful or injured or sprained ligaments, tendons, muscles, knee meniscus, shoulder or hip labrum, and sciatica—as well as joint osteoarthritis (OA)—are generally all problems that can be considered for treatment. However, the specifics of each patient history and issue need to be evaluated on an individual basis to determine if a person is a good candidate to receive Prolotherapy treatment.

How long do treatments last? Are they permanent, or will I need maintenance?

Prolotherapy is a regenerative treatment that stimulates repair. Think of a skin cut that has healed. Once the skin has healed, it has healed. After a treatment course is completed, the patient is "graduated," and maintenance is not required. However, this does not make the person bionic!

It is possible to re-injure the site, and that does sometimes occur; in those cases, a person would come back for a "tune-up." In some cases, the problem treated has a structural abnormality to begin with, and we can only go so far with treatment. In those cases, a patient may want to come back periodically for treatment. However, in most cases, patients do not need to come back for maintenance; when they are done with a course of treatment, they are done. During the time I have been practicing this procedure (over twenty years), I have had patients come back after several years have gone by; however, in the majority of cases, these patients are coming back to consult and treat a *different* problem area; in most cases, the originally treated joint is still doing well.

What if I have been told I am "bone on bone?" Can I still be a candidate for treatment?

The diagnosis of "bone on bone" is unfortunately given to many patients, but can mean different things. Often, this term refers to a small portion of a joint, with most of the joint in good shape, and this person may very well be an excellent candidate for Prolotherapy treatment. Other factors are which joint is affected by the "bone on bone" situation. The knee, for instance, is a very forgiving joint; it can have a large portion of "bone on bone" and still do very well with Prolotherapy treatment. On the other hand, the hip is a very unforgiving joint, so even a small amount of "bone on bone" may make this patient difficult to treat. The bottom line is not to feel discouraged if you are told "bone on bone," and you have an interest in Prolotherapy treatment; it is usually worthwhile to get a consultation and evaluation.

Does medical insurance cover this treatment?

As discussed earlier, with a few exceptions, most insurance companies do not cover regenerative injection therapies such as Prolotherapy. If you have a PPO insurance plan that pays for out-of-network physicians, you might (I repeat, "might") be able to get some reimbursement for a portion of the office visit, depending on the terms of your policy (PPO stands for "Preferred Provider Organization," a type of insurance with more flexibility). Other insurers, such as Medicare, have made it clear that they will not cover any aspect of Prolotherapy treatment. However, even though standard medical insurance coverage itself does not generally cover these procedures, payment with health savings accounts is almost always accepted.

There are some exceptions. As mentioned earlier, Arkansas now grants medical coverage for orthopedic regenerative injection therapies for government employees and teachers under the Emerging Therapies Act of 2017.[1] There is also Unity Health in Madison, Wisconsin, which will grant coverage for some preauthorized injections. I have also heard of some Kaiser Permanente facilities offering Dextrose Prolotherapy and/or PRP, depending on the medical staffing at those facilities. Over the years, I have also seen random insurance companies and even workers' compensation on occasion reimbursing patients for treatments; however, this seems to be on an individual per patient basis.

How much does Prolotherapy cost?

The cost of Prolotherapy treatment varies between doctors within a given area and also between different states, but to offer a ballpark figure for 2017, the price ranges nationwide are consultation $300 to $500; Dextrose Prolotherapy for one joint is $200 to $500; Platelet-Rich Plasma (PRP) Prolotherapy for one joint area $800 to $1,200; Biocellular (Stem Cell–Rich) Prolotherapy for one joint $4,000 to $6,000, with *some* physicians treating additional joint areas at a discount if done during the same procedure. Note that costs in larger metropolitan areas will be on the higher end of these ranges.

Will I need to take time off from work after the treatment?

This will depend on the area being treated, the type of Prolotherapy used, and the type of job you have (physical or not). In most cases, it is a good idea to be able to have the option to rest the day after the procedure. However, as long as the job is not physical, a person can return to work almost immediately. If there is a physical aspect to the job that may re-injure the treated area, this can be discussed with the physician and a specified period of time, usually a few days to a week, can be arranged to be taken off after a procedure.

How long will my appointment be?
How long do procedures take?

The initial consultation is scheduled for 90 minutes. This allows time for the doctor to take a thorough history, do the diagnostic ultrasound, and then go over the findings/results and options. Time for the actual procedure will depend on which formula is used. Dextrose

Prolotherapy treatments are scheduled for half an hour; however, the actual procedure time can be as little as 5 minutes if just one joint is being injected and up to 20 minutes if several joints are being treated. PRP procedure appointments are scheduled for one hour, as blood needs to be drawn, centrifuged, and then injected. Biocellular procedure appointments are scheduled for two hours, as there is the added step of tissue extraction.

Do you give pain medication before a treatment?

A fast-acting, local anesthetic is used prior to each injection for PRP or Biocellular Prolotherapy. For Dextrose Prolotherapy, there is also a local anesthetic that is mixed into the formula. In most cases, that is all that is needed for patients to tolerate procedures well, without sedation or other pain medication. However, if a patient is particularly anxious or pain intolerant, a light oral sedative or pain medication can be given prior to treatment. Be sure to discuss this with the physician providing your treatment if you feel you will need to take something prior to the procedure.

Will I be able to drive myself home?

In most cases, yes (unless you have taken medication prior to treatment). However, for your first treatment, we recommend having someone accompany you to drive you home afterward. This is because while most people feel fine and will have no problem driving home after a treatment, other individuals may have some discomfort and prefer not to have to drive. After the first treatment, you will then see what is involved and how you feel, and decide if you need a driver afterward.

Does Prolotherapy stimulate cartilage repair?

In the past, the answer to this was unclear. However, over the past ten years, evidence has emerged that supports that Prolotherapy can indeed stimulate cartilage growth and repair. A 2016 study of patients with moderately severe knee osteoarthritis (OA) demonstrated evidence of cartilage building effects after Dextrose Prolotherapy.[2] Platelet-rich plasma has also been shown to protect against cartilage damage[3] and to play a part in its regeneration, as well as slow the progression of OA.[4] And multiple investigations, in both basic research and clinical studies, have demonstrated the effectiveness of using adult stem cells for cartilage repair.[5]

Can Prolotherapy make a condition worse?

In over 20 years of performing this procedure—and in knowing many other physicians who offer it—I have not seen or heard of a patient whose condition worsened as a result of Prolotherapy treatment when performed by a properly trained physician. Some individuals experience a significant level of temporary after-treatment pain or discomfort and may feel as though they are worse for a while after a treatment, before they get better. This is somewhat expected; however, I have always seen after-treatment discomfort resolve, and when it does, most people feel improvement, with only a small percentage experiencing no change (however, ultimately not worse than prior to treatment).

That said, every patient is different, and in all medical procedures, there is always some risk. So be sure to ask your physician about both the likely and unlikely potential consequences of Prolotherapy treatment. It's also important that you are comfortable with the physician doing the procedure. I am a big believer in trusting your gut. Don't be afraid to ask questions; it's OK to "doctor shop" until you find a doctor whom you feel has the right level of experience to treat your specific problem and also that you are comfortable with.

I've heard that lidocaine (a local anesthetic) can be toxic to platelet-rich plasma or adult stem cells and should not be used. Is this true?

The answer is not clear-cut; however, there has been concern in recent years that lidocaine might reduce the effectiveness of platelet-rich plasma[6] or be toxic to stem cells.[7] Because of this, many practitioners use more cell-friendly local anesthetics (such as procaine or ropivacaine) when doing advanced Prolotherapy procedures. Also, the local anesthetic is not, in most cases, mixed directly with the platelet-rich plasma or adipose/bone marrow cells when doing advanced Prolotherapy, but rather injected separately. Therefore, there is reduced risk that the anesthetic will interact directly with the formula.

I see a lot of advertisement about clinics offering platelet-rich plasma and stem cell therapies. Are all these treatments the same?

The use of regenerative therapies has exploded in the last ten years, and in some ways, it is like the "Wild West." Although many orthopedic and sports clinics and doctors now offer these therapies, there is a wide variation of methods practiced. One issue is that while treatment should be tailored for each individual, some facilities offer more of a "one-size-fits-all" approach. This can be effective in simple, straightforward cases; however, the more complex a case is, the more important it is that the physician analyzes pain referral patterns and gets a correct diagnosis before proceeding to treatment. Other issues are that protocols vary, as well as the type and method of preparation of platelet-rich plasma used, or what type of stem cell source is being used. The bottom line is not all facilities offer the same treatment; therefore, do your homework to determine which facility and method you are most comfortable with.

I've heard of star athletes getting PRP treatments overseas, for instance going to Germany. Do they do it better there?
Before PRP Prolotherapy was well known in the United States, it was popular for elite athletes (such as Kobe Bryant of the Los Angeles Lakers) to go to Germany for a similar treatment known as "Orthokine." Orthokine treatment involves a processing method that is approved in Germany but not in the United States. With this method, the patient's blood is heated overnight before being centrifuged; this process eliminates the inflammatory proteins while concentrating the anti-inflammatory proteins, which are then used for the injection. Yearly injections are usually needed.[8] A version of this treatment done in the United States is called "Regenokine."

Since inflammation is needed for healing, the question arises regarding which result is preferable: short-term, anti-inflammatory relief or longer-term, pro-inflammatory healing. Of course, if an athlete needs to get back in the game, receiving a natural anti-inflammatory regenerative-oriented technique from one's own blood certainly has its appeal over cortisone. However, since yearly injections are typically needed, it is unclear what the long-term regenerative effect of this treatment is. There is also no good way to make a detailed comparison between Orthokine/Regenokine, or PRP since there are limited studies that compare them long term.

What if I'm taking aspirin or anti-inflammatory medications (NSAIDs) when I begin treatment?

Because all the various forms of Prolotherapy are intended to stimulate inflammation in order to promote healing, the recommendation is to not take NSAIDs while getting treatment. If you are taking a baby aspirin for your heart, this can continue during Prolotherapy treatment, as the low dose will not affect treatment results. If you are taking a higher dose, this should be discussed with your physician prior to treatment. Regarding other NSAID medication, some patients may need to take these for some other reason, such as headaches that, for that person, may only respond to that type of medication. The advanced formulas (platelet-rich plasma and biocellular) seem to be more forgiving of briefly taking NSAIDs, especially if timed so that they are not taken during the most critical periods of healing. Of course, this should be discussed with your treating physician prior to treatment so a plan of action can be determined.

What if I'm taking a blood thinner or other anti-platelet medication? Will these interfere?

There is some controversy regarding whether anti-platelet medications interfere with the therapeutic ability of PRP. Many studies indicate no effect or minimal effect;[9] others indicate a negative effect.[10] Regardless, most physicians agree that it is not wise to discontinue these medications and that Prolotherapy, including PRP and Biocellular Prolotherapy, may usually still be done as long as there is no excessive bleeding time. If the patient is taking coumadin, a blood thinner which requires monitoring, we ask for a copy of the last 6 to 12 months of your blood monitoring testing (called an "INR," which stands for International Normalized Ratio") to see that your levels are stable. If there are any questions about a patient's history or ability to go through a Prolotherapy treatment, the patient may be asked to clear the procedure with his/her primary care physician, internist, or specialist prior to treatment.

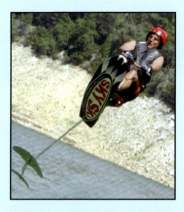

Chiropractic Physician

I am a 60-year-old chiropractic physician. Twenty-five years ago, when I was in my 30s, I injured my left shoulder while golfing on frozen ground. We were moving residences at the time, and I remember being unable to lift anything. From that point on, I was not able to sleep on my left shoulder. I had periodic pain in my left shoulder blade, especially while golfing or lifting. As I aged, lifting became even more difficult, so I refrained from doing it. I also adapted how I did activities such as driving. As the years went by, I lost range of motion in my shoulder and was unable to put my kids, or later my grandkids, on my shoulders to carry them. Over the years, I had my shoulder worked on by chiropractors as well as practitioners of massage, acupuncture, and other alternative methods; however, the problem continued. The final straw came a few years ago after carrying lawn furniture overhead to store it in our pool house. That night, I was in so much pain, I couldn't sleep.

I got an MRI, which indicated I had a 90 percent tear in one of my rotator cuff tendons, so I consulted a local orthopedic surgeon who was a friend of mine. My friend told me I would need surgical repair and that the recovery time was about three months—with my left arm in a sling, with no motion at all, for the first month. As I was the sole doctor at my busy practice, this was not a good option. I have also talked to many patients, and others, over the years who have had shoulder surgery and who, in spite of this, still continue to experience pain. So it wasn't clear-cut to me that surgery would resolve my issue. A man I attend church with had surgery on both his shoulders and still can't raise his arms very high; he is now on permanent disability. I decided to check into other possible nonsurgical options first. I knew about Dextrose Prolotherapy but did not think it would be strong enough for my problem. I consulted with Dr. Alderman about regenerative treatment alternatives.

I liked what she proposed, especially the possibility of repair without surgery, scar tissue, or much downtime. She did a diagnostic musculoskeletal ultrasound in the office, which revealed more information than had been on the MRI. After discussing the pros and cons with her, and understanding that there was no way to guarantee the procedure would work, it seemed like the most reasonable next step, so I decided to move forward. I received my first treatment, Biocellular (Stem Cell–Rich) Prolotherapy, the same day as my consultation. There was pain after the treatment, as expected, but it was manageable, and after four days off work, I was back in the office treating patients.

The shoulder gradually began to improve; other than the initial few days, I was able to continue working. Approximately three months after my first treatment, I went in for a follow-up evaluation, and we could see improvement on the diagnostic ultrasound. That day, I had a PRP Prolotherapy treatment, and then ten months after that, I had a second Biocellular treatment. I estimate that I was 90 percent improved after one year and relatively pain free. My shoulder has continued to improve since my last treatment a year ago. I was able to return to my passion of hydrofoil waterskiing the following summer. The hydrofoil weighs approximately 40 pounds, and there is resistance from the water when you lift it back onto the boat. That summer, I was able to lift it out of the water and hang it up on the tower of the boat—something I was unable to do before the treatments. And I can now sleep on my left shoulder most nights! I can also now carry my grandkids on my shoulders. The most beneficial thing has been that I was able to continue to work and not lose months just to recover—not to mention avoiding the increased risk of general anesthesia and surgery. I also now have full range of motion in my shoulder. I am thrilled with my improvement.

Dennis Harding, DC
Chiropractic Physician

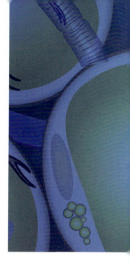

CHAPTER 18

What to Expect during Treatment and Related FAQs

T his chapter will go over what to expect from an evaluation and the details on how treatments are typically done, with related frequently asked questions. However, remember every patient is different, so while this section can give you a general idea of what is involved with treatments, questions concerning your specific condition should be addressed directly with your physician prior to treatment.

PROCEDURE FAQS

Where is the Prolotherapy treatment performed?

Prolotherapy is usually done in the office setting, not a hospital. It is done typically in the procedure room by a doctor who has been trained in Prolotherapy, platelet-rich plasma or biocellular, injections.

What kind of doctors are able to do these procedures, and where can I find one?

Several different types of practitioners are doing these injections: family physicians, sports medicine physicians, orthopedists, rheumatologists, podiatrists, and even some dentists (for temporomandibular joint, for instance). However, it goes without saying that the level of training and scope of practice and experience can vary widely among different practitioners. There are multiple training organizations offering courses in these procedures (see Chapter 8: "Prolotherapy Regenerative Medicine Is Evidence Based") and even some certifications available now in the field of Prolotherapy and Orthopedic Regenerative Medicine. If you are seeking a practitioner, contacting one of these organizations or checking the organization website for a listing of members may be helpful. There is also a website, http://www.getprolo.com, where practitioners trained in Prolotherapy can be found.

How many injections are given in a Prolotherapy treatment?

Any one Prolotherapy treatment may involve multiple injections; exactly how many depends on the area(s) being treated and the type of Prolotherapy being done. Most Dextrose Prolotherapy injections are made at the fibro-osseous junction (*fibro* for "fiber," *osseous* for "bone"), which is where ligaments and tendons attach to the bone. This is because that is where blood supply is good and where growth can be best stimulated. With Dextrose Prolotherapy the area is generally "peppered" with multiple injections. Since the advanced Prolotherapy (platelet-rich plasma, adipose (fat), or bone marrow) formulas contain one's own blood and cells, which contain natural growth factors, fewer injections are needed. Also, the advanced formulas are often administered with the assistance of ultrasound guidance, therefore more targeted injections can be made.

Does Prolotherapy treatment hurt?

Most patients tolerate the procedure very well; however, a shot is a shot, and there is a certain amount of discomfort involved. To help with discomfort, a local anesthetic is used. Also, the needles used are very thin, which helps with pain. The procedure is also relatively quick. In spite of this, some individuals may feel anxiety about having this type of procedure, especially if they have a low pain tolerance; therefore, oral anti-anxiety or pain medication can be taken prior to the procedure (be sure to discuss with your doctor if you think this may be needed). In the large majority of cases, no medication is needed.

How will I feel after the treatment?
How much pain will I be in?

All individuals respond to treatment differently, so there is no way to predict *exactly* what your experience or degree of pain will be. However, in general, patients are somewhat sore for a day or two, with some individuals very sore for several days—or, in rare cases, longer—then begin to feel better. Other patients, amazingly, have very little discomfort at all. The severity of after-treatment discomfort depends on several factors, including individual pain tolerance, which sites are injected, and which formula is utilized.

Because a local anesthetic is used, many patients do not feel much discomfort immediately after the procedure. In fact, for the first hour or so afterward, it is even possible to feel a decrease in the pain one came in for. After the local anesthetic wears off, the treatment area will generally feel stiff and sore, and may progress to moderate pain and discomfort. For this reason, a short course of pain medication may be prescribed after a treatment. As for the injection sites: some joint locations are less "forgiving" than others and so tend to be more uncomfortable after treatment. Shoulders and elbows, for instance, are almost always very sore for a few days; knees tend to be moderately sore; low backs tend to be the least sore.

Also, different formulas have different typical after-treatment patterns. Dextrose, in my experience, is the least aggravating (even with its additional "peppering"). It also tends to be uncomfortable for the least amount of time afterwards. The platelet-rich plasma and biocellular formulas tend to be more aggravating initially, and also seem to cause an "ebb-and-flow" phenomenon, not usually seen with dextrose. This involves initial discomfort for a day or two, with the person then starting to feel better. However, a week or so later, and seemingly out of the blue, there seems to be the return of a weaker version of the initial discomfort, which is also much shorter in duration. This type of brief discomfort may continue to occur every week or so, for several weeks after treatment, decreasing in intensity each time it occurs. The reason for this phenomenon is unclear, however because these formulas are living cells which communicate and signal for other cells, it is likely that multiple waves of healing are occurring as new cells arrive to continue the healing process, causing this "ebb and flow" pattern. Therefore, it may feel like four steps forward and two steps backwards, but it is important to understand this phenomenon, have patience, and realize that progress is being made.

Is the procedure for Biocellular Prolotherapy (using adipose or bone marrow) more painful than the one for Platelet-Rich Plasma (PRP) Prolotherapy (using blood)?

When doing a Biocellular procedure, there is an additional step: that of extracting either adipose (fat) or bone marrow. This does make this procedure more involved and, yes, more uncomfortable than just doing a PRP treatment; however, in general, the extraction procedures are well tolerated. Once extraction is done, the injection process, whether its platelet-rich plasma or biocellular, is almost identical and feels about the same for most people.

Is there any chance I will feel immediate improvement after a treatment?

Sometimes the pain goes away completely for several hours, days, or longer immediately after a treatment, especially in the low back. There are a few reasons for this. One is that the injected formula itself, along with the initial fluid and positive inflammation that are induced, provide stability to the joint. Another reason is that "trigger points" (muscle knots surrounding weak joints) might have been released by the injections. In some cases, the release of these trigger points (usually in the low back) is so profound that the individual can experience a long-term relief of pain. However, because instability of the joint (ligament laxity) is the true cause of the problem in most cases, and muscle spasm is just the body's response, the pain usually eventually returns, until there has been enough time for actual connective tissue healing to occur.

How many treatments will I need, and how often are they given?

The number of treatments and the time between them will vary from case to case. The idea is to stimulate the body's natural "stimulus-response" repair mechanism and then give the body enough time to heal. An average number of treatments for Dextrose or PRP Prolotherapy is four-to-six treatments. Since connective tissue takes an average of four to six weeks to heal after an injury, the general protocol is to repeat treatments every four to six or eight weeks for both Traditional and PRP Prolotherapy, with intervals starting closer together in the beginning and then increasing over the course of treatment. With Biocellular Prolotherapy (using adipose or bone marrow), fewer treatments are needed, in many cases just one, sometimes two, and the intervals between treatments is usually longer—6 to 12 months.

Other variables to the number of treatments and length of intervals include how rapidly a person tends to heal and how active he/she is. Note too that sometimes the doctor will start with one formula and then move on to another after the improvement from the first has leveled off. I am conservative and like to start with the least invasive formula I believe will work and then see within a treatment or two if it's necessary to advance to the next level of treatment. The treatment plan will depend on response to treatment and was previously laid out in the treatment algorithm in Chapter 10 (see Figure 10.5), which also provides information on why a specific formula may be used over another.

How long will it take before I see improvement?

It usually takes at least two treatments before improvement is noticed. Although factors such as the changing of medication and routines can play a part, the main reason it takes a while to notice improvement is because it takes time for connective tissue to grow and heal. There are time frames the body needs to make tissue; for instance, it takes nine months to make a baby. Maybe you can get a very small premature baby at five or six months, but you will not be able to get a viable baby after two months! It takes six weeks to make new collagen, so you will be into your second treatment, usually, before there has been enough time for change to start showing up. That said, there are patients who notice improvement sooner, even after the first treatment, or who may not notice much change until after the third or even fourth treatment. There are also other factors, such as prior NSAID use and an increase or change in activity or life demands, that may affect perception of improvement. Therefore, I recommend patience; it's better to expect it to take a while and then be pleasantly surprised if you are better sooner than expected.

How will I measure improvement?

Sometimes, there will be improvement in objective measurements, such as orthopedic testing to measure range of motion and strength. Similarly, ultrasound images of the problem site from before and after treatment may also show improvement in tissue quality or repair; however, these visual changes do not always show up right away. The most important measure of progress is subjective improvement: how the patient feels—i.e., decreased pain and increased activity. Change may show up gradually; the comments I hear are "I feel stronger," "I have less overall pain," "The joint feels more stable," "I'm able to sit longer," and "I need less pain medication." These are all signs of improvement.

When can I resume my normal physical activity after a treatment?

Complete rest of the treated area is recommended for 24 hours after a treatment. This is especially true for the advanced formulas, because we want the blood and cells to "stay put" and activate within the injected location. But after that initial resting period, your body needs normal motion so it knows where to lay down new tissue based on the activities that will be expected of it. Therefore, it is good to start moving the treated area in its normal range of motion. That said, it's important to not "load" that joint too soon. Movement is good, loading or stressing the joint is not. So no heavy lifting! The rule on exercise, in general, is that a person can begin doing whatever exercise has not historically caused any of the pain that is being treated. That is, you should avoid any exercise or routine that has aggravated the treated area in the past, but you can resume activities that did not historically cause pain. When starting back to these activities (the ones that previously did not cause pain), it is best to start at about half the exercise/activity/intensity, see how you do, and then slowly increase until back to normal, again avoiding lifting or loading on the treated joint as much as possible. This general rule applies to the first treatment or two. After this, since that joint has had time to get stronger, you will usually be able to introduce the original exercises that had been the most difficult or challenging, but when you do, again, start at a lower level than you were doing previously, increasing the intensity slowly.

Should I use ice or heat after a treatment?

Many individuals are in the habit of using ice almost continually before and after exercise, or after an injury. While there are times when ice can be helpful, if used continually, it may slow down healing. Think of a person who falls in a frozen lake, his/her circulation slows down significantly after a time; healing is not occurring while the person is frozen in the lake! Yet ice can sometimes be helpful if there is an exceptional amount of swelling or pain after a treatment and is certainly better than taking a drug if applied briefly. As I tell my patients, do not "marry" the ice! Regarding heat, that is usually the go-to remedy to help with healing in between treatments. However heat can be overdone too, and if too much heat is used, it can aggravate the area and pain can flare. Do not marry the heating pad either! Usually I tell patients no heat, no ice for the first 24 hours after a treatment since the treatment itself is aggravating. After the first 24 hours then use heat if needed, but do not sleep with it. Use ice very briefly if the need is felt and that is the person's usual habit. Heat is also best used if moist. Ways to do this are a hot bath, jacuzzi, or a moist heating pad. In any case, it is always to discuss the specifics of your situation, activity, and usual use of ice/heat, with your physician so that the two of you decide on the best after-treatment plan for you.

Why Isn't One Treatment Enough?

In explaining why multiple Prolotherapy treatments are needed, Dr. Ross Hauser uses the analogy of getting children to clean their rooms when told to. There's a slight chance it will happen on the first request, but that's not likely. Usually, the task requires a gradual stimulus-response process, which goes something like this:

First stimulus: "Clean your room."

First response: Child just stares at you.

Second stimulus: *"Clean your room!"*

Second response: Some toys are picked up and put back in their bins.

Third stimulus: **"Clean your room!"**

Third response: The bed gets made.

Fourth stimulus: *"CLEAN! YOUR! ROOM!"*

Fourth response: Everything is put away, and all the surfaces are tidied.

In other words, the idea in Prolotherapy is to get the body to heal by stimulating repair with repetition and an increase in the level of coaxing, as well as formula strength if required. Like the tortoise and the hare, the expectation should be slow-and-steady progress.

What are trigger points?

Trigger points are painful knots in a muscle where a spasm is occurring. After a muscle has been working for a while to hold in a weak joint, it can develop constant and automatic tight areas that help it secure the weak joint without the body having to "think about it." Trigger points can be released in a variety of ways; sometimes, pressure or massage helps, but the ultimate way to release a trigger point is to shoot it with a needle and local anesthetic. While Prolotherapy injections are not directed to those trigger points themselves, because the injections go through the muscle to get to the targeted joint, sometimes these trigger points release, bringing immediate relief. Trigger point injection therapy is sometimes done as a stand-alone pain treatment; it was the basis of the research by Dr. Janet Travell, John F. Kennedy's personal physician, in the 1950s. But, in general, unless the underlying joint weakness is resolved, the trigger point will return with time. That is why a treatment, such as Prolotherapy, which stimulates repair of the underlying joint is important, rather than just trigger point release itself. When the joint heals, these trigger points generally just go away on their own. In some cases, however, trigger points persist after Prolotherapy treatments. I believe this occurs because the body is so used to having these "knots" that it doesn't easily let go of them. If trigger points continue after the joint has repaired, the doctor can easily inject them directly to release them.

How is platelet-rich plasma made in the doctor's office?

To make platelet-rich plasma, a portion of the patient's blood is drawn into a syringe that contains a small amount of an anticlotting agent. The blood is then processed to concentrate the platelets. The most common method uses a special FDA-cleared centrifuge that separates the blood into layers based on weight—a process that takes approximately 15 to 20 minutes. The platelet-poor plasma layer is the lightest; the red blood cell layer is the heaviest, and in between is a yellowish layer called the "buffy coat," which contains a concentration of platelets (see Figure 18.1: How Platelet-Rich Plasma (PRP) is done).

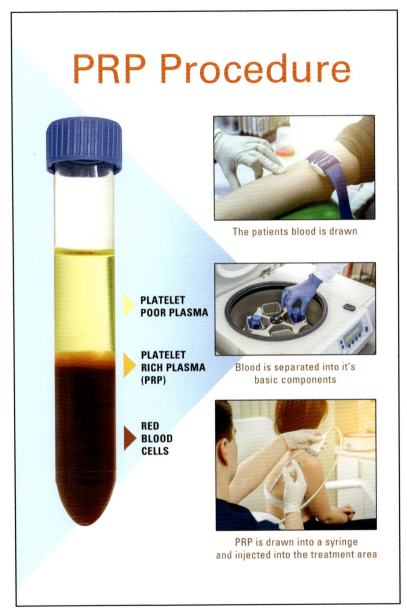

Figure 18.1: How Platelet-Rich Plasma (PRP) Prolotherapy is done

How is adipose-derived Biocellular Prolotherapy done?

The first step in Biocellular Prolotherapy using adipose is the removal of fat from the patient. In conjunction with adipose, PRP is usually done so blood is drawn first. Then the adipose extraction is done. This involves a sterile procedure similar to liposuction but on a *much* smaller scale. (Note that since the amount of fat needed is very small, its removal does not noticeably affect the patient's shape.) The fat is extracted with a thin, blunt (not sharp), tube-like syringe instrument called a "microcannula" (from the Latin *micro*, meaning "small," and *cannula*, meaning "little reed"). A pinhole-sized opening is made in the skin. The doctor inserts the cannula and gently moves the microcannula back and forth to slowly distribute the fluid and break up the adipose. After that, a small amount of suction is created by pulling the syringe plunger back and then adipose is extracted. The adipose is then separated by either gravity or more commonly now by putting it in a centrifuge, which then spins it, removes excess fluids, and concentrates the adipose (see Figure 18.2: Adipose extraction). The Biocellular formula is then made, and treatment proceeds, typically using ultrasound to guide the injection precisely into the injured tendon or joint location.

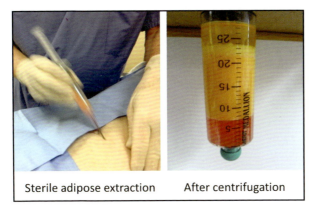

| Sterile adipose extraction | After centrifugation |

Figure 18.2: Adipose extraction

How is bone marrow–derived Biocellular Prolotherapy done?

The first step in Biocellular Prolotherapy using bone marrow is extraction of the bone marrow itself. This is a sterile procedure done in a procedure room, typically using a collection kit made by one of several manufacturers. The usual site of extraction is along the upper back portion of the pelvic bone (see Figure 18.3 Bone marrow extraction). Prior to the extraction, a local anesthetic is injected through the skin to the top of the bone at the extraction site; this enables a relatively comfortable extraction. If a patient is anxious about the procedure, pain or anti-anxiety medication is often offered in advance.

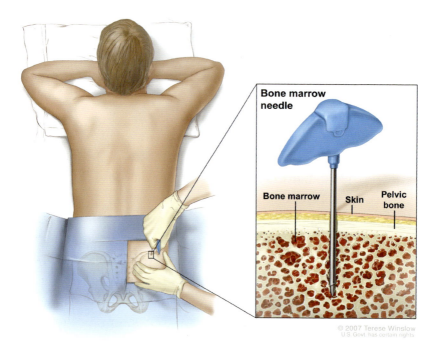

© 2007 Terese Winslow
U.S. Govt. has certain rights

Figure 18.3: Bone marrow extraction. Once the bone marrow needle is placed, a syringe is attached and marrow withdrawn.

The bone marrow is then put into a centrifuge which spins it, removes excess fluids, and concentrates it. By this process, the extracted bone marrow has become "bone marrow aspirate concentrate" ("BMAC") and is ready to be injected into the injured ligament, tendon, or joint—usually using ultrasound guidance to assist in precisely determining the injection sites.

Are there any contraindications to Prolotherapy treatment?

A contraindication is a reason why treatment should not be done. One of the biggest contraindications is if the problem is determined to be one for which

Prolotherapy will likely have no, or minimal, results, Another contraindication is an active underlying infection or illness. For instance, if a patient is not feeling well with a cold or flu, treatment should be delayed until he/she is better. Or if someone is currently receiving treatment for an active chronic illness or cancer, Prolotherapy would not be done, as we do not want to interfere with that treatment. However, if the cancer was in the past, and now considered cured, this would generally not be a problem. Other examples would be a patient with active/acute gout or rheumatoid arthritis (meaning flared at the moment); however, someone can have rheumatoid, gout, or another autoimmune issue that is controlled and not currently flared, and still be a candidate for treatment. The same is true for diabetes; if controlled, this is generally not a problem; however, if blood sugar is high and out of control, Prolotherapy would be postponed until this is stable.

A contradiction can be "absolute," meaning no matter what, or "relative," meaning treatment can still be done depending on the specifics of the issue. An example of an absolute contraindication would be known allergy to any of the ingredients in the Prolotherapy formula or unwillingness to experience possible after-treatment discomfort. Patients should understand the course of the Prolotherapy treatment and be participants in their treatment plan. Relative contraindications include current, long-term use of high doses of opioid medications, because, as previously discussed, these medications can lower the immune system and response to treatment, but might be allowable under some circumstances. Current use of systemic corticosteroids or NSAIDS (anti-inflammatory medication) are also relative contraindications, as these are counterproductive to the inflammatory process, but, again, patients may still be able to receive treatment under some circumstances. Other relative contraindications include central canal spinal stenosis, if it is a known cause of the pain, and severe degenerative hip OA with loss of range of motion, as these can be difficult conditions to treat and should be carefully evaluated prior to treatment to ensure a reasonable probability of success before starting. If any of these types of conditions are known to exist, these should always be discussed with the physician prior to treatment to determine if treatment is recommended and will be beneficial.

What are the risks of Prolotherapy procedure treatments?

Prolotherapy is a medical procedure. Although there are risks associated with all medical procedures, the risk with Prolotherapy is considered to be low. The most common (expected) risk is that you will feel worse before you feel better, and some joint areas may be profoundly sore for a few days after a treatment. In some cases, there may be little or minimal soreness, and that is normal too. Most of the risk has to do with the fact that these are injections and the risk associated with that, which would be bruising and soreness from the injection itself. However, the remaining risks that could result from an injection are rare headache; infection;

temporary irritation of a nearby nerve; pneumothorax (collapse of lung) if doing injections near there, although this is extremely rare; and allergic reaction to the formula ingredients. As for the latter, in a few rare cases, people with corn allergies have reacted to dextrose. It's also possible that someone has a previously unknown allergy to local anesthetic. It's theoretically possible that someone could have a reaction to his/her own blood platelets or cells, but there have been no reports of such a response happening. There may also be risks related to a patient's medical history. It is essential that a patient thoroughly understands all possible risks before starting a course of Prolotherapy treatment. There are also specific risks mentioned in the chapters on PRP and Biocellular Prolotherapy. And, finally, since no medical treatment can be guaranteed, there is the risk that Prolotherapy will not work. Although it has a high success rate (around 90 percent for appropriate conditions), for some individuals, it does not work.

What are the reasons Prolotherapy does not work?

As mentioned earlier, there seems to be a small percentage of Prolotherapy patients who do not respond to a course of treatment. In my experience, there are four reasons Prolotherapy would not work.

1. The patient's inability to heal: Some people just have trouble healing, especially in making new, strong collagen. Other factors could include taking anti-inflammatory or other medications that interfere with treatment,

overactivity resulting in re-injury or reag-gravation of the treatment area, poor nutri-tion including insufficient protein, smoking (which interferes with collagen repair), or an underlying metabolic or disease process preventing healing, low testosterone, thy-roid or other hormone imbalance, or severe sleep disturbance.

2. Too much damage, such as a severely degen-erated joint, a completely ruptured tendon, or bone degeneration: Most of the time, these findings are obvious, and no treat-ment is attempted. However, in some cases, the damage may be worse than it appears, either in the exam or on images.

3. Wrong diagnosis: In some cases, a patient's presentation is very complex, and getting an exact and specific diagnosis can be challeng-ing. The doctor does a thorough evaluation and comes up with a working diagnosis, which, if correct, will lead to positive treat-ment results most of the time. However, if the diagnosis is not correct, for instance, if some-one is diagnosed with a knee problem, but that pain is actually referring from a prob-lem in the hip, then treatment on the knee will fail to resolve the problem. Or, worse, if the pain is coming from the progression of an unknown disease, for instance, pros-tate cancer causing low back pain, then

Prolotherapy treatment of the low back will not resolve the pain. Fortunately, this last possibility is rare, but however unusual it may be, sometimes, there are issues that are unknown at the start of treatment. That is why after a few treatments, if no change is achieved, the doctor usually does a reevaluation of some sort to make sure he/she is on the right track.

4. No known reason: This is a very small percentage of cases, about 1 or 2 percent. There is no known reason why the treatment isn't working—health status is good, no red flags—and yet there is no or limited response to treatment.

Again, remember, these are general questions and general answers. Also, different doctors may perform treatments in slightly different ways. All concerns, questions, and specifics relating to your personal history, expectations, pain tolerances, or treatment issues should be addressed directly to the physician who is planning your Prolotherapy care.

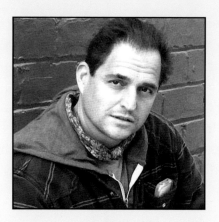

Actor

Over ten years ago, my left ankle mysteriously became tender, and I foolishly assumed it would heal right away. I continued to use it and ended up re-injuring it time after time, including fracturing one of the bones in my foot and eventually finding myself with joint osteoarthritis and plantar fasciitis, to the point that I was disabled. Just crossing a room required a lot of thought because it was so difficult. Trips to the bathroom at night were no fun either. I needed to use a cane because the pain became so chronic and severe that I worried I would not be able to walk at all. I got MRIs. I went to orthopedists, rheumatologists, rehabilitation specialists, physical therapists, acupuncturists, and chiropractor after chiropractor. I tried scores of supplements as well as every new age, positive-minded, sonic-laser-cure-all salve suggested to me.

Encouragingly, some of these treatments would work a little, but most not at all. I began to believe that being without chronic pain was not in the cards for me. It hurt to walk—every step—and then it progressed to where I had pain even at rest. I saw another leading orthopedist at Cedars-Sinai Medical Center who advised fusion surgery for my ankle but said I could be left with possible lifetime chronic pain and an expected awkward, hobbling gait, with a year of surgery recovery. Not a very attractive proposition.

Then I found out about Prolotherapy and started on a treatment course of PRP Prolotherapy, using ultrasound imaging for added accuracy. This helped, but my results leveled off, so I eventually received Biocellular (Stem Cell–Rich) Prolotherapy using my bone marrow because of the extensive cartilage degeneration in my ankle joint. I had some hesitation about the idea of going through a bone marrow extraction procedure, but in comparison to the doubtful, last-resort, fused-ankle surgery with irreversible repercussions, it seemed much less risky and certainly was only a fraction of the cost of what that surgery would be.

As it turned out, the Biocellular Prolotherapy procedure itself was manageable, and the results were wonderfully positive. This took me light-years ahead—and within a few months after the treatment. Because I had such a severe degenerative issue, I decided to repeat the treatment several months later for further improvement. It has been over a year since my last treatment, and I can walk without discomfort. I do not need a cane anymore, and I'm back to doing the things I enjoy. I am exceedingly grateful for my results.

Michael DeLuise
Actor, son of late comedian Dom DeLuise, noted for the TV series *NYPD Blue*, *SeaQuest 2032*, *Brooklyn South*, *Gilmore Girls*, and the film *Encino Man* (Endnotes)

CHAPTER 19

Joint Pain: The Nutrition Connection

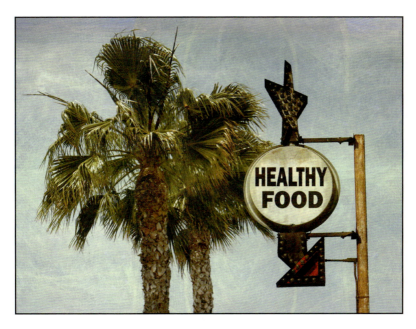

Let food be thy medicine,
and let thy medicine be food.

~ Hippocrates, Father of Medicine (460–377 BC)

I t is hard to deny that nutrition plays a role in healing and joint pain. In years past, nutritional deficiency diseases were common, especially in children when the demand for nutrients is higher. Among these diseases, rare today in the United States, are "rickets" (softening of bones because of inadequate vitamin D); scurvy (poor wound healing, joint pain, caused by inadequate vitamin C); beriberi (poor muscle coordination, nerve degeneration, caused by lack of vitamin B1), and the list goes on. If you think about it, these are really magnified problems which can occur at a lower level if the deficiency is small. Symptoms might not be as severe as these disease states, however just enough to affect the quality of healing. Other situations may also occur, such as the need for a particular nutrient has increased because of lifestyle, stress, or injury. In those cases, blood testing for known "deficiencies" will show normal results, however there really is a shortfall. This may then impact healing or create other unfavorable phenomena.

It is certainly clear that specific essential minerals and micronutrients play a role in the ability to repair injured connective tissue and joints properly, and their absence will result in a less than ideal healing environment. However, there is controversy as to what degree nutrition is important. Part of the controversy is a result of genetic differences between individuals that make responses to nutritional treatment or diet variable—i.e., some people seem to eat whatever they want without adverse consequences, where others are extremely sensitive. However it is undeniable that since we put food in our mouths every day, and certain nutrients are required by our bodies for good health, nutrition should not be ignored or overlooked.

Different opinions exist as to what is the best diet. It has also been suggested that lack of enough fruits and vegetables, and too many refined foods and sweets can create a "pro-inflammatory" condition, making a person more susceptible to pain.[1] Lack of enough dietary protein has also been linked to pain conditions. [2] And certain foods or food allergies are known to aggravate arthritic or pain conditions in some people. This chapter will go over some nutritional facts and theories that have been linked to pain and nutritional approaches that have been shown to improve it.

MICRONUTRIENTS ARE NEEDED FOR JOINT REPAIR AND THE IMPORTANCE OF SILICON

Nutrients and micronutrients necessary for connective tissue and joint repair include copper, calcium, manganese, magnesium, molybdenum, potassium, vitamin C, zinc, and silicon; however, silicon is often overlooked in many formulations designed for joints.

Silicon is the third-most abundant trace element in the human body[3] and essential for proper healing and repair of injured ligaments, tendons and joints. This is believed to be because of its role in the making of collagen in the body.[4] Silicon exists in various forms, with most of the silicon in the body in a form called "orthosilicic acid." [5] When stabilized with choline (a vitamin-like essential nutrient), orthosilicic acid is the safest and most orally bioavailable (meaning easily absorbable) form of silicon.[6] Multiple studies have shown favorable correlations between intake of orthosilicic acid and the health of connective tissue,[7] as well as other potential health benefits to the immune system, including possible prevention of osteoporosis and Alzheimer's disease, and the improved health of hair, skin, and nails.[8]

The Story of LigaGenix®

It is important that patients receiving Prolotherapy treatment get adequate nutritional support after their procedures. Over the years, I had recommended various brands and types of nutritional supplements for this purpose. At one point, I thought I had found a good supplement and was recommending it to patients, but then the manufacturer changed it from capsules to hard tablets, which were not as easily absorbable. I began getting negative feedback about this product from my patients and so called the representative for the supplement company, who I knew fairly well, to give him my input. He listened politely, then said, "I'm sorry, Dr. Alderman, thanks for your opinion, but we're not changing the tablet; it's a money thing." That bothered me. I thought "Really?" This was a moderately sized company, and it didn't make sense to me that they wouldn't be willing to spend a few more cents to get a better product. I started looking for another brand to recommend, but other than this last supplement, which wasn't perfect either, I had not found any one specific supplement that had all the ingredients needed in one formula—with some formulas having extra and unneeded ingredients. Since many of my patients were already taking basic vitamins, I was reluctant to recommend a number of *additional* supplements. So, I decided then to develop a comprehensive, better product, using the nutritional training I had received as a student at Cornell, and in 2010, LigaGenix® was born. This all-in-one supplement has the nutrients and micronutrients needed to support collagen repair, including the very important choline-stabilized silicon. Specifically tailored for patients receiving Prolotherapy regenerative injections to optimize healing afterwards, LigaGenix® is also taken, at lower doses, for maintenance of connective tissue health in general, and has had excellent patient feedback since its development (for more information, see www.ligagenix.com).

THE IMPORTANCE OF DIETARY PROTEIN

There is a relationship between inadequate protein consumption and chronic pain. In fact, patients with chronic pain often have a diet high in carbohydrates and low in protein.[9] This lack of protein in the diet can lead to an inability of our bodies to maintain enough of the building blocks (amino acids—a component of protein) needed to rebuild collagen. On top of that, amino acids are used to make our bodies' own "natural" painkillers, such as "endorphins," which you may have heard about. Endorphins (from "endogenous" meaning "contained within" and "morphine," which is a strong painkiller) are "morphine like substances originating from within the body."[10] We naturally make endorphins in response to pain or stress, after vigorous exercise (i.e., endorphins are responsible for "runners" high), or after eating certain foods such as chocolate. If there is too much pain or stress, the body can use up available endorphins, and if there is a lack of the right kind of protein in the diet to keep up and make more endorphins, then pain levels increase. Other natural painkillers our bodies make from protein amino acids are serotonin and gamma amino butyric acid (known as "GABA"), both important for relaxation, sleep, and mood. The bottom line is that taking the right type of amino acids, either in the diet or supplement form, may be able to help reduce pain.[11] For more information on the importance of protein for chronic pain, see the article by Julia Ross in *Practical Pain Management Journal* found at https://www.practicalpainmanagement.com/treatments/nutraceutical/amino-acids-diet-chronic-pain-management.

ENDORPHIGEN®

Almost forty years ago, a researcher at Chicago Medical School found that adding a certain amino acid to pain patients' diets lowered that patients' need for opiate pain medications.[12] As it turns out, the amino acid he added was found to increase the patient's natural endorphin levels, so that their need for pain medication decreased. The way that works is complicated, but the short explanation is that this particular amino acid works to block the breakdown of our own natural endorphins so these are available longer. This discovery eventually resulted in the formulation of a commercially available supplement called "EndorphiGen®" made by Lidkte Labs that contains an amino acid similar to the one used in that Chicago Medical study.[13] This supplement is designed to raise one's natural endorphin levels and has been found to be very helpful for reducing pain in some patients.

FOOD ALLERGIES AND JOINT PAIN

Food sensitivities and allergies seem to play a part in the development of joint pain.[14] Individuals can be allergic to foods eaten on a regular basis without showing any obvious symptoms. This type of allergic reaction is more subtle, but can eventually result in joint inflammation and pain. The trouble is that these symptoms might emerge days or even weeks after the offending foods were eaten, which makes these type of food allergies more difficult to diagnose.

Fortunately, there are remedies. Anti-inflammatory foods, food-allergy blood testing, and change in dietary patterns have all been used successfully to treat pain syndromes.[15] It has been well established that gluten, a protein present in grains such as wheat, rye, and barley, can produce a range of negative reactions, including skin responses such as hives or rashes, as well as other allergy-type reactions—from minor sinus congestion and sneezing to much more serious sudden, potentially fatal, allergic responses. While many of these reactions might occur immediately after ingesting gluten, severe autoimmune (the body fighting itself) reactions often emerge *years* after the initial gluten exposure.[16] Gluten sensitivity has also been linked to arthritis,[17] low back pain,[18] and other joint and muscle pain.[19]

If you have persistent joint pain, consider getting blood tested for food and gluten allergies, which can be done through a simple blood test. One company, Immuno Laboratories, offers a very comprehensive food and gluten allergy analysis (www.immunolabs. com). Even without a specific blood test, a person could try a gluten-free diet to see if pain improves. While not always easy to be "gluten-free" in today's world, aware- ness of this condition is increasing, and more options are available in restaurants and grocery stores.

NIGHTSHADES AND JOINT PAIN

A particular family of foods known as "nightshades" (because of these plants preference to grow in the shade and flower at night) has been recognized for many years to cause debilitating arthritis in animals.[20] Similar phenomena have been observed in some (but not all) humans. This family of foods includes eggplant, peppers (all kinds except black), potatoes, tobacco, tomatoes, and spices such as cayenne, chili, curry, paprika, and ground red pepper. The nightshade family has been implicated in muscle spasm as well as in joint pain and stiffness.[21] In patient studies, avoiding these foods resulted in some improvement—or even marked improvement—in joint pain and arthritis symptoms for some patients.[22] Of course, these foods are integrated into much of the American lifestyle, and so they are rather difficult to avoid. However, if you've had persistent joint or muscle pain, you could try eliminating these foods from your diet for four to six weeks just to see how you respond.

OTHER NATURAL REMEDIES FOR JOINT PAIN

Glucosamine: In 2001, the well-respected medical journal *The Lancet* published a long-term study that looked at the effect of glucosamine in slowing the progression of osteoarthritis (OA), showing significant improvement in pain for the group taking 1,500 mg of glucosamine sulfate per day.[23] Of course, again, there was controversy, with other authors contesting those results and contending no benefit existed.[24] However, the anti-inflammatory medication celecoxib (Celebrex), an NSAID, was compared to a combination of glucosamine and chondroitin. In that study both the supplement combination and the NSAID were concluded to have "comparable efficacy in reducing pain, stiffness, functional limitation, and joint swelling/effusion" in knee OA.[25]

Cetyl myrisoleate (CM): In 1962, arthritis research done at the National Institutes of Health brought about the accidental discovery of another potentially effective supplement. A certain type of mouse was found to be resistant to developing arthritis. Further investigation revealed that this mouse had something the other lab animals did not: a fatty acid named cetyl myrisoleate (CM).[26] CM was then extracted for use in humans, studied, and found to safely offer significant benefit for some, but not all, people with arthritis.[27]

Green-lipped mussel: Another arthritis remedy was uncovered when it was noted that coastal-dwelling natives in New Zealand have an extremely low incidence of joint pain and arthritis as compared to individuals living further inland.[28] It was found that the coastal group heavily consumed the green-lipped mussel, which happens to contain omega-3 polyunsaturated fatty acids. Multiple studies have shown these mussels (or their oil extract) to safely decrease joint pain with no real side effects.[29] As with CM, the magic of the green-lipped mussel may not work for all people.

SAM-e: Still another potentially helpful supplement is SAM-e (short for S-adenosyl methionine)—a substance found naturally in the body. Used since the mid-1970s for arthritis, SAM-e also seems to have a positive effect on mood. A double-blind study of 734 patients, including 582 with OA of the hip or knee, compared taking SAM-e to the NSAID naproxen (Aleve). In that study, SAM-e was shown to be as effective as naproxen but with fewer side effects.[30] Another double-blind study of patients with OA showed SAM-e to be as effective as the anti-inflammatory medication ibuprofen (Advil, Motrin) for reducing pain and increasing mobility.[31] The report, published in the *Journal of Family Practice*, concluded, "SAMe appears to be as effective as NSAIDs in reducing pain and improving functional limitation in patients with osteoarthritis without the adverse effects often associated with NSAID therapies."[32]

Omega-3 Fatty Acids: Finally, omega-3 essential fatty acids (EFAs) have shown promise in helping with pain. One study of arthritis patients compared using omega-3 EFAs versus the NSAID ibuprofen and found EFAs were as effective as ibuprofen in reducing arthritic pain.[33] As an added bonus, omega-3 EFAs have been associated with other health benefits, such as lower cholesterol[34] and blood pressure,[35] and, most recently, improved cognitive function.[36]

The bottom line is, as Hippocrates appropriately advised, "Let food be thy medicine, and let thy medicine be food." While not the complete answer, nutrition plays an important role in healing, joint health and pain conditions. Improving one's diet and/or nutritional support is a low-risk endeavor: usually little is to be lost. While making positive changes or trying a particular nutritional approach may not work for everyone or every situation, when a change does help, it has the potential to make an impact on the quality of one's life.

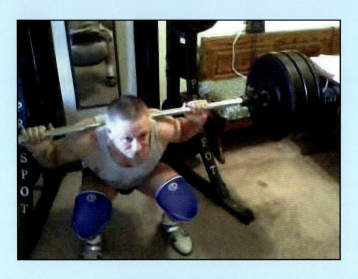

Lifetime Bodybuilder

At age 26, I underwent ACL (anterior cruciate ligament) reconstruction knee surgery for an injury sustained during a gymnastics training session. After two years of rehab, I was able to return to gymnastics competition for a couple more years. I then took a 14-year hiatus, returning to weightlifting and fitness training at age 44. When I started training again, it became clear that there was something wrong with my knee. I was told I suffered from patellar tendonitis due in part to the surgical technique used in my ACL operation years earlier, which utilized the central portion of my patellar tendon as the replacement for the ACL (modified Jones technique). This tendonitis became worse as I continued to train, and I developed compensatory additional joint pain and symptoms, primarily in the iliotibial band and its attachments around my knee.

One day, I was squatting 400 pounds and my knee wobbled. There was no immediate pain, and I was able to rack the bar, but two weeks later, while on the leg press, after just two repetitions with a moderate weight, I felt a sharp pain on the outside of the right knee and heard a loud snap. From that point on, my right knee continued to suffer, and my leg started to get progressively weaker. After a year of trying rest and rehab, it was no better.

I had heard of Prolotherapy and finally decided to give it a try; after all, I had very little to lose. At that point, I was not able to do the sport I loved and had tried everything else. Since seeing Dr. Alderman and receiving Prolotherapy, my knee has gotten progressively better. She began conservatively with a few Dextrose Prolotherapy treatments, followed by three PRP Prolotherapy treatments, and then one Biocellular (Stem Cell–Rich) Prolotherapy treatment using my fat as the source of cells. So in case anyone asks, yes, I have had liposuction!

My knee has made steady progress and continues to be good, pain free, and stable over three years since my last treatment. I just recently squatted 400 pounds with no problems. That was my touchstone to know if my knee had been rehabilitated. I would say to anyone who asks that it has! I am very grateful.

Barry Taft
Lifetime Bodybuilder

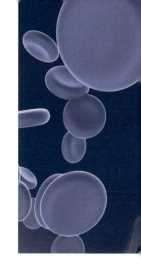

CHAPTER 20

Conclusion:
The Road You Walk

L ife is full of choices. Granted, you may not have chosen to be in a motor vehicle accident that left you with years of neck and back pain, or to twist an ankle while playing basketball that never quite healed. But even if you didn't choose your situation, you do have a choice about what to do now. After all, it is your body. Far too often, we let the medical community tell us what to do and tell us what is best for us. Maybe the advice we get is good, but maybe it isn't. Medical treatment must make sense to you because you are the one taking the risks. While you cannot always predict the outcome, you can do enough research to make an intelligent decision that seems right for you. Ultimately, what medical treatment you receive is your choice, and you will experience the consequences of that choice. Let me tell you about Mike.

Mike walked into my office using a cane, bent over like a thin twig that had been hit hard in a torrid snowstorm. A mere 40 years old, he was ragged and worn from pain and moved like he was 80. He had trouble getting up from a chair and walking for very long, as well as sitting. Mike told me he had been this way for several months. He experienced terrible low back pain on his left side, which shot down the back of his leg and into his foot. Because of the pain, he often was unable to sleep.

Mike had been to another clinic, where he was pre-scribed opioid painkillers. He had started physical therapy, been scheduled for an MRI, and told that he would probably need surgery. Mike worked as a col-lege professor at a local university, but, incapable of standing for very long, he had not been able to teach. What bothered Mike the most was his inability to lift or play with his six-month-old daughter, Jessica.

After examining Mike and determining that he was a candidate for Prolotherapy, I told him that it was his choice which direction to go. I could see the road he was walking down—one sure to be filled with stron-ger and stronger painkilling medication that would not only lower his immune system but also reduce his mental capacity and clarity. Since painkillers do noth-ing to cure pain—they only temporarily cover it up—these drugs would not heal him. Because depression often accompanies pain and a diminished way of life, Mike would probably be prescribed antidepressants at some point as well. However, the antidepressants wouldn't solve the problem either. Mike was walking down a road filled with these mind-weakening drugs, more pain, and then likely a surgery that he might not need but would be desperate enough to undergo.

Don't get me wrong, sometimes people do need surgery. Far too often, however, the surgeon relies on an MRI alone for his diagnosis, and, as you know by now, MRIs by themselves are not enough to determine that surgery is needed. As you will recall from Chapter 7: "The Importance of a Correct Diagnosis," abnormal findings on MRIs in people with low back pain might be coincidental and not the actual cause of their pain.[1] Time and time again in my practice, I have found this to be true.

An MRI needs to be correlated to the individual. To simply look at the MRI and say, "This disc is herniated, so it must be the problem. Let's cut it out," will not resolve the problem if the problem is not the disc. And because I have seen patients who have undergone multiple surgeries for back pain that did not resolve the pain, I consider surgery a last resort unless it is truly indicated.

Mike was a conservative guy who was brought up to respect authority and wanted to follow his other doctor's advice for the time being. He said he would think about his options and come back if he wanted to try Prolotherapy. I did not see Mike again for several months, until one day he showed up for an appointment. I was shocked to see how much worse he had become. He had almost doubled his intake of painkillers and reported that, in spite of everything, he was still in constant pain and unable to work. He had received the MRI and been told he needed surgery, but had been putting it off. He asked for my help, and we started

Prolotherapy treatments that day. Three months later, he was walking without a cane, and six months later, he was playing with, and lifting Jessica, now a toddler. Mike went back to work and was able to stop taking painkillers. The day I "graduated" him from treatment, he practically danced out of the office, happy and smiling. And he never did have that surgery.

This story may not be yours, for truly every experience is different. However, the bottom line is that each of us has a choice of which road to walk and when to walk it. I hope this book has been useful to you in your journey. Well wishes to you on whatever road you choose!

PART III:
MORE PATIENT STORIES

*Everyone you will ever meet
knows something you don't.*

—Bill Nye ("the Science Guy")

American science communicator
and television presenter

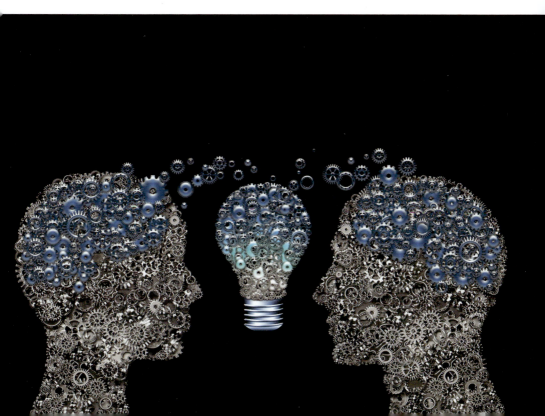

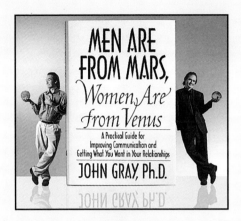

Writer

After 25 years as a professional writer and many hours at the computer, my neck and back were beginning to feel like a pretzel. My frequent traveling didn't help, and I often felt that my head was in a tight vise. My posture was worsening, and I began to get low back pain, sometimes with sciatic nerve pain down my leg. My ankle, as well, had been bothering me for over ten years, a consequence of aggressive physical activity in my youth. Over the years, I had tried chiropractic and acupuncture, but I was still in pain, and it wasn't getting any better. Then, through a friend, I heard about Prolotherapy.

After just one Prolotherapy treatment, I felt immediate improvement. After five treatments, my neck is fantastic, and I am virtually pain free. My posture has improved, and I feel stronger. I no longer have low back pain; the pain down my leg is gone, and my ankle has more bounce and doesn't click like it used to.

Prolotherapy is something you can do to take control of the downward spiral of aging and chronic pain. You have the power to do something positive to improve your physical condition, without drugs, without surgery. It worked for me.

John Grey, PhD
Author of *Men Are from Mars, Women Are from Venus*,
and multiple other books

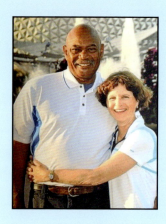

Retired Army Officer/Dedicated Golfer

For most of my life, I have been a very active person and have participated in a variety of sports. In my 20s, I was an Army paratrooper in Vietnam and survived being shot down in a helicopter. In my 30s, I was running 50-plus miles per week, but after five years, I was forced to stop running because of gradually increasing knee pain. At age 45, I began playing golf, and I was immediately hooked on the most difficult athletic activity in which I've ever been involved. During the next 20-plus years, I played hundreds of rounds of golf. Not only did I play the usual 18 holes, but I routinely played 36 holes or more in a single outing, even enjoying 54 holes on occasion—nonstop.

About two years ago, escalating chronic pain in my left knee forced me to abandon golf and most other activities that require the use of two good knees. After six months of traditional orthopedic care, my doctor informed me that, other than a knee replacement, there was nothing that could be done for my specific ailment: patellar osteoarthritis (arthritis under the kneecap). Fortunately, for me, my wife was familiar with Prolotherapy, and her osteopathic physician suggested that Dr. Alderman might be able to treat my problem without surgery, as I really did not want a knee replacement.

Now, I must admit that my first reaction to this alternative was unfavorable, because it sounded a bit like voodoo to me. But I figured, "What the hell, go check it out." Man, I am so glad I did! After three treatments of PRP Prolotherapy, I was back on the golf course. In fact, two weeks after my third treatment, my wife and I were off to Maui for a much-needed vacation. Needless to say, I played a lot of golf! During our two-week stay, I was able to play 11 rounds of golf pain free! Since then, I have been able to enjoy golf again without the constant, excruciating knee pain I endured before I knew about Prolotherapy.

Walter Thomas
Retired Army Officer/Dedicated Golfer

Registered Nurse and Mother

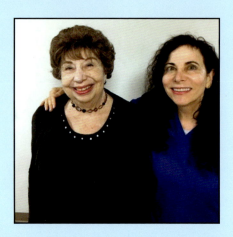

Dr. Alderman with her mother, one happy customer, after traditional Prolotherapy eliminated her knee pain 20 years ago, and then 2 years ago Platelet-Rich Plasma (PRP) Prolotherapy resolved her low back pain after a severe fall

I am Dr. Alderman's mother. I am an R.N., and grew up in an era where traditional medicine was considered the only valid approach. I love my daughter, but didn't understand her approach to medicine and considered what she did as "voodoo." However, in 1997, right before a trip to Europe, I twisted and hurt my knee, and was unable to walk without pain. Because of my medical orientation towards traditional approaches, Donna wasn't the first doctor I called. I consulted with my internist, then an orthopedist, a neurologist, and even my son, a kidney specialist. They all said my options were to limit activities, take pain medication, live with the pain—or consider surgery, which had no guarantees. Since I had a trip to Europe planned soon that would involve a lot of walking, I became desperate and asked Donna to help. I'll admit, I was skeptical, but felt I really didn't have much to lose. I received a Dextrose Prolotherapy treatment on my very painful knee. Less than two weeks later I was walking without pain. This was truly a miracle for me, and I was able to travel to Europe and enjoy myself without pain. When I returned home I received another treatment on that knee, and that was all I needed. That was over 20 years ago and that knee continues to be pain free to this day.

Years later, in 2016, still very active at the age of 87, I had a very severe fall after tripping on stairs. I was rushed to the emergency room where it was determined I had fractured my pelvis in five locations, and bedrest was ordered for eight weeks! I was transferred to a nursing home where I had nothing to do but wait and see if these fractures would heal. My doctors were telling me I would never walk again with a walker, but I decided they were wrong. I may be older, but I was determined to live the rest of my life as active as I can be. After eight boring weeks in bed, I began physical therapy and was able to eventually walk with a cane. Yet I still had annoying, lingering pain on one side of my back which didn't go away. After six months of putting up with that pain, I asked Donna to check me out. A diagnostic ultrasound revealed injury to my pelvic ligaments—not surprising considering the severity of the fall. While the bones in my pelvis had healed well, the ligaments had not. We did a Platelet-Rich Plasma Prolotherapy treatment that day, and I'm happy to report my pain went away completely. Almost two years have passed since then, and I continue to walk pain free and without a cane, and without a walker!

Bess Alderman, RN
Registered Nurse and Mother

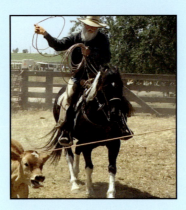

Organic Farmer

As organic farmers, we see the miracles of life every day. We see the wonder of birth and the splendor of life, from the microbes in the soil to the birds in the sky. To see and feel the miracle of your own body's ability to heal is to experience life at the fullest. Prolotherapy has given us the ability to live fully again. When my husband, Ward, was in his 50s, he had a horse accident and broke his pelvis—split it down the center. We were very grateful for the medical help we were given at Stanford University Medical Center, but after months of healing, something wasn't right. Ward still could not stand or walk. Even after exhausting referrals to all different kinds of specialists, Ward still had excruciating pain that prevented him from doing anything but lying flat in bed.

Our chiropractor recommended Prolotherapy, and Ward has received both Dextrose and PRP Prolotherapy for his low back. This has allowed him to be able to work on the farm he loves so much and also to continue to enjoy riding and roping at brandings. This summer, we took some of our grandkids on a pack trip to the Sierras. Words cannot express our gratitude to be able to enjoy and live life. We have recommended this treatment to everyone we hear of who has similar problems. Our bodies have the remarkable ability to heal, and we believe that Prolotherapy should be the first choice for people with unresolved pain.

Rose Marie and Ward Burroughs
Organic Farmers

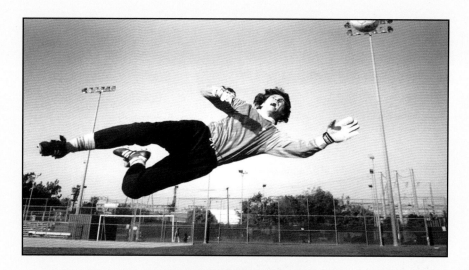

Sports Body Therapist

For five years, I had been pushing my body way too hard doing the work I love: helping athletes. I began noticing spine and joint pain while working, which made it difficult to perform my job. Eventually, I felt pain even when I wasn't working. My left knee had a torn meniscus and would often swell; I also had a hip labral tear and low back pain, which was becoming progressively more painful. I also had a feeling of instability in my neck, which compromised my sense of well-being, causing headaches and discomfort. For two years, this situation continued and was getting worse, with no end in sight.

I realized it was time to do something about my own body if I was going to be able to continue helping others. In 2016, I received Biocellular Prolotherapy to multiple joints of my body, using my own fat. Several weeks later, I received a Platelet-Rich Plasma Prolotherapy treatment. The results have been amazing! The knee that used to bother me so much now has no more swelling, no more pain! The pain in my back and pelvis, which used to bother me so much when I was working, is gone. And the hip labral pain and iliopsoas (hip tendon) pain is also gone. I used to feel weakness in the thoracic (upper-back) area and the thoracic/lumbar junction (upper- /low-back transition area), which did not allow me to sleep on my right side without pain. Now that's gone, and my sleep is so much better. My neck feels stable, and I no longer experience headaches. And the wrists and thumb areas are healed also; I no longer feel pain in these areas when working. It has been over a year since I was last seen, and I continue to feel amazing.

Thank you for giving me another chance at being pain free and for significantly extending my career working with athletes. And special thanks for your, and your team's, genuine kindness. Much love and big thanks.

Ivan Novak
Sports Body Therapist

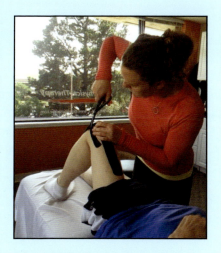

Physical Therapist

A few years ago, I injured my shoulder rotator cuff from repetitive stress while working out, doing a lot of over-head lifting and pull-ups. I treated it conservatively with physical therapy, Rolfing, and craniosacral therapy, and then tried cortisone—none of which gave me much relief. An MRI revealed rotator cuff and labral tears, as well as joint degenera-tion. I went ahead and had arthroscopic shoulder surgery, and I seemed to be recovering as expected until I developed frozen shoulder about three months after surgery. For ten months, I worked very hard to get through the frozen shoulder, and I was able to recover about 80 percent of my range of motion, but I was still struggling with pain and limited function. I couldn't sleep, put on a shirt, or reach for my seatbelt without pain—not to mention being unable to work out. At this time, I consult-ed with Dr. Alderman. She was extremely thorough, and her extensive knowledge about, and experience with, the various forms of Prolotherapy was evident. As a physical therapist, I have been very familiar with these regenerative procedures since 2003; I also have a good friend who was one of the first doctors in the country performing these procedures, so I felt comfortable going in this direction.

Based on my clinical evaluation, MRI, diagnostic ultrasound, and past medical history, Dr. Alderman recommended that I start with PRP to see how I respond. I received a PRP treatment (this was one year after the arthroscopic surgery) and soon after experienced about 20 percent reduction in pain and increased function. She also did osteopathic techniques to help release the frozen shoulder. Two months later, I had a second round of PRP. Since that produced very little further improvement, on my third visit, we decided to proceed with Biocellular (Stem Cell–Rich) Prolotherapy using adipose. A few weeks later, I started seeing reduced pain and increased range of motion. With continued bodywork and some simple manual resistance exercises, I continued to see progress week after week, month after month. Now, seven months after the Biocellular procedure, I am thrilled to report that I am 98 percent better, and I expect to reach 100 percent in the very near future. I can sleep through the night on my affected shoulder; I can put on my seatbelt and jacket without pain; I can swim, work all day, and even work out now without problem. I couldn't be happier, and I highly recommend this course of treatment.

Jill McCormick
Physical Therapist

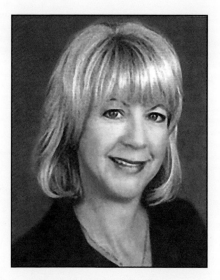

Former Court Reporter

I was a court reporter for 22 years, and experienced repetitive trauma to both my elbows. Finally, I was diagnosed with chronic epicondylitis and tendonitis. I tried NSAIDs, braces, cortisone; however, my elbows continued to hurt 24/7. I experienced a constant penetrating ache and my elbows felt bruised or like they had been slammed with a hammer.

After Prolotherapy, I have regained the use of my elbows and have more endurance. I no longer have burning and tightness in my forearms and the constant pain I had before. Two years after finishing my Prolotherapy treatments, I am still 95 percent improved. I am able to live life now without chronic pain. I recommend this treatment highly.

Brenda Falvi
Former Court Reporter

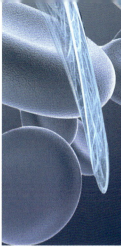

Bibliography of Medical Studies, Research Articles, and Books, Prolotherapy Regenerative Medicine

Facts are stubborn things; and whatever may be our wishes, our inclinations, or the dictates of our passions, they cannot alter the state of facts and evidence.

—John Adams, 2nd President of the United States

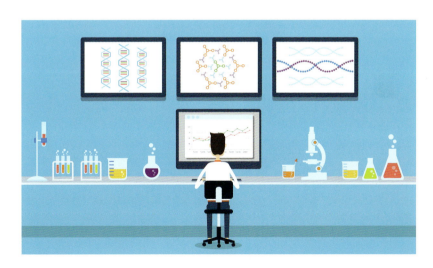

Traditional Dextrose Prolotherapy

Ahmet M, Yavuz F. Treatment of a medial collateral ligament sprain using prolotherapy: a case study. *Alternative Therapies in Health and Medicine*. 2015; 21(4): 68–71.

Ahn KH, Kim HS, Lee WK, Kim HW, Yun DH, Kim DH. The effect of prolotherapy on the injured Achilles tendon in a rat model. *Journal of Korean Academy of Rehabilitation Medicine*. 2002; 26(3): 332–336.

Alderman DD. State of the art: prolotherapy regenerative medicine. *Pain Week Journal*. 2016; 4(Q4): 44–52.

Alderman DD. Regenerative injection therapies for pain: traditional, platelet-rich plasma and biocellular prolotherapy. In *Integrative Pain Management*, eds. Bonakdar A, Sukiennik A (pp. 345–360). New York, New York: Oxford University Press; 2016.

Alderman DD. The new age of prolotherapy, *Practical Pain Management*. 2010; 10 (May): 54–68.

Alderman DD. A history of the American Osteopathic College of Schlerotherapeutic pain management, the oldest prolotherapy organization. *Journal of Prolotherapy*. 2009; 1(4): 200–204.

Alderman DD. *Free Yourself from Chronic Pain: How Prolotherapy Can Help You Become Pain Free*. Glendale, California: Family Doctor Press; 2008.

Alderman DD. Prolotherapy for golfing injuries and pain. *Practical Pain Management*. 2008; 8(5): 56–64.

Alderman DD. Prolotherapy for musculoskeletal pain. *Practical Pain Management*. 2007; 7(1): 10–15.

Alderman DD. Prolotherapy for low back pain. *Practical Pain Management*. 2007; 7(4): 58–63.

Alfredson H, Ohberg L. Sclerosing injections to areas of neovascularization reduce pain in chronic Achilles tendinopathy: a double-blind randomized trial. *Knee Surgery, Sports Traumatology, Arthroscopy*. 2005; 13(4): 338–344.

Aloi A. Is regenerative injection therapy (prolotherapy) effective at reducing pain associated with knee osteoarthritis? PA Studies Student dissertation, Philadelphia College of Osteopathic

Medicine, 2015 [cited 2017 April 2] https://digitalcommons.pcom. edu/cgi/viewcontent.cgi?referer=&httpsredir=1&article=1202&-context=pa_systematic_reviews.

Banks A. A rationale for prolotherapy. *Journal of Orthopaedic Medicine.* 1991; 13(3): 54–59.

Banner R, Batson GM, Werstine R, Smith F. The resolution of grade I lumbar retrolisthesis with prolotherapy: a case study. *Journal of Prolotherapy.* 2010; 2(2): 352–355.

Bertrand H, Reeves KD, Bennett CJ, Bicknell S, Cheng A. Dextrose prolotherapy versus control injections in painful rotator cuff tendinopathy. *Archives of Physical Medicine and Rehabilitation.* 2016; 97(1): 17–25.

Brody JE. Injections to kickstart tissue repair. *New York Times.* 2007 Aug 7: D8.

Bronston GJ. The strengthening of chronically strained ankle ligaments with injections of sodium psylliate. *Journal of American Podiatric Medical Association.* 1958; 48(11): 511–516.

Bronston GJ. Injection therapy for ligamentous strain. *Journal of the National Association of Chiropodists Journal.* 1957; 42(12): 614–615.

Bowne K, Ross M.D.. Physical therapy combined with prolotherapy in a recreationally active middle-aged man with knee pain and chondromalacia patella. *Journal of Orthopaedic & Sports Physical.* 2017 Jan 1; 47(1): A68-9.

Centeno CJ, Elliot J, Elkins WL, Freeman M. Fluoroscopically guided cervical prolotherapy for instability with blinded pre and post radiographic reading. *Pain Physician.* 2005; 8(1): 67–72.

Cezairli B, Sivrikaya EC, Omezli MM, Ayranci F, Seyhan Cezairli N. Results of combined, single-session arthrocentesis and dextrose prolotherapy for symptomatic temporomandibular joint syndrome: A case series. *The Journal of Alternative and Complementary Medicine.* 2017 Oct 1; 23(10): 771–777.

Chan O, Havard B, Morton S, Pritchard M, Maffulli N, Crisp T, Padhiar, N, Perry, JD, King, J, Morrissey, D. Outcomes of prolotherapy for intra-tendinous Achilles tears: a case series. *Muscles, Ligaments and Tendons Journals.* 2017; 7(1): 78–87.

Chase RH. Basic sclerotherapy. *Osteopathic Annals.* 1978; 6(12): 16–20.

Chen H, Yuan A. Prolotherapy treatment for Dequervain's teno-synovitis and intersection syndrome. *Journal of Pain*. 2015; 15(4): S113.

Chiou HJ. Ultrasound Guided Prolotherapy. *Ultrasound in Medicine and Biology*. 2017 Jan 1; 43: S242.

Clark G. Building a rational for evidence-based prolotherapy in orthopedic medicine practice: part III: a case series report for chronic back pain associated with sacroiliac joint dysfunction treated by prolotherapy—a six-year prospective analysis. *Journal of Prolotherapy*. 2011; 3(2): 644–671.

Clayton MI, Weir GJ. Experimental investigations of ligamentous healing. *American Journal of Surgery*. 1950; 98(3): 373–378.

Clinkscales C. Alternative treatments for tennis elbow: acupuncture, prolotherapy, and shock wave lithotripsy. In *Tennis Elbow: Clinical Management*, ed. Wolf JM (pp. 85–92). New York, New York: Springer US; 2015.

Conaway E, Browning B. Neural prolotherapy for neuralgia. *Journal of Prolotherapy*. 2014; 6: e928–e931.

Conti GV. The unstable low back: causes and treatment. *Osteopathic Annals*. 1978; 6(12): 36–41.

Covey CJ. Prolotherapy: can it help your patient? *Journal of Family Practice*. 2015; 64(12): 763–769.

Curtin M, Crisp T, Malliaras P, Padhiar N. The effectiveness of prolotherapy in the management of recalcitrant medial tibial stress syndrome: a pilot study. *British Journal of Sports Medicine*. 2011; 45(2): e1

Cusi M, Saunders J, Hungerford B, Wisbey-Roth T, Lucas P, Wilson S. The use of prolotherapy in the sacroiliac joint. *British Journal of Sports Medicine*. 2010; 44(2): 100–104.

Cyriax J, Russel G. *Textbook of Orthopaedic Medicine: Vol. 2. Treatment by Manipulation, Massage and Injection*. Baltimore, Maryland: Williams & Wilkins; 1977.

Dagenais S, Mayer J, Haldeman S, Borg-Stein J. Evidence-informed management of chronic low back pain with prolotherapy. *Spine Journal*. 2008; 8(1): 203–212.

Dagenais S, Haldeman S, Wooley JR. Intra-ligamentous injection of sclerosing solutions (prolotherapy) for spinal pain: a critical review of the literature. *Spine Journal*. 2005; 5(3): 310–328.

Darrow M. *Prolotherapy: The Hollywood Pain Solution*. Los Angeles, California: Protex Press; 2003.

Darrow M. *The Collagen Revolution: Living Pain Free*. Los Angeles, California: Protex Press; 2002.

DeChellis M.D., Cortazzo MH. Regenerative medicine in the field of pain medicine: prolotherapy, platelet-rich plasma therapy, and stem cell therapy—theory and evidence. *Techniques in Regional Anesthesia and Pain Management*. 2011; 15(2): 74–80.

Dechow E, Davies RK, Carr AJ, Thompson PW. A randomized, double-blind, placebo-controlled trial of sclerosing injections in patients with chronic low back pain. *Rheumatology*. 1999; 38(12): 1255–1259.

Dorman TA. Pelvic mechanics and prolotherapy. *Townsend Letter for Doctors and Patients*. 2001; 215: 90–93.

Dorman, TA. Introducing prolotherapy and orthopedic medicine. *Fact, Fiction & Fraud in Modern Medicine*. 1996; 1(5).

Dorman TA. Back pain, a misunderstood, often misdiagnosed 20th century scourge. *Fact, Fiction & Fraud in Modern Medicine*. 1996; 1(4).

Dorman TA. *Prolotherapy in the Lumbar Spine and Pelvis*. Philadelphia, Pennsylvania: Hanley & Belfus; 1995.

Dorman TA, Cohen RE, Dasig D, Jeng S, Discher N, de Jong A. Energy efficiency during human walking: before and after prolotherapy. *Journal of Orthopedic Medicine*. 1994; 15(3): 64–67.

Dorman TA Prolotherapy: a survey. *Journal of Orthopedic Medicine*. 1993; 15(2): 49–50.

Dorman TA. Treatment for spine pain arising in ligaments using prolotherapy: a retrospective study. *Journal of Orthopedic Medicine*. 1991; 13(1): 13–19.

Dorman TA, Ravin T. *Diagnosis and Injection Techniques in Orthopedic Medicine*. Philadelphia, Pennsylvania: Williams & Wilkins; 1991.

Dumais R, Benoit C, Dumais A, Babin L, Bordage R, de Arcos C, Bélanger M. Effect of regenerative injection therapy on function and pain in patients with knee osteoarthritis: a randomized crossover study. *Pain Medicine.* 2012; 13(8): 990–999.

Ekinci S, Tatar O, Akpancar S, Turgut H, Seven MM. A new treatment option in osteoarthritis: prolotherapy injections. *Journal of Orthopedic Research.* 2016; 26: 816–823.

Eslamian F, Amouzandeh B. Therapeutic effects of prolotherapy with intra-articular dextrose injection in patients with moderate knee osteoarthritis: a single-arm study with 6 months follow up. *Therapeutic Advances in Musculoskeletal Disease.* 2015; 7(2): 35–44.

Faber WJ. Biological reconstruction: solution for refractory head and neck pain. *Journal of Neuro Orthopedic Med Surgery.* 1991; 12: 6–11.

Faber WJ. Non-surgical tendon, ligament and joint reconstruction. *Townsend Letter for Doctors.* 1993; 118: 428.

Faber WJ, Walker M. *Pain, Pain Go Away.* Mountain View, California: ISHI Press International; 1990.

Faber WJ, Walker M. *Instant pain relief.* Milwaukee, Wisconsin: Biological Publications; 1991.

Frost Jr. WW. Case study: sacro-iliac problems and the benefit of prolotherapy over time. *Journal of Orthopaedic Medicine.* 1994; 16(3) [cited 2015 July 1].

http://www.rejuvmedical.com/pages/Orthopedic-Research.

Fullerton BD. Prolotherapy for the Thoracolumbar Myofascial System. *Physical Medicine and Rehabilitation Clinics.* 2018 Feb 1; 29(1): 125–138.

Fullerton BD. High-resolution ultrasound and magnetic resonance imaging to document tissue repair after prolotherapy: a report of 3 cases. *Archives of Physical Medicine and Rehabilitation.* 2008; 89(2): 377–385.

Fullerton BD, Reeves KD. Ultrasonography in regenerative injection (prolotherapy) using dextrose, platelet-rich plasma, and other injectants. *Physical Medicine and Rehabilitation Clinics of North America.* 2010; 21(3): 585–605.

Gedney EH. The application of sclerotherapy in spondylolisthesis and spondylolysis. *The Osteopathic Profession.* 1954b September; 66–69, 102–105.

Gedney EH. Progress report on use of sclerosing solutions in low back syndromes. *The Osteopathic Profession.* 1954 August; 21(11): 18–21, 40–44.

Gedney EH. Technic for sclerotherapy in the management of hypermobile sacroiliac. *The Osteopathic Profession.* 1952 August; 19(11); 16–19, 37–38.

Gedney EH. Sclerosing solution may change therapy in vertebral disk problem. *The Osteopathic Profession.* 1952 April; 19(7); 11–13, 34, 36, 38, 40–41.

Gedney EH. Disc syndrome. *The Osteopathic Profession.* 1951 September; 18(12): 11–15, 38, 40, 44,46.

Gedney EH. The hypermobile joint—Further reports on injection method. Paper presented at *Osteopathic Clinical Society of Pennsylvania*, February 13, 1938.

Gedney EH. Special Technic: hypermobile joint: a preliminary report. *Osteopathic Profession.* 1937; 4(9): 30–31.

George J. Chn'g LS, Jaafar Z, Hamid MSA. Comparative effectiveness of ultrasound guided intratendinous prolotherapy injection with conventional treatment to treat focal supraspinatus tendinosis: randomised control study. In *ISI Conference Proceedings 13th Asian Federation of Sports Medicine Congress*, 2014 [cited 2017 March 8] https://umexpert.um.edu.my/file/publication/00000816_99538.pdf.

Ghasemi M, Behnaz F, Sajjadi MM, Zandi R, Hashemi M. The effect of Hypertonic Dextrose injection on the control of pain associated with knee osteoarthritis. *Middle East Journal of Family Medicine.* 2017 Oct; 15(8): 193–200.

Gracer R. A study suggesting an algorithm describing the place of proliferative therapy in the treatment of ligamentous pain. Paper presented at the Institute of Orthopaedic Medicine, Schonreid, Switzerland; 1987. *Journal of Orthopaedic Medicine*; 1988.

Gordin K, Hauser R. The case for utilizing prolotherapy as a promising stand-alone or adjunctive treatment for over-manipulation syndrome. *Journal of Applied Research*. 2013; 13(1): 1–28.

Gordin K. Case for prolotherapy. *Patients*. 2011; 3(2): 601–609.

Gordin K. A publication for regenerative medicine techniques. *Journal of Prolotherapy*. 2011; 3(4): 813–825.

Gross L. An innovative solution for aching joints? *Muscle and Fitness*. 2002: 92–98.

Grote W, Delucia R, Waxman R, Zgierska A, Wilson J, Rabago D. Repair of a complete anterior cruciate tear using prolotherapy: a case report. *International Musculoskeletal Medicine* 2009; 31(4): 159–165.

Hackett GS, Hemwall GA, Montgomery GA. *Ligament and Tendon Relaxation Treated by Prolotherapy*, ed. Thomas CC. Springfield, Illinois: 5th Edition Institute in Basic Life Principles; 1991.

Hackett GS. Prolotherapy for headache. *Headache*. 1962; 2(2): 20–28.

Hackett GS. Huang TC, Raftery A. Prolotherapy for headache, pain in the head and neck and neuritis. *Headache*. 1962; 2(1): 20–28.

Hackett GS, Huang TC. Prolotherapy for sciatica from weak pelvic ligaments and bone dystrophy. *Clinical Medicine*. 1961; 8(12): 2301–2316.

Hackett GS. Back pain following trauma and disease— prolotherapy. *Military Medicine*. 1961; 126: 517–525.

Hackett GS. Prolotherapy in whiplash and low back pain. *Postgraduate Medical Journal*. 1960; 27(2): 214–219.

Hackett GS. Low back pain. *British Journal of Physical Medicine*. 1956; 19(2): 25–35.

Hackett GS. Joint stabilization: an experimental, histologic study with comments on the clinical application in ligament proliferation. *American Journal of Surgery*. 1955; 89(5): 968–973.

Hackett GS. Henderson DG. Joint stabilization. *American Journal of Surgery*. 1955; 89(5): 968–973.

Hackett GS. Shearing injury to the sacroiliac joint. *Journal of the International College of Surgeons*. 1954; 22(6): 631–642.

Hakala R, Ledermann KM. The use of prolotherapy for temporomandibular joint dysfunction. *Journal of Prolotherapy.* 2010; 2(3): 439–446.

Hassan F, Trebinjac S, Murrell WD, Maffullii N. The effectiveness of prolotherapy in treating knee osteoarthritis in adults: a systematic review. *British Medical Bulletin.* 2017; 122(1): 91–108.

Hauser RA, Lackner JB, Steilen-Matias D, Harris DK. A systematic review of dextrose prolotherapy for chronic musculoskeletal pain. *Clinical Medicine Insights. Arthritis and Musculoskeletal Disorders.* 2016; 9: 139–159.

Hauser RA, Steilen D, Gordin K. The biology of prolotherapy and its application in clinical cervical spine instability and chronic neck pain: a retrospective study. *European Journal of Preventive Medicine.* 2015; 3(4): 85–102.

Hauser RA, Steilen DR, Fisher P. Upper cervical instability of traumatic origin treated with dextrose prolotherapy: a caser report. *Journal of Prolotherapy.* 2015; 7: e932–e935.

Hauser RA, Steilen DR, Schaefer Sprague I. Cervical instability as a cause of Barré-Liéou syndrome and definitive treatment with prolotherapy: a case series. *European Journal of Preventive Medicine,* 2015 Sept; 3(5): 155-166.

Hauser RA, Schaefer Sprague I. Outcomes of prolotherapy in chondromalacia patella patients: improvements in pain level and function. *Clinical Medicine Insights. Arthritis and Musculoskeletal Disorders.* 2014; 7: 13–20.

Hauser RA, Woldin B. Treating osteoarthritic joints using dextrose prolotherapy and direct bone marrow aspirate injection therapy. *Open Arthritis Journal.* 2014; 7(1): 1–9.

Hauser RA, Blakemore PJ, Wang J, Steilen D. Structural basis of joint instability as cause for chronic musculoskeletal pain and its successful treatment with regenerative injection therapy (prolotherapy). *Open Pain Journal.* 2014; 7(1): 9–22.

Hauser RA, Dolan E, Orlofsky A. Prolotherapy: a non-invasive approach to lesions of the glenoid labrum: a non-controlled questionnaire based study. *Open Rehabilitation Journal.* 2013; 6(1): 69–76.

Hauser RA, Feister WA. Treatment of basal thumb osteoarthritis: a retrospective study of dextrose prolotherapy injections as an alternative treatment. *Journal of Prolotherapy.* 2013; 5: e913–e921.

Hauser RA, Orlofsky A. Regenerative injection therapy (prolotherapy) for hip labrum lesions: rationale and retrospective. *Open Rehabilitation Journal.* 2013; 6(1): 59–68.

Hauser RA, Ostergaard S, Santilli S. Stabilization of rheumatoid thumb interphalangeal boutonniere deformity and severe subluxation with splinting and prolotherapy: a case report. *Journal of Prolotherapy.* 2012; 4: e849–e854.

Hauser RA, Feister WA. Dextrose prolotherapy with human growth hormone to treat chronic first metatarsophalangeal joint pain. *Foot and Ankle Online Journal.* 2012; 5(9): 1–9.

Hauser RA, Feister WA, Brinker DK. Dextrose prolotherapy treatment for unresolved "Morton's Neuroma" pain. *Foot and Ankle Online Journal.* 2012 June; 5(6): 1.

Hauser RA, Ostergaard S. Direct bone marrow injections for avascular necrosis of the talus: a case report. *Journal of Prolotherapy.* 2012; 4: e891–e894.

Hauser RA, Hauser MA, Baird NM. Evidence-based use of dextrose prolotherapy for musculoskeletal pain: a scientific literature review. *Journal of Prolotherapy.* 2011; 3(4): 765–789.

Hauser RA, Dolan EE. Ligament injury and healing: an overview of current clinical concepts. *Journal of Prolotherapy.* 2011; 3(4): 836–846.

Hauser RA. Prolotherapy as an alternative treatment for osteochondritis dissecans: two cases of young baseball players. *Journal of Prolotherapy.* 2011; 3(1): 568–571.

Hauser RA, Hauser MA, Cukla J. A retrospective observational study on Hackett-Hemwall dextrose prolotherapy for unresolved foot and toe pain at an outpatient charity clinic in rural Illinois. *Journal of Prolotherapy.* 2011; 3: 543–551.

Hauser RA, Maddela HS, Alderman DD, Baehnisch G, Banner R, Blakemore PJ, Calderón JE, Clark GB, DeLaurntis M, Fauley S, Funck J, Gladstein B, Johnson ML, Kramer GH, Neustadt J, Resk J, Salazar JH, Swetlikoff G, Van Pelt RS, Wheaton MT. Journal of Prolotherapy international medical editorial board consensus statement on the use of prolotherapy for musculoskeletal pain. *Journal of Prolotherapy.* 2011; 3(4): 744–764.

Hauser RA. Treatment of joint hypermobility syndrome, including Ehlers-Danlos syndrome with Hackett-Hemwall prolotherapy. *Journal of Prolotherapy.* 2011; 3(2): 612–629.

Hauser RA, Baird NM, Cukla JJ. A retrospective observational study on Hackett-Hemwall dextrose prolotherapy for unresolved hand and finger pain at an outpatient charity clinic in rural Illinois. *Journal of Prolotherapy.* 2010; 2(4): 480–486.

Hauser RA, Hauser M, Cukla JJ. Dextrose Prolotherapy injections for chronic ankle pain. *Practical Pain Management.* 2010; 10(1): 70–76.

Hauser RA. The acceleration of articular cartilage degeneration in osteoarthritis by nonsteroidal anti-inflammatory drugs. *Journal of Prolotherapy.* 2010; 2(1): 305–322.

Hauser RA, Hauser M, Baird NM, Martin D. Prolotherapy as an alternative to surgery: a prospective pilot study of 34 patients from a private medical practice. *Journal of Prolotherapy.* 2010; 2(1): 272–281.

Hauser RA, Phillips HJ, Maddela HS. The case for utilizing prolotherapy as first-line treatment for meniscal pathology: a retrospective study shows prolotherapy is effective in the treatment of MRI-documented meniscal tears and degeneration. *Journal of Prolotherapy.* 2010; 2(3): 416–437.

Hauser RA, Hauser M, Cukla JJ. Dextrose prolotherapy injections for chronic ankle pain. *Practical Pain Management.* 2010; 10(1): 70–76.

Hauser RA, Philips HJ. The case for utilizing prolotherapy as first-line treatment for meniscal pathology. *Journal of Prolotherapy.* 2010; 2(3): 416–437.

Hauser RA, Greun KA. The use of prolotherapy in the treatment of chronic overuse shoulder and neck pain, neurogenic pain, and hip degeneration in an incomplete C-4-C-5 spinal cord injury patient. *Journal of Prolotherapy.* 2009; 1(3): 166–171.

Hauser RA. It isn't about pain management, it is about pain resolution. *Journal of Prolotherapy.* 2009; 1(4): 197–199.

Hauser RA. The regeneration of articular cartilage with prolotherapy. *Journal of Prolotherapy.* 2009; 1(1): 39–44.

Hauser RA. The deterioration of articular cartilage in osteoarthritis by corticosteroid injections. *Journal of Prolotherapy.* 2009; 1(2): 107–123.

Hauser RA, Batson GM, Ferrigno C. Non-operative treatment of cervical radiculopathy: a three part article from the approach of a physiatrist, chiropractor, and physical therapists. *Journal of Prolotherapy.* 2009; 1(4): 217–231.

Hauser RA, Cukla JJ. Standard clinical x-ray studies document cartilage regeneration in five degenerated knees after prolotherapy. *Journal of Prolo*therapy. 2009; 1(1): 22–28.

Hauser RA, Greun KA. The use of prolotherapy in the treatment of chronic overuse shoulder and neck pain, neurogenic pain and hip degeneration in incomplete C4–C5 spinal cord injury patient. *Journal of Prolotherapy.* 2009; 1(3): 166–171.

Hauser RA, Hauser MA. A retrospective study on Hackett-Hemwall dextrose prolotherapy for chronic hip pain at an outpatient charity clinic in rural Illinois. *Journal of Prolotherapy.* 2009; 1(2): 76–88.

Hauser RA, Hauser MA. A retrospective study on dextrose prolotherapy for unresolved knee pain. *Journal of Prolotherapy.* 2009; 1(1): 11–21.

Hauser RA, Hauser MA. Dextrose prolotherapy for unresolved low back pain. *Journal of Prolotherapy.* 2009; 1(3): 145–155.

Hauser RA, Hauser M, Holian P. Dextrose prolotherapy for unresolved wrist pain. *Practical Pain Management.* 2009; 9(9): 72–89.

Hauser RA, Hauser M, Holian P. Hackett-Hemwall dextrose prolotherapy for unresolved elbow pain. *Practical Pain Management.* 2009; 9(8): 14–26.

Hauser RA, McCullough H. Dextrose prolotherapy for recurring headache and migraine pain. *Practical Pain Management.* 2009; 9(5): 58–65.

Hauser RA, Hauser M. A retrospective study on Hackett-Hemwall dextrose prolotherapy for chronic shoulder pain at an outpatient charity clinic in rural Illinois. *Journal of Prolotherapy.* 2009: 1(4): 205–216.

Hauser RA, Hauser M. Dextrose prolotherapy for unresolved neck pain. *Practical Pain Management.* 2007; 7(8): 56–60.

Hauser RA, Hauser M, Blakemore K. Dextrose prolotherapy for TMJ dysfunction. *Practical Pain Management.* 2007; 7(9): 49–57.

Hauser RA, Hauser M. *Prolotherapy: An Alternative to Knee Surgery.* Oak Park, Illinois: Beulah Land Press; 2004.

Hauser RA, Hauser M. *Prolo Your Sports Injuries Away!* Oak Park, Illinois: Beulah Land Press; 2001.

Hauser RA, Punishing the pain. Treating chronic pain with pro-lotherapy. *Rehab Management.* 1999; 12(2): 26–28, 30.

Hauser RA, Hauser M. *Prolo Your Pain Away!* Oak Park, Illinois: Beulah Land Press; 1998.

Hauser RA, Hauser M, Pottinger K. *Prolo Your Fibromyalgia Pain Away!: Curing Chronic Pain with Prolotherapy.* Oak Park, Illinois: Beulah Land Press; 1998.

Hemwall G. Barré-Liéou syndrome. *Journal of Orthopaedic Medicine.* 2007; 29(3): 95–97.

Hooper RA, Ding M. Retrospective case series on patients with chronic spinal pain treated with dextrose prolotherapy. *Journal of Alternative and Complementary Medicine.* 2004; 10(4): 670–674.

Hooper RA. Frizzell JB, Faris P. Case series on chronic whiplash related neck pain treated with intraarticular zygapophysial joint regeneration injection therapy. *Pain Physician Journal.* 2007; 10(2): 313–318.

Howes RG, Isdale IC. The loose back: an unrecognized syndrome. *Rheumatology and Physical Medicine.* 1971; 11(2): 72–77.

Hung CY, Hsiao MY, Chang KV, Han DS, Wang TG. Comparative effectiveness of dextrose prolotherapy versus control injections and exercise in the management of osteoarthritis pain: a systematic review and meta-analysis. *Journal of Pain Research.* 2016; 9: 847–857.

Hung CY, Chang KV, Özçakar L. Snapping hip due to gluteus medius tendinopathy: ultrasound imaging in the diagnosis and guidance for prolotherapy. *Pain Medicine*. 2015; 16(10): 2040–2041.

Inklebarger J, Petrides S. Prolotherapy for lumbar segmental instability associated with degenerative disc disease. *Journal of Prolotherapy*. 2016; 8: e971–e977.

Itkin A. Treatment of trigeminal neuralgia utilizing neural prolotherapy: a case report. *Journal of Prolotherapy*. 2016; 8: e961–e965.

Jacks A, Edgeworth A. A retrospective audit of patients with osteo-arthritic knees treated with prolotherapy in a general practice. *International Musculoskeletal Medicine*. 2008; 30(2): 61–66.

Jahangiri A, Moghaddam FR, Najafi S. Hypertonic dextrose versus corticosteroid local injection for the treatment of osteoarthritis in the first carpometacarpal joint: a double-blind randomized clinical trial. *Journal of Orthopaedic Science*. 2014; 19(5): 737–743.

Jain S, Rajesh J, Arora KK. Prolotherapy for early osteoarthritis knee. *International Journal of Medical Research and Review*. 2014; 2(4): 279–282.

Jeelani S, Krishna S, Reddy J, Reddy V. Prolotherapy in temporomandibular disorders: an overview. *Open Journal of Dentistry and Oral Medicine*. 2013; 1(2): 15–18.

Jensen K. *Dissertation: Healing Response of Knee Ligaments to Prolotherapy in a Rat Model*. Madison, Wisconsin: Biomedical Engineering, University of Wisconsin; 2006.

Jensen KT, Rabago DP, Best TM, Patterson JJ, Vanderby R. Early inflammatory response of knee ligaments to prolotherapy in a rat model. *Journal of Orthopaedic Research*. 2008; 26(6): 816–823.

Jensen KT, Rabago DP, Best TM, Patterson JJ, Vanderby Jr. R. Response of knee ligaments to prolotherapy in a rat injury model. *American Journal of Sports Medicine*. 2008; 36(7): 1347–1357.

Jo CH, Lee YG, Shin WH, Kim H, Chai JW, Jeong EC, Kim JE, Shim H, Shin JS, Shin IS, Ra JC, Oh S, Yoon KS. Intra-articular injection of mesenchymal stem cells for the treatment of osteoarthritis of the knee: a proof-of-concept clinical trial. *Stem Cell*. 2014; 32(5): 1254–1266.

Jo D, Kim M. Effects of prolotherapy on knee joint pain due to ligament laxity. *Journal of Korean Pain Society*. 2004; 17(1): 47–50.

Jo D, Ryu K, Yang S, Kim M. The effects of prolotherapy on shoulder pain. *Korean Journal of Anesthesiology*. 2004; 46(5): 589–592.

Jo D, Yang SJ, Lee SW, Kim MH. The effects of prolotherapy on the lumbar herniated nucleus pulposus. *Journal of Korean Pain Society*. 2003; 16(1): 68–72.

Johnson ML. Prolotherapy and connective tissue damage syndrome. *Journal of Prolotherapy*. 2009; 1(1): 45–53.

Jonely H, Brismée J, Desai MJ, Reoli R. Chronic sacroiliac joint and pelvic girdle dysfunction in a 35-year-old nulliparous woman successfully managed with multimodal and multidisciplinary approach. *Journal of Manual & Manipulative Therapy*. 2015; 23(1): 20–26.

Jones K. Irritation to make the pain go away: prolotherapy for knee osteoarthritis. *Evidence-Based Practice*. 2014: 17(9): 5.

Kang SH, Seo KM, Kim DK, Shin JY, Song IS. Ultrasonographic findings of chronic lateral epicondylitis with partial tear before and after prolotherapy. *Journal of Korean Academy of Rehabilitation Medicine*. 2004; 28(1): 88–93.

Karam C, Ibrahim V, Pohlman D, Saini V, Parag S. Poster 160 prolotherapy in Charcot-Marie-Tooth disease to relieve pain and stabilize the lateral ankle ligaments: a case report. *PM&R Journal*. 2012; 4(10): S245.

Kayfetz D.O.. Occipito-cervical (whiplash) injuries treated by prolotherapy. *Medical Trial Technique Quarterly*. 1963; 9: 9–29.

Kayfetz D.O., Blumenthal LS, Hackett GS, Hemwall GA, Neff FE. Whiplash injury and other ligamentous headache—its management with prolotherapy. *Headache*. 1963; 3(1): 21–28.

Kesikburun S, Yasar E, Aras B, Kelle B, Yilmaz B. The effect of prolotherapy on hemiplegic shoulder pain due to rotator cuff tendinopathy: a pilot study. *Cukurova Medical Journal*. 2017; 42(1): 13–18.

Kim BK, Shin JY, Seo KM. The effect of prolotherapy for the chronic pain of musculoskeletal system. *Journal of Korean Academy of Rehabilitation Medicine*. 2001; 25(1): 128–133.

Khan SA, Kumar A, Varshney MK, Trikha V, Yadav CS. Dextrose prolotherapy for recalcitrant coccygodynia. *Journal of Orthopaedic Surgery-Hong Kong.* 2008; 16(1): 27–29.

Kidd RF. Indications for low back prolotherapy. *Australasian Musculoskeletal Medicine.* 2005 May; 10(1): 20.

Kidd RF. Treatment of Osgood-Schlatter disease by prolotherapy: a case report. *Journal of Orthopaedic Medicine.* 1993; 15(3): 62–63.

Kiliç SC, Güngörmüş M. Is dextrose prolotherapy superior to placebo for the treatment of temporomandibular joint hypermobility? A randomized clinical trial. *International Journal of Oral and Maxillofacial Surgery.* 2016; 45(7): 813–819.

Kim WJ, Shin HY, Koo GH, Park HG, Ha YC, Park YH. Ultrasound-guided prolotherapy with polydeoxyribonucleotide sodium in ischiofemoral impingement syndrome. *Pain Practice.* 2014; 14(7): 649–655.

Kim E, Lee JH. Autologous platelet-rich plasma versus dextrose prolotherapy for the treatment of chronic recalcitrant plantar fasciitis. *PM&R Journal.* 2014; 6(2): 152–158.

Kim HS, Jung KH, Park IH, Ryu JK, Sun KJ, Lim KJ, Jo DH. Diagnosis and treatment of sacral asymlocation in back pain patients: clinical application of prolotherapy. *Korean Journal of Pain.* 2007; 20(2): 130–137.

Kim HS, Ahn KH, Lee JH, Lee KT, Yoon JS. Comparison between the effect of local steroid injection and prolotherapy on iliac crest pain syndrome. *Journal of Korean Academy of Rehabilitation Medicine.* 2007; 31(1): 20–24.

Kim JM. The effect of prolotherapy for osteoarthritis of the knee. *Journal of Korean Academy of Rehabilitation Medicine.* 2002; 26(4): 445–448.

Kim SA, Kim EH, Kim SY. The effects of hyperosmolar dextrose and autologous serum injection in the experimental articular defect of rabbit. *Archives of Physical Medicine and Rehabilitation.* 2006; 30(2): 173–178.

Kim SR, Stitik TP, Foye PM, Greenwald BD, Campagnolo DI. Critical review of prolotherapy for osteoarthritis, low back pain, and other musculoskeletal conditions: a physiatric perspective. *American Journal of Physical Medicine & Rehabilitation*. 2004; 83(5): 379–389.

Kim W, Lee HG, Jeong CW, Kim CM, Yoon MH. A randomized controlled trial of intra-articular prolotherapy versus steroid injection for sacroiliac joint pain. *Journal of Alternative and Complementary Medicine*. 2010; 16(12): 1285–1290.

Kim SH, Jeon YH, Park JW. Effects of prolotherapy on chronic musculoskeletal disease. *The Korean Pain Society*. 2002; 15(2): 121–125.

Kim BK, Shin JY, Seo KM. The effect of prolotherapy for the chronic pain of musculoskeletal system. *Journal of Korean Academy of Rehabilitation Medicine*. 2001; 25(1): 128–133.

Kim SR, Stitik TP, Foye PM, Greenwald BD, Campagnolo DI. Critical review of prolotherapy for osteoarthritis, low back pain, and other musculoskeletal conditions: a physiatric perspective. *American Journal of Physical Medicine & Rehabilitation*. 2004; 83(5): 379–389.

Kiter E, Celikbas E, Akkaya S, Demirkan F, Kilic BA. Comparison of injection modalities in the treatment of plantar heel pain: a randomized controlled trial. *Journal of the American Podiatric Medical Association*. 2006; 96(4): 293–296.

Klein RG, Dorman TA, Johnson CE. Proliferant injections for low back pain: histologic changes of injected ligaments and objective measurements of lumbar spine mobility before and after treatment. *Journal of Neuro Orthopedic Med Surgery*. 1989; 10(2): 123–126.

Klein RG, Eek BC, Delong WB, Mooney V. A randomized double-blind trial of dextrose-glycerine-phenol injections for chronic, low back pain. *Journal of Spinal Disorders & Techniques*. 1993; 6(1): 23–33.

Klein RG, Eek BC, O'Neill CW, Elin C, Mooney V, Derby RR. Biochemical injection treatment for discogenic low back pain: a pilot study. *Spine Journal*. 2003; 3(3): 220–226.

Koudele CJ. Treatment of joint pain. *Osteopathic Annals*. 1978; 6(12): 42–45.

Krstičević M, Jerić M, Došenović S, KadićAJ, Puljak L. Proliferative injection therapy for osteoarthritis: a systematic review. *International Orthopaedics*. 2017; 41(4) 671–679.

Kumar AV, Jaishanklar HP, Kavitha AP, Roa Naik P. Prolotherapy: a new hope for temporomandibular joint pain. *Indian Journal of Pain*. 2013; 27(2): 49–52.

Kung SC, Su DC, Chou W. Poster 234: Treatment of First Metacarpophalangeal Joint Instability and Snapping Thumb Using Ultrasound-guided Prolotherapy and Hydrodissection: A Case Report. *PM&R*. 2017 Sep 30; 9(9): S206.

Lam SK. Three cases of chronic pain relieved with prolotherapy in Hong Kong clinic. *Journal of Prolotherapy*. 2009; 1(3): 163–165.

Lazzara MA. The non-surgical repair of a complete Achilles tendon rupture by prolotherapy: biological reconstruction. A case report. *Journal of Orthopaedic Medicine*. 2005; 27(3): 128–132.

Lee CW, Jim Ys, Ahn JK, Song BH, Jung Ds, Hwang HE. Clinical experience of prolotherapy for chronic musculoskeletal disease: a report of 5 cases. *Journal of Korean Pain Society*. 2001; 14(1): 114–117. Korean.

Lee DH, Kawck KS, Rah UW, Yoon SH. Prolotherapy for refractory rotator cuff disease: retrospective case-control study of 1-year follow up. *Archives of Physical Medicine and Rehabilitation*. 2015; 96(11): 2027–2032.

Leedy RF. Applications of sclerotherapy to specific problems. *Osteopathic Reporter*. 1977; 2: 79–97.

Leedy RF. Basic techniques of sclerotherapy. *Osteopathic Medicine*. 1977; 15–22, 109–114.

Linetsky FS, Alfredson H, Crane D, Centeno CJ. Treatment of Chronic Painful Musculoskeletal Injuries and Diseases with Regenerative Injection Therapy (RIT): Regenerative Injection Therapy Principles and Practice. In *Treatment of Chronic Pain by Integrative Approaches* (pp. 145–168). New York, NY: Springer; 2015.

Linetsky F, Stanton-Hicks M, Saberski, L. Regenerative injection therapy aka prolotherapy. In *Pain Medicine and Management—Just the Facts, Second Edition* (pp. 443–449). New York, NY: McGraw & Hill Education; 2015.

Linetsky FS, Trescot AM, Wiederholz MH. Regenerative injection therapy. In *Pain Management and Palliative Care* (pp. 369–375). New York, NY: Springer; 2015.

Linetsky F, Torres F. An assessment on the ultrasound guided dextrose prolotherapy for persistent coccygeal pain: a case series and review of literature. *Alternative & Integrative Medicine.* 2014; 3(2).

Linetsky F, Alfredson H, Crane D, Centeno CJ. Treatment of chronic painful musculoskeletal injuries and diseases with regenerative injection therapy (RIT): regenerative injection therapy principles and practice. In *Comprehensive Treatment of Chronic Pain by Medical Interventional and Integrative Approaches, the American Academy of Pain Medicine Textbook on Patient Management* (pp. 889–912). New York, NY: Springer; 2013.

Linetsky FS, Botwin K, Gorfine L, Jay GW, Miguel R, Mikulinksy A, Parris W, Pollack S, Ray A, Saberski L, Taraschi P, Torress F, Trescot A. Position Paper of the Florida Academy of Pain Medicine on Regenerative Injection Therapy: Effectiveness and Appropriate Usage. *The Pain Clinic.* 2002 June; 4(3): 38–45.

Linetsky FS, Derby R, Miguel R, Saberski L, Stanton-Hicks M. Pain management with regenerative injection therapy. In *Weiner's Pain Management: A Practical Guide (pp. 939-962).* 2006.

Linetsky FS, Manchikanti L. Regenerative injection therapy for axial pain. *Techniques in Regional Anesthesia and Pain Management.* 2005 Jan 31; 9(1): 40–49.

Linetsky FS, Miguel R, Torres F. Treatment of cervicothoracic pain and cervicogenic headaches with regenerative injection therapy. *Current Pain and Headache Reports.* 2004; 8(1): 41–48.

Linetsky FS, Miguel R, Saberski L. Pain management with regenerative injection therapy (RIT). In *Pain Management,* ed. Weiner RS (pp. 381–402). Boca Raton, Florida: CRC Press; 2002.

Liu YK, Tipton CM, Matthes RD, Bedford TG, Maynard JA, Walmer HC. An in situ study of the influence of a sclerosing solution in rabbit medial collateral ligaments and its junction strength. *Connective Tissue Research.* 1983; 11(2–3): 95–102.

Lone AH, Khursheed O, Rashid S, Mir BA, Nazeefa. Management of chronic plantar fasciitis using hyperosmolar dextrose injection. *Journal of Medical Science and Clinical Research.* 2015; 3(1): 3931–3935.

Louw F. The occasional prolotherapy for lateral epicondylosis (tennis elbow). *Canadian Journal of Rural Medicine*. 2014; 19(1): 31–34.

Lyftogt J. Subcutaneous prolotherapy treatment of refractory knee, shoulder, and lateral elbow pain. *Australasian Musculoskeletal Medicine*. 2007; 12(2): 110–112.

Lyftogt J. Prolotherapy for recalcitrant lumbago. *Australasian Musculoskeletal Medicine*. 2008; 13(1): 18–20.

Majumdar SK, Krishna S, Chatterjee A, Chakraborty R, Ansari N. Single injection technique prolotherapy for hypermobility disorders of TMJ using 25% dextrose: a clinical study. *Journal of Maxillofacial and Oral Surgery*. 2017; 16(2): 226–230.

Maniquis-Smigel L, Reeves KD, Rosen HJ, Lyftogt J, Graham-Coleman C, Cheng AL, Rabago D. Short term analgesic effects of 5% dextrose epidural injections for chronic low back pain: a randomized controlled trial. *Anesthesiology and Pain Medicine*. 2017 Feb; 7(1): e42550.

Mauermann ML, Watson JC. A Novel Treatment for Carpal Tunnel Syndrome? *Mayo Clinic Proceedings*. 2017 Aug 1; 92(8): 1173–1175.

Mayo Clinic Health Letter. Alternative treatments: Dealing with chronic pain. 2005 April; 23(4). http://www.prolotherapy.com/Mayo-Clinic-Prolo%202005.pdf.

Maxwell NJ. Ryan MB, Taunton JE, Gillies JH, Wong AD. Sonographically guided intratendinous injection of hyperosmolar dextrose to treat chronic tendinosis of the Achilles tendon: a pilot study. *American Journal of Roentgenology*. 2007; 184(4): W215–W220.

Merriman JR. Prolotherapy versus operative fusion in the treatment of joint instability of the spine and pelvis. *Journal of the International College Surgeons*. 1964; 42(2): 150–159.

Miller MR, Mathews RS, Reeves KD. Treatment of painful advanced internal lumbar disc derangement with intradiscal injection of hypertonic dextrose. *Pain Physical*. 2006; 9(2): 115–121.

Mitchell B, Rose R, Barnard A. Prolotherapy for sacroiliac joint pain—12 months outcomes. *Journal of Science and Medicine in Sport*. 2014; 18: e90.

Morath O, Kubosch EJ, Taeymans J, Zwingmann J, Kostantinidis L, Südkamp NP, Hirschmüller A. The effect of sclerotherapy and prolotherapy on chronic painful Achilles tendinopathy–a systematic review including meta-analysis. *Scandinavian Journal of Medicine & Science in Sports.* 2017; 1–12.

Murphy M. Road to prolotherapy: an athlete's prolotherapy story. *Journal of Prolotherapy.* 2009; 1(2): 96–98.

Myers A. Prolotherapy: a treatment of low back pain and sciatica. *Bulletin of the Hospital for Joint Diseases.*1961; 22(1):48–55.

Naeim F, Froetscher L, Hirschberg GG. Treatment of the chronic iliolumbar syndrome by infiltration of the iliolumbar ligament. *The Western Journal of Medicine.* 1982; 136(4): 372–374.

Nourani B, Rabago D. Prolotherapy for knee osteoarthritis: a descriptive review. *Current Physical Medicine and Rehabilitation Reports.* 2016; 4(1): 42–49.

Ojofeitimi S, Bronner S, Becica L. Conservative management of second metatarsophalangeal joint instability in a professional dancer: a case report. *Journal of Orthopedic & Sports Physical Therapy.* 2016; 46(2): 114–123.

Ongley MJ, Dorman TA, Eek B, Lundgren D, Klein R. Ligament instability of knees: a new approach to treatment. *Journal of Manual & Manipulative Therapy.*1998; 3: 152–154.

Ongley MJ, Dorman TA, Klein R, Eek B, Hubert L. A new approach to the treatment of chronic low back pain. *Lancet.* 1987; 330(8551): 143–146.

Ojofeitimi S, Bronner S, Becica L, Conservative management of second metatarsophalangeal joint instability in a professional dancer. A case report. *Journal of Orthopaedic & Sports Physical Therapy.* 2016: 46(2):114–123.

Örsçelik A, Yasar H, Köroglu O, Seven MM. P-75 Prolotherapy for carpal tunnel syndrome: a case report. *British Journal of Sports Medicine.* 2016; 50(1): A73.

Park JH, Song IS, Lee JB, Lee HY, Yoo SM, Yang SJ, Seo KM, Kim DG. Ultrasonographic findings of healing of torn tendon in the patients with lateral epicondylitis after prolotherapy. *Journal of Korean Society of Ultrasound in Medicine.* 2003; 22(3): 177–183.

Park JY. Nonsurgical management of chronic low back pain. *Journal of the Korean Medical Association.* 2007; 50(6): 507–522.

Patel DN; Strauss EJ. Alternative therapeutic modalities in sports medicine. *Bulletin of the NYU Hospital for Joint Diseases.* 2015; 73(2): 122–122.

Polukhin E. Prolotherapy, myths and the truth. *Alternative & Integrative Medicine.* 2013; 2(3): 1–3.

Rabago D, Nourani B. Prolotherapy for osteoarthritis and tendinopathy: a descriptive review. *Current Rheumatology Reports.* 2017 June 1; 19(6): 34.

Rabago D, van Lueven L, Benes L, Fortney L, Slattegren A, Grettie J, Mundt M. Qualitative assessment of patients receiving prolotherapy for knee osteoarthritis in a multimethod study. *Journal of Alternative and Complementary Medicine.* 2016; 22(12): 983–989.

Rabago D, Lam SKH, Reeves KD. Dextrose prolotherapy for chronic temporomandibular pain and dysfunction: results of a pilot-level randomized controlled study. *Archives of Physical Medicine and Rehabilitation.* 2016; 97(10): e139.

Rabago D, Mundt M, Zgierska A, Grettie J. Hypertonic dextrose injection (prolotherapy) for knee osteoarthritis: long term outcomes. *Complementary Therapies in Medicine.* 2015; 23(3): 388–395.

Rabago D, Patterson JJ, Mundt M, Zgierska A, Fortney L, Grettie J, Kijowski R. Dextrose and morrhuate sodium injections (prolotherapy) for knee osteoarthritis: a prospective open-label trial. *Journal of Alternative and Complementary Medicine.* 2014; 20(5): 383–391.

Rabago D, Patterson JJ, Mundt M. Feature article prolotherapy: a nontraditional approach to knee osteoarthritis dextrose injections into the knee can reduce pain and improve a patient's quality of life. *Journal of Family Practice.* 2014; 63(4): 206–208.

Rabago D, Patterson JJ, Mundt M, Kijowski R, Grettie J, Segal NA, Zgierska A. Dextrose prolotherapy for knee osteoarthritis: a randomized controlled trial. *Annals of Family Medicine.* 2013; 11(3): 229–237.

Rabago D, Lee KS, Ryan M, Chourasia AO, Sesto ME, Zgierska A, Kijowski R, Grettie J, Wilson, J, Miller, D. Hypertonic dextrose and morrhuate sodium injections (prolotherapy) for lateral epicondylosis (tennis elbow): results of a single-blind, pilot-level randomized controlled trial. *American Journal of Physical Medicine & Rehabilitation/ Association of Academic Physiatrists.* 2013; 92(7): 587–596.

Rabago D, Kijowski R, Woods M, Patterson JJ, Mundt M, Zgierska A, Grettie J, Lyftogt J, Fortney L. Association between disease-specific quality of life and magnetic resonance imaging outcomes in a clinical trial of prolotherapy for knee osteoarthritis. *Archives of Physical Medicine and Rehabilitation*. 2013; 94(11): 2075–2082.

Rabago D, Patterson JJ, Mundt M, Kijowski R, Grettie J, Segal NA, Zgierska A. Dextrose prolotherapy for knee osteoarthritis: a randomized controlled trial. *Annals of Family Medicine*. 2013; 11(3): 229–237.

Rabago D, Patterson JJ. Prolotherapy: an effective adjunctive therapy for knee osteoarthritis. *Journal of the American Osteopathic Association*. 2013; 113(2): 122–123.

Rabago D, Ryan M, Lee K, Chourasia A, Sesto M, Zgierska A, Miller D, Kijowski R, Wilson J. The efficacy of prolotherapy using dextrose-morrhuate for lateral epicondylosis: a pilot randomized controlled trial. *BMC Complementary and Alternative Medicine*. 2012; 12(1): 79.

Rabago D, Zgierska A, Fortney L, Kijowski R, Mundt M, Ryan M, Grettie J, Patterson J. Hypertonic dextrose injections (prolotherapy) for knee osteoarthritis: results of a single-arm uncontrolled study with one-year follow-up. *Journal of Alternative and Complementary Medicine*. 2012; 4(18): 408–414.

Rabago D. Prolotherapy for chronic musculoskeletal pain. *Complementary and Alternative Therapies in the Aging Population*. 2011: 15.

Rabago D, Miller DJ, Zgierska AE, Mundt M, Kijowski R, Jessica B, Patterson JJ. Dextrose prolotherapy for knee osteoarthritis: results of a randomized controlled trial [abstract 308]. *Osteoarthritis and Cartilage*. 2011; 19(1): S142–S143.

Rabago D, Yelland M, Patterson JJ, Zgierska A. Prolotherapy for chronic musculoskeletal pain. *American Family Physician*. 2011; 84(11): 1208–1210.

Rabago D, Kijowski R, Zgierska A, Yelland M, Scarpone M. Magnetic resonance imaging outcomes in a randomised, controlled trial of prolotherapy for lateral epicondylosis. *International Musculoskeletal Medicine*. 2010; 32(3): 117–123.

Rabago D, Slattengren A, Zgierska A. Prolotherapy in primary care practice. *Primary Care: Clinics in Office Practice.* 2010; 37(1): 65–80.

Rabago D, Best TM, Zgierska AE, Zeisig E, Ryan M, Crane D. A systematic review of four injection therapies for lateral epicondylosis: prolotherapy, polidocanol, whole blood and platelet-rich plasma. *British Journal of Sports Medicine.* 2009; 43(7): 471–481.

Rabago D, Best TM, Beamsley M, Patterson JJ. A systematic review of prolotherapy for chronic musculoskeletal pain. *Clinical Journal of Sports Medicine.* 2005; 15(5): 376–380.

Ravin T, Cantieri M, Pasquarello G. *Principles of Prolotherapy.* Denver, Colorado: American Academy of Musculoskeletal Medicine; 2008.

Reeves KD, Sit R, Rabago D. Dextrose prolotherapy: a narrative review of basic science, clinical research, and best treatment recommendations. *Physical Medicine and Rehabilitation Clinics of North America.* 2016; 27(4): 783–823.

Reeves KD, Fullerton BD, Topol G. Chapter 50: Evidence-based regenerative injection therapy (prolotherapy) in sports medicine. In *The Sports Medicine Resource Manual 1st Edition.* (pp. 611–619). Philadelphia, Pennsylvania: Saunders; 2008.

Reeves KD. Sweet relief. *Journal of Biomechanics.* 2004; 9: 25–35.

Reeves KD, Hassanein KM. Long-term effects of dextrose prolotherapy for anterior cruciate ligament laxity: a prospective and consecutive patient study. *Alternative Therapies in Health and Medicine.* 2003; 9(3): 58–62.

Reeves KD, Hassanein KM. Long term effects of dextrose prolotherapy for anterior cruciate ligament laxity. *Alternative Therapies in Health and Medicine.* 2003; 9(3): 58–62.

Reeves KD. Prolotherapy: basic science, clinical studies, and technique. In *Pain Procedures in Clinical Practice, 2nd Edition,* ed. Lennard TA. Philadelphia, Pennsylvania: Hanley and Belfus; 2000: 172–190.

Reeves KD. Prolotherapy: present and future applications in soft-tissue pain and disability. *Physical Medicine & Rehabilitation Clinics of North America.* 1995; 6(4): 917–926.

Reeves KD, Hassanein KM. Randomized prospective double-blind placebo-controlled study of dextrose prolotherapy for knee osteo-arthritis with or without ACL laxity. *Alternative Therapies in Health and Medicine*. 2000; 6(2): 68–80.

Reeves KD, Hassanein KM. Randomized, prospective, place-bo-controlled double-blind study of dextrose prolotherapy for osteoarthritic thumb and finger (DIP, PIP, and trapeziometacar-pal) joints: evidence of clinical efficacy. *Journal of Alternative and Complementary Medicine*. 2000; 6(4): 311–320.

Reeves KD, Hassanein KM. Randomized prospective double-blind placebo-controlled study of dextrose prolotherapy for knee osteo-arthritis with or without ACL laxity. *Alternative Therapies in Health and Medicine*. 2000; 6(2): 68–79.

Reeves KD. Prolotherapy: basic science, clinical studies, and tech-nique. In *Pain Procedures in Clinical Practice, 2nd Edition* (pp. 172–190). Philadelphia, Pennsylvania: Hanley and Belfus; 2000.

Reeves KD. Technique of Prolotherapy. In *Pain Procedures in Clinical Practice*, ed. Lennard TA (pp. 57–70). Philadelphia, Pennsylvania: Hanley & Belfus, Inc.; 1994.

Reeves KD. Treatment of consecutive severe fibromyalgia patients with prolotherapy. *Journal of Orthopaedic Medicine*. 1994; 16(3): 84–89.

Refai H. Long-term therapeutic effects of dextrose prolotherapy in patients with hypermobility of the temporomandibular joint: a single-arm study with 1–4 years' follow up. *British Journal of Oral and Maxillofacial Surgery*. 2017; 55(5): 465–470.

Refai H, Altahhan O, Elsharkawy R. The efficacy of dextrose pro-lotherapy for temporomandibular joint hypermobility: a prelim-inary prospective, randomized, double-blind, placebo-controlled clinical trial. *Journal of Oral and Maxillofacial Surgery*. 2011; 69(12): 2962–2970.

Rezasoltani Z, Taheri M, Mofrad MK, Mohanjerani SA. Periarticular dextrose prolotherapy instead of intra-articular injection for pain and functional improvement in knee osteoar-thritis. *Journal of Pain Research*. 2017; 10: 1179–1187.

Rose R, Barnard A. Efficacy of prolotherapy treatment for sacro-iliac joint instability and pain. *Journal of Science and Medicine in Sport*. 2015; 19: e70.

Ryan MB, Wong AD, Gillies JH, Wong J, Taunton JE. Sonographically guided intratendinous injections of hyperosmolar dextrose/lido-caine: a pilot study for the treatment of chronic plantar fasciitis. *British Journal of Sports Medicine*. 2009; 43(4): 303–306.

Ryan M, Wong A, Taunton J. Favorable outcomes after sonograph-ically guided intratendinous injection of hyperosmolar dextrose for chronic insertional and midportion Achilles tendinosis. *AJR American Journal of Roentgenology*. 2010; 194(4): 1047–1053.

Ryan M, Wong A, Rabago D, Lee K, Taunton J. Ultrasound-guided injections of hyperosmolar dextrose for overuse patellar tend-inopathy: a pilot study. *British Journal of Sports Medicine*. 2011: bjsports81455.

Sanderson LM, Bryant A. Effectiveness and safety of prolother-apy injections for management of lower limb tendinopathy and fasciopathy: a systematic review. *Journal of Foot and Ankle Research*. 2015; 8(1): 1–15.

Scarpone M, Rabago DP, Zgierska A, Arbogast G, Snell E. The efficacy of prolotherapy for lateral epicondylosis: a pilot study. *Clinical Journal of Sports Medicine*. 2008; 18(3): 248–254.

Schapiro A, Lee K, Rabago D, Wilson J. Platelet-rich plasma and hyperosmolar dextrose (prolotherapy) for lateral epicondylosis: power Doppler sonographic assessment of tendon neovascular-ity as a measure of healing response. *Ultrasound in Medicine and Biology*. 2015; 41(4): S88–S89.

Seenauth C, Inouye V, Langland JO. Dextrose Prolotherapy for Chronic Shoulder Pain: A Case Report. *Alternative Therapies in Health and Medicine*. 2017 Nov 4. Epub ahead of print [cited 2017 Dec 9); https://www.ncbi.nlm.nih.gov/pubmed/29101774

Şentürk E, Şahin E, Serter S. Prolotherapy: an effective therapy for Tietze syndrome. *Journal of Back and Musculoskeletal Rehabilitation*. 2017 Sept 22; 30(5): 975–978.

Schultz LW. Treatment for subluxation of the temporomandibular joint. *JAMA*. 1937; 109(13): 1032–1035.

Schwartz R. Prolotherapy: a literature review and retrospective study. *Journal of Neurology, Orthopedic Medicine, and Surgery*. 1991; 12: 220–223.

Seven MM, Ersen O, Akpancar S, Ozkan H, Turkkan S, Yıldız Y, Koca K. Effectiveness of prolotherapy in the treatment of chronic rotator cuff lesions. *Orthopaedics & Traumatology: Surgery & Research*. 2017; 103(3): 427–433.

Sharma GS, Jayakar R, Pham Q. Poster 448: Prolotherapy for the Treatment of interspinous ligament injury: a case report. *PM&R*. 2017 Sep 30; 9(9): S3274–S275.

Shin JY, Seo KM, Kim DK, Kim BK, Kang SH. The effect of prolotherapy on lateral epicondylitis of elbow. *Journal of Korean Academy of Rehabilitation Medicine Korean*. 2002; 26(6): 764–768.

Shuman D. Ambulation, osteopathic manipulative therapy, and joint sclerotherapy in the management of common low-back disorders. *Journal of the American Osteopathic Association*. 1967; 67(1): 52–59.

Shuman D. Sclerotherapy. *Osteopathic Annals*. 1978; 6(12): 10–14.

Singh V. Trescot A, Nishio I. Injections for chronic pain. *Physical Medicine & Rehabilitation Clinics of North America*. 2015; 26(2): 249–261.

Sit RWS, Chung VCH, Reeves KD, Rabago D, Chan KKW, Chan DCC, Wu X, Ho RST, Wong SYS. Hypertonic dextrose injections (prolotherapy) in the treatment of symptomatic knee osteoarthritis: a systematic review and meta-analysis. *Scientific Reports*. 2016; 6: 25247.

Slattengren AH, Christensen T, Prasad S, Jones K. PURLs: Prolotherapy: a nontraditional approach to knee osteoarthritis. *Journal of Family Practice*. 2014; 63(4): 206–208.

Soliman DM. Advantages of dextrose, platelet rich plasma and stem cells over the traditional conventional methods in treatment of sports injuries and joint osteoarthritis. *Journal of Sports Science*. 2017; 5: 113–118.

Soliman D. Management of musculoskeletal pain. *Journal of Physical Science and Application*. 2017; 7(2): 27–30.

Solmaz I, Deniz S, Cifci OT. Treatment of advanced stage gonarthrosis with prolotherapy: case report. *Anesthesiology and Pain Medicine.* 2014; 4(1): e9171.

Stein A, Mcaleer S, Hinz M. Microperforation prolotherapy: a novel method for successful nonsurgical treatment of atraumatic spontaneous anterior sternoclavicular subluxation, with an illustrative case. *Open Access Journal of Sports Medicine.* 2011; 2: 47–52.

Steilen D, Hauser R, Woldin B, Sawyer S. Chronic neck pain: making the connection between capsular ligament laxity and cervical instability. *Open Orthopaedics Journal.* 2014; 8: 326.

Stovitz SD, Johnson RJ. NSAIDs and musculoskeletal treatment: What is the clinical evidence? *Physician and Sportsmedicine.* 2003; 31: 1

Strauchman MN, Morningstar MW. Prolotherapy injections for diastasis recti: a case report. *Case Reports in Clinical Medicine.* 2016; 5(9): 342-346.

Tolbert G, Roy D, Walker V. Ultrasound guided dextrose prolotherapy and platelet rich plasma therapy in chronic low back pain: three case reports. *International Journal of Physical Medicine & Rehabilitation.* 2013; 1(6).

Topol GA, Podesta LA, Reeves KD, Giraldo MM, Johnson LL, Grasso R, Jamin A, Clark T, Ragago D. Chondrogenic effect of intra-articular hypertonic-dextrose (prolotherapy) in severe knee osteoarthritis. *PM&R.* 2016; 8(11): 1072–1082.

Topol GA, Podesta LA, Reeves KD, Raya MF, Fullerton BD, Yeh HW. Hyperosmolar dextrose injection for recalcitrant Osgood-Schlatter disease. *Pediatrics.* 2011; 185(5): e1121–e1128.

Topol GA, Reeves KD. Regenerative injection of elite athletes with career-altering chronic groin pain who fail conservative treatment. *American Journal of Physical Medicine & Rehabilitation.* 2008; 87(11): 890–902.

Topol GA, Reeves KD, Hassanein KM. Efficacy of dextrose prolotherapy in elite male kicking-sport athletes with chronic groin pain. *Archives of Physical Medicine and Rehabilitation.* 2005; 86(4): 697–702.

Trebinjac S, Kitchbi H. Long-term effect of prolotherapy on symptomatic rotator cuff tendinopathy. *Journal of Health Sciences.* 2015; 5(3): 93–98.

Tsatsos G, Mandal R. Prolotherapy in the treatment of foot problems. *Journal of the American Podiatric Medical Association.* 2002; 92(6): 366–368.

Ungor C, Atasoy KT, Taskesen F, Cezairli B, Dayisoylu EH, Tosun E, Senel FC. Short-term results of prolotherapy in the management of temporomandibular joint dislocation. *Journal of Craniofacial Surgery.* 2013; 24(2): 411–415.

Van ark M, Zwerver J, Van den Akker-Scheek I. Injection treatments for patellar tendinopathy. *British Journal of Sports Medicine.* 2011; 45(13): 1068–1076.

Vankdoth S, Adamala SR, Talla H, Vijayalaxmi N, Madhulatha G. Prolotherapy—a venturing treatment for temporomandibular joint disorder. *International Journal of Solids and Structures.* 2014; 1(7): 27-30.

Vora A, Borg-stein J, Nguyen RT. Regenerative injection therapy for osteoarthritis: fundamental concepts and evidence-based review. *PM&R.* 2012; 4(5): S104–S109.

Walmer HC. A comprehensive, nonsurgical approach to the low-back problem. *Osteopathic Annals.* 1978; 6(12): 29–34.

Watson JD, Shay BL. Treatment of chronic low-back pain: a 1-year or greater follow-up. *Journal of Alternative and Complementary Medicine.* 2010; 16(9): 951–958.

Weglein AD. Neural prolotherapy. *Journal of Prolotherapy.* 2001; 3(2): 639–643.

Westminster CO, Centeno CJ. Sclerotherapy of Baker's cyst with imaging confirmation of resolution. *Pain Physician.* 2008; 11: 257–261.

Wheaton MT, Jensen N. The ligament injury-osteoarthritis connection: the role of prolotherapy in ligament repair and the prevention of osteoarthritis. *Journal of Prolotherapy.* 2011; 3(4): 790–812.

Wheaton MT, Jensen N. The ligament injury connection to osteoarthritis. *Journal of Prolotherapy.* 2010; 2(1): 294–304

Wheaton MT, Manley J. Prolotherapy gets college basketball player back on the court. *Journal of Prolotherapy.* 2009; 1(1): 32–35.

Wilkinson HA. Injection therapy for enthesopathies causing axial spine pain and the "failed back syndrome": a single blinded, randomized and cross-over study. *Pain Physician.* 2005; 8(2): 167–173.

Woldin B, Hauser R. Pain in osteoarthritis: can prolotherapy help? *The Pain Practitioner.* 2014; 24(3): 16–22.

Woldin B, Hauser R. Prolotherapy: under-recognized treatment for osteoarthritis pain. *Academy of Integrative Pain Management.* 2015 [cited 2015 July 29] http://www.aapainmanage.org/pain-practitioner/prolotherapy-under-recognized-treatment-for-osteoarthritis-pain/.

Wu J, Zhou J, Liu C, Zhang J, Xiong W, Lv Y, Liu R, Wang R, Du Z, Zhang G, Lui Q. A prospective study comparing platelet-rich plasma and local anesthetic (LA)/corticosteroid in intra-articular injection for the treatment of lumbar facet joint syndrome. *Pain Practice.* 2017; 17(7): 914–924.

Wu D, Hu K, Zhou H. Modified dextrose prolotherapy for the treatment of recurrent temporomandibular joint dislocation. *Chinese Journal of Stomatology.* 2015; 50(2): 113–114.

Yaman H, Vural R. Prolotherapy: a new method for chronic pain management in family medicine. *Ankara Medical Journal.* 2016; 16(2).

Yavuz F, Kibar S, Balaban B. Hypertonic dextrose injection for the treatment of a baker's cyst. *Journal of Clinical and Diagnostic Research: JCDR.* 2016; 10(2): YD01.

Yelland MJ. Review of prolotherapy for musculoskeletal pain and disability. *Australasian Musculoskeletal Medicine Journal.* 2002; 7(2): 69–77.

Yelland MJ, Del Mar C, Pirozzo S, Schoene ML. Prolotherapy injections for chronic low back pain: a systematic review. *Spine Journal.* 2004; 29(19): 2126–2133.

Yelland MJ, Del Mar C, Pirozzo S, Schoene ML, Vercoe P. Prolotherapy injections for chronic low-back pain. *The Cochrane Database of Systematic Reviews.* 2004; 2: CD004059.

Yelland MJ, Glasziou PP, Bogduk N, Schluter PJ, McKernon M. Prolotherapy injections, saline injections, and exercises for chronic low-back pain: a randomized trial. *Spine Journal*. 2004; 29(1): 9–16.

Yelland MJ, Sweeting KR, Lyftogt JA, Ng SK, Scuffham PA, Evans KA. Prolotherapy injections and eccentric loading exercises for painful Achilles tendinosis: a randomised trial. *British Journal of Sports Medicine*. 2011; 45(5): 421–428.

Yelland MJ, Yao M, Schluter P. Prolotherapy injections for chronic low back pain: results of a pilot comparative study. *Australasian Musculoskeletal Medicine Journal*. 2000; 5(2): 20–30.

Zeisig E, Fahlström M, Ohberg L, Alfredson H. A two-year sonographic follow-up after intratendinous injection therapy in patients with tennis elbow. *British Journal of Sports Medicine*. 2010; 44(8): 584–587.

Zhou H, Hu K, Ding Y. Modified dextrose prolotherapy for recurrent temporomandibular joint dislocation. *British Journal of Oral and Maxillofacial Surgery*. 2014; 52(1): 63–66.

Platelet-Rich Plasma (PRP) Prolotherapy

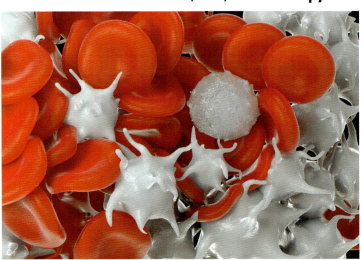

Ahmad Z, Brooks R, Kang SN, Weaver H, Nunney I, Tytherleigh-Strong G, Rushton N. The effect of platelet-rich plasma on clinical outcomes in lateral epicondylitis. *Arthroscopy*. 2013; 29(11): 1851–1862.

Akman B, Güven M, Bildik C, Şaylı U, Parnianfard A, Rahimli M. MRI Documented Improvement in Patient with Juvenile Osteochondritis Dissecans Treated with Platelet Rich Plasma. *Journal of Prolotherapy*. 2016; 8: e966–e970.

Alderman DD. State of the art: prolotherapy regenerative medicine. *Pain Week Journal*. 2016; 4(4): 44–52.

Alderman DD. Regenerative injection therapies for pain: traditional, platelet rich plasma and biocellular prolotherapy. In *Integrative Pain Management* (pp. 345–360). New York, New York: Oxford University Press; 2016.

Alderman DD. Platelet rich plasma in prolotherapy. *Practical Pain Management*. 2009: 68–69.

Alderman DD. The new age of prolotherapy. *Practical Pain Management*. 2010; 10(4): 54–68.

Alderman DD, Robbins SC. Platelet rich plasma for rotator cuff tears. *Practical Pain Management.* 2012; 12(8): 21–23.

Andia I, Maffulli N. Biological therapies in regenerative sports medicine. *Sports Medicine.* 2017; 47(5): 807–828.

Arirachakaran A, Sukthuayat A, Sisayanarane T, Laoratanavoraphong S, Kanchanatawan W, Kongtharvonskul J. Platelet-rich plasma versus autologous blood versus steroid injection in lateral epicondylitis: systematic review and network meta-analysis. *Journal of Orthopaedics and Traumatology.* 2016; 17(2): 101–112.

Aufiero D, Vincent H, Sampson S, Bodor M. Regenerative injection treatment in the spine: review and case series with platelet rich plasma. *Journal of Stem Cells Research, Reviews & Reports.* 2015; 2(1): id1019.

Bashir J, Panero AJ, Sherman AL. The emerging use of platelet-rich plasma in musculoskeletal medicine. *Journal of the American Osteopathic Association.* 2015; 115(1): 24–31.

Barile A, La Marra A, Arrigoni F, Mariani S, Zugaro L, Splendiani A, Di Cesare E, Reginelli A, Zappia M, Brunese L, Duka E, Carrafiello G, Masciocchi C. Anaesthetics, steroids and platelet-rich plasma (PRP) in ultrasound-guided musculoskeletal procedures. *British Journal of Radiology.* 2016; 89: 20150355.

Bava ED, Barber FA. Platelet-rich plasma products in sports medicine. *Physician and Sports Medicine.* 2011; 39(3): 94–99.

Bava SS, Sonone S, Dahapute A, Virani S, Gautham S. Local injection of platelet rich plasma versus corticosteroids for treatment of lateral epicondylitis of humerus. *International Journal of Scientific Research.* 2016; 5(9).

Bertrand H, Reeves KD, Bennett CJ, Bicknell S, Cheng A. Dextrose prolotherapy versus control injections in painful rotator cuff tendinopathy. *Archives of Physical Medicine and Rehabilitation.* 2016; 97(1): 17–25.

Bhatia R, Chopra G. Efficacy of platelet rich plasma via lumbar epidural route in chronic prolapsed intervertebral disc patients—a pilot study. *Journal of Clinical and Diagnostic Research: JCDR.* 2016; 10(9): UC05.

Bocanegra-Pérez S, Vicente-Barrero M, Knezevic M, Castellano-Navarro JM, Rodríguez-Bocanegra E, Rodríguez-Millares J, Pérez-Plasencia D, Ramos-Macías A. Use of platelet-rich plasma in the treatment of bisphosphonate-related osteonecrosis of the jaw. *International Journal of Oral and Maxillofacial Surgery*. 2012; 41(11): 1410–1415.

Brossi PM, Moreira JJ, Machado TS, Baccarin RY. Platelet-rich plasma in orthopedic therapy: a comparative systematic review of clinical and experimental data in equine and human musculo-skeletal lesions. *BMC Veterinary Research*. 2015; 11: 98.

Brkljac M, Kumar S, Kalloo DH. The effect of platelet-rich plasma injection on lateral epicondylitis following failed conservative management. *Journal of Orthopaedics*. 2015; 12: S166–S170.

Brown MN, Shiple BJ, Scarpone M. Regenerative approaches to tendon and ligament conditions. *Physical Medicine and Rehabilitation Clinics of North America*. 2016; 27(4): 941–984.

Cameron JA, Thielen KM. Autologous platelet rich plasma for neck and lower back pain secondary to spinal disc herniation: Midterm results. *Spine Research*. 2017 Aug 30; 3(2): Article ID 100030: 5 pages.

Cavallo C, Filardo G, Mariani E, Kon E, Marcacci M, Pereiera Ruiz MT, Facchinin A, Grigolo B. Comparison of platelet-rich plasma formulations for cartilage healing: an in vitro study. *Journal of Bone and Joint Surgery*. 2014; 96(5): 423–429.

Chang RG, Hurwitz NR, Harrison JR, Jennifer C, Lutz GE. Ankylosing Spondylitis Versus Internal Disc Disruption: A Case Report Treated Successfully with Intradiscal Platelet-Rich Plasma Injection. *Spine Research*. 2017 Apr 28; 3(1): 4.

Chao L, Murray MM, Vavken P. Platelet-rich plasma (PRP) in ligament and tendon repair. In *Platelet-Rich Plasma*. (pp. 215–230). Berlin, Heidelberg: Springer; 2014.

Chen L, Dong SW, Liu JP, Tao X, Tang KL, Xu JZ. Synergy of tendon stem cells and platelet-rich plasma in tendon healing. *Journal of Orthopaedic Research*. 2012; 30(6): 991–997.

Cole BJ, Karas V, Hussey K, Pilz K, Fortier LA. Hyaluronic acid versus platelet-rich plasma: a prospective, double-blind random-ized controlled trial comparing clinical outcomes and effects of intra-articular biology for the treatment of knee osteoarthritis. *American Journal of Sports Medicine.* 2017 Feb; 45(2): 339–346.

Cong GT, Carballo C, Camp CL, Album Z, Lebaschi A, Zong J, Zong J, Rodeo SA. Platelet-rich plasma in treating patellar tendinopathy. *Operative Techniques in Orthopaedics.* 2016; 26(2): 110–116.

Crane D, Oliver K. Platelet-rich plasma and biocellular grafts. In *Platelet-Rich Plasma* (pp. 249–264). Berlin, Heidelberg: Springer; 2014.

Crane D, Everts P. Platelet rich plasma (PRP) matrix grafts. *Practical Pain Management.* 2008; 8(1): 12–26.

Crane DM, Oliver KS, Bayes MC. Orthobiologics and knee osteoarthritis: a recent literature review, treatment algorithm, and pathophysiology discussion. *Physical Medicine and Rehabilitation Clinics of North America.* 2016; 27(4): 985–1002.

Creaney L, Hamilton B. Growth factor delivery methods in the management of sports injuries: the state of play. *British Journal of Sports Medicine.* 2008; 42(5): 314–320.

Creaney L, Wallace A, Curtis M, Connell D. Growth factor-based therapies provide additional benefit beyond physical therapy in resistant elbow tendinopathy: a prospective, single-blind, randomized trial of autologous blood injections versus plate-rich plasma injections. *British Journal of Sports Medicine.* 2011; 45: 966–971.

Dallari D, Stagni C, Rani N, Sabbioni G, Pelotti P, Torricelli P, Tschon M, Giavaresi G. Ultrasound-guided injection of platelet-rich plasma and hyaluronic acid, separately and in combination for hip osteoarthritis: a randomized controlled study. *American Journal of Sports Medicine.* 2016; 44(3): 664–671.

Dallaudiere B, Louedec L, Paule M, Lenet J, Pesquer L, Blaise E, Perozziello A, Michel JB, Moinard M, Meyer P, Serfaty JM. The molecular systemic and local effects of intra-tendinous injection of platelet rich plasma in tendinosis: preliminary results on a rat model with ELISA method. *Muscles, Ligaments and Tendons Journal.* 2015; 5(2): 99–105.

Davenport KL, Campos JS, Nguyen J, Saboeiro G, Adler RS, Moley PJ. Ultrasound-guided intratendinous injections with platelet-rich plasma or autologous whole blood for treatment of proximal hamstring tendinopathy: a double-blind randomized controlled trial. *Journal of Ultrasound Medicine.* 2015; 34(8): 1455–1463.

Deal JB, Smith E, Heard W, O'Brien MJ, Savoie III FH. Platelet-Rich Plasma for Primary Treatment of partial ulnar collateral ligament tears: MRI correlation with results. *Orthopaedic Journal of Sports Medicine.* 2017 Nov 8; 5(11) [cited December 26, 2017]. http://journals.sagepub.com/doi/full/10.1177/2325967117738238.

De Almeida AM, Demange MK, Sobrado MF, Rodrigues MB, Pedrinelli A, Hernandez AJ. Patellar tendon healing with platelet-rich plasma: a prospective randomized controlled trial. *American Journal of Sports Medicine.* 2012; 40(6): 1282–1288.

DeChellis DM, Cortazzo MH. Regenerative medicine in the field of pain medicine: prolotherapy, platelet-rich plasma therapy, and stem cell therapy—theory and evidence. *Techniques in Regional Anesthesia and Pain Management.* 2011; 15(2): 74–80.

De Jonge S, De Vos RJ, Weir A. One-year follow-up of platelet-rich plasma treatment in chronic Achilles tendinopathy: a double-blind randomized placebo-controlled trial. *American Journal of Sports Medicine.* 2011; 39(8): 1623–1629.

Del Buono A, Papalia R, Denaro V, Maccauro G, Maffulli N. Platelet rich plasma and tendinopathy: state of the art. *International Journal of Immunopathology and Pharmacology.* 2011; 4(2): 79–83.

Diehl JW. Platelet-rich plasma therapy in chronic Achilles tendinopathy. *Techniques in Foot & Ankle Surgery.* 2011; 1(10): 2–6.

.Dhillon MS, Sandeep P, Rakesh J. PRP in OA knee–update, current confusions and future options. *Sociéte Internationale de Chirurgie Orthpédique et de Traumatologie.* 2017; 3: 27.

Di Matteo B, Filardo G, Kon E, Marcacci M. Platelet-rich plasma: evidence for the treatment of patellar and Achilles tendinopathy—a systematic review. *Musculoskeletal Surgery.* 2015; 99(1): 1–9.

Di Matteo B, Kon E, Filardo G. Intra-articular platelet-rich plasma for the treatment of osteoarthritis. *Annals of Translational Medicine.* 2016; 4(3): 63.

Dojode CM. A randomized control trial to evaluate the efficacy of autologous blood injection versus local corticosteroid injection for treatment of lateral epicondylitis. *Bone & Joint Research.* 2012; 1: 192–197.

Dragoo JL, Wasterlain AS, Braun HJ, Nead KT. Platelet-rich plasma as a treatment for patellar tendinopathy: a double-blind, randomized controlled trial. *American Journal of Sports Medicine.* 2014; 42(3): 610–618.

Engebretsen L, Steffen K, Alsousou J, Anitua E, Bachl N, Devilee R, Everts P, Hamilton B, Huard J, Jenoure P, Kelberine F, Kon E, Maffulli N, Matheson G, Mei-Dan O, Menetrey J, Philippon M, Randelli P, Schamasch P, Schwellnus M, Vernec A, Verrall G. IOC consensus paper on the use of platelet-rich plasma in sports medicine. *British Journal of Sports Medicine.* 2010; 44: 1072–1081.

Fader RR, Mitchell JJ, Traub S, Nichols R, Roper M, Mei-Dan O, McCarty EC. Platelet-rich plasma treatment improves outcomes for chronic proximal hamstring injuries in an athletic population. *Muscles Ligaments and Tendons Journal.* 2014; 4(4): 461–466.

Ferrero G, Fabbro E, Orlandi D, Martini C, Lacelli F, Serafini G, Silvestri E, Sconfienza LM. Ultrasound-guided injection of platelet-rich plasma in chronic Achilles and patellar tendinopathy. *Journal of Ultrasound.* 2012; 15(4): 260–266.

Filardo G, Di Matteo B, Kon E, Dhillon MS, Patel S, Marwaha N. Platelet-rich plasma for knee osteoarthritis. *American Journal of Sports Medicine.* 2013; 41(9): NP42–NP43.

Filardo G, Kon E, Buda R, Timoncini A, Di Martino A, Cenacchi A, Fornasari PM, Giannini S, Marcacci M. Platelet-rich plasma intra-articular knee injections for the treatment of degenerative cartilage lesions and osteoarthritis. *Knee Surgery, Sports Traumatology, Arthroscopy.* 2011; 19(4): 528–535.

Filardo G, Kon E, Della Villa S, Vincentelli F, Fornasari PM, Marcacci M. Use of platelet-rich plasma for the treatment of refractory jumper's knee. *International Orthopaedics.* 2010; 34(6): 909–915.

Filardo G, Kon E, Di Matteo B, Di Martino A, Tesei G, Pelotti P, Cenacchi A, Marcacci M. Platelet-rich plasma injections for the treatment of refractory Achilles tendinopathy: results at 4 years. *Blood Transfusion.* 2014; 12(4): 533–540.

Filardo G, Kon E, Di Matteo B, Di Martino A, Sessa A, Merli ML, Marcacci M. Leukocyte-poor PRP application for the treatment of knee osteoarthritis. *Joints.* 2013; 1(3): 112–120.

Filardo G, Kon E, Di Matteo B, Pelotti P, Di Martino A, Marcacci M. Platelet-rich plasma for the treatment of patellar tendinopathy: clinical and imaging findings at medium-term follow-up. *International Orthopaedics*. 2013; 37(8): 1583–1589.

Filardo G, Kon E, Di Martino A, Di Matteo B, Merli ML, Cenacchi A, Fornasari PM, Marcacci M. Platelet-rich plasma vs hyaluronic acid to treat knee degenerative pathology: study design and preliminary results of a randomized controlled trial. *BMC Musculoskeletal Disorders*. 2012; 13: 229.

Filardo G, Kon E, Pereira Ruiz MT, Vaccaro F, Guitaldi R, Di Martino A, Cenacchi A, Fornasari PM, Marcacci M. Platelet-rich plasma intra-articular injections for cartilage degeneration and osteoarthritis: single- versus double-spinning approach. *Knee Surgery, Sports Traumatology, Arthroscopy*. 2012; 20(10): 2082–2091.

Filardo G, Kon E, Roffi A, Di Matteo B, Merli ML, Marcacci M. Platelet-rich plasma: why intra-articular? A systematic review of preclinical studies and clinical evidence on PRP for joint degeneration. *Knee Surgery, Sports Traumatology, Arthroscopy*. 2013; 23(9): 2459–2474.

Fitzpatrick J, Bulsara M, Zheng MH. The effectiveness of platelet-rich plasma in the treatment of tendinopathy: a meta-analysis of randomized controlled clinical trials. *American Journal of Sports Medicine*. 2017; 45(1): 226–233.

Ford RD, Schmitt WP, Lineberry K, Luce P. A retrospective comparison of the management of recalcitrant lateral elbow tendinosis: platelet-rich plasma injections versus surgery. *Hand (N Y)*. 2015; 10(2): 285–291.

Foster TE, Puskas BL, Mandelbaum BR, Gerhardt MB, Rodeo SA. Platelet-rich plasma: from basic science to clinical applications. *American Journal of Sports Medicine*. 2009; 37(11): 2259–2272.

Franceschi F, Papalia R, Franceschetti E, Paciotti M, Maffulli N, Denaro V. Platelet-rich plasma injections for chronic plantar fasciopathy: a systematic review. *British Medical Bulletin*. 2014; 112(1): 83–95.

Grambart ST. Sports medicine and platelet-rich plasma: nonsurgical therapy. *Clinics in Podiatric Medicine and Surgery*. 2015; 32(1): 99–107.

Gamradt ST. PRP as a treatment alternative for symptomatic rotator cuff tendinopathy for patients failing conservative treatments. *Techniques in Orthopaedics*. 2007; 22(1): 26–33.

Gautam VK, Verma S, Batra S, Bhatnagar N, Arora S. Platelet-rich plasma versus corticosteroid injection for recalcitrant lateral epicondylitis: clinical and ultrasonographic evaluation. *Journal of Orthopaedic Surgery*. 2015; 23(1): 1–5.

Gaweda K, Tarczynska M, Krzyzanowski W. Treatment of Achilles tendinopathy with platelet-rich plasma. *International Journal of Sports Medicine*. 2010; 31(8): 577–583.

Geaney LE, Arciero RA, DeBerardino TM, Mazzocca AD. The effects of platelet-rich plasma on tendon and ligament: basic science and clinical application. *Operative Techniques in Sports Medicine*. 2011; 19(3): 160–164.

Georgy JS, Lai LP, Stitik TP, Desai RD, Koon C, Kumbar S, Chen B, Foye PM. Role of PRP in the treatment of knee osteoarthritis. *Current Physical Medicine and Rehabilitation Reports*. 2016; 4(2): 138–144.

Gill SPS, Singh J, Raj M, Singh P, Mittal A, Vishwakarma R. A randomized controlled study to evaluate the effectiveness of local platelet rich plasma (PRP) injection for the management of the cases of planter fasciitis – final outcome of 179 cases at 12 months. *Indian Journal of Applied Research*. 2016; 6(11): 59–64.

Glanzmann MC, Audigé L. Efficacy of platelet-rich plasma injections for chronic medial epicondylitis. *Journal of Hand Surgery (European Volume)*. 2015; 40(7): 744–745.

Gordin K. Comprehensive scientific overview on the use of platelet rich plasma prolotherapy (PRP). *Journal of Prolotherapy*. 2011; 3(4): 813–825.

Görmeli G, Görmeli CA, Ataoglu B, Çolak C, Aslantürk O, Ertem K. Multiple PRP injections are more effective than single injections and hyaluronic acid in knees with early osteoarthritis: a randomized, double-blind, placebo-controlled trial. *Knee Surgery, Sports Traumatology, Arthroscopy*. 2017; 25(3): 958–965.

Gosens T, Den Oudsten BL, Fievez E, van 't Spijker P, Fievez A. Pain and activity levels before and after platelet-rich plasma injection treatment of patellar tendinopathy: a prospective cohort study and the influence of previous treatment. *International Orthopaedics*. 2012; 36(9): 1941–1946.

Gosens T, Peerbooms JC, van Laar W, Den Oudsten BL. Ongoing positive effect of platelet-rich plasma versus corticosteroid injection in lateral epicondylitis: a double-blind randomized controlled trial with 2-year follow-up. *American Journal of Sports Medicine*. 2011; 36(6): 1200–1208.

Georgy JS, Lai LP, Stitik TP, Desai RD, Koon C, Kumbar S, Chen B, Foye PM. Role of PRP in the treatment of knee osteoarthritis. *Current Physical Medicine and Rehabilitation Reports*. 2016; 4(2): 138–144.

Groner C. Platelet-rich plasma: more than a last resort? *Lower Extremity Review Magazine*. 2011: 1–9.

Hall MP, Band PA, Meislin RJ, Jazrawi LM, Cardone DA. Platelet-rich plasma: current concepts and application in sports medicine. *Journal of the American Academy of Orthopaedic Surgeons*. 2009; 17(10): 602–608.

Halpern BC, Chaudhury S, Rodeo SA. Clinical and MRI outcomes after platelet-rich plasma treatment for knee osteoarthritis. *Clinical Journal of Sports Medicine*. 2013; 23(3): 238–239.

Halpern BC, Chaudhury S, Rodeo SA. The role of platelet-rich plasma in inducing musculoskeletal tissue healing. *Musculoskeletal Journal of Hospital Special Surgery*. 2012; 8(2): 137–145.

Hamid AMS, Mohamed Ali MR, Yusof A, George J, Lee LP. Platelet-rich plasma injections for the treatment of hamstring injuries: a randomized controlled trial. *American Journal of Sports Medicine*. 2014; 42(10): 2410–2418.

Hamid M, Yusof A, Ali M. Platelet-rich plasma (PRP) for acute muscle injury: a systematic review. *PLOS One*. 2014; 9(2): 1–7.

Hammond JW, Hinton RY, Curl LA, Muriel JM, Lovering RM. Use of autologous platelet-rich plasma to treat muscle strain injuries. *American Journal of Sports Medicine*. 2009; 37(6): 1135–1142.

Hart R, Safi A, Jajtner P, Puskeiler M, Hartová P, Komzák M. Tibiofemoral chondromalacia treated with platelet-rich plasma and hyaluronic acid. *Current Orthopaedic Practice*. 2017; 28(1): 58–65.

Hauser RA, Maddela HS, Alderman DD, Baehnisch G, Banner R, Blakemore PJ, Calderón JE, Clark GB, DeLaurentis M, Fauley S, Funck J, Gladstein B, Johnson ML, Kramer GH, Neustadt J, Resk J, Salazar JH, Swetlikoff G, Van Pelt RS, Wheaton MT. Journal of Prolotherapy international medical editorial board consensus statement on the use of prolotherapy for musculoskeletal pain. *Journal of Prolotherapy.* 2011; 3(4): 744–764.

Hauser R, Phillips HJ, Maddela H. Platelet rich plasma prolotherapy as first-line treatment for meniscal pathology. *Practical Pain Management.* 2010; 10(6): 53–64.

Hauser RA, Hauser MA. PRP injection technique. *Journal of Prolotherapy.* 2009; 3(12) [cited 2007 May 19] http://www.journalof-prolotherapy.com/pdfs/issue_03/issue_03_12_platelet_rich_plasma.pdf.

Haynesworth SE, Kadiyala S, Liang LN, Bruder SP. Mitogenic stimulation of human mesenchymal stem cells by platelet releasate suggests a mechanism for enhancement of bone repair by platelet concentrate. In *Transactions of the Annual Meeting-Orthopaedic Research Society* (p. 462). 2002; Boston, Massachusetts: Orthopaedic Research Society.

Hossameldin RH, McCain JP. Efficacy of platelet-rich plasma versus hyaluronic acid intraarticular injection in arthroscopic management of Wilkes V temporomandibular joint patients. *International Journal of Oral and Maxillofacial Surgery.* 2017 Mar 1; 46: 229-30.

Hussein M, Hussein T. Effect of autologous platelet leukocyte rich plasma injections on atrophied lumbar multifidus muscle in low back pain patients with monosegmental degenerative disc disease. *International Society of Orthopaedic Surgery and Traumatology.* 2016; 2: 12.

Ihm J, Mautner K, Blazuk J, Singh JR. Platelet-rich plasma versus an eccentric exercise program for recalcitrant lateral elbow tendinopathy. *American Journal of Physical Medicine and Rehabilitation.* 2015; 7(6): 654–661.

Jacobson JA, Yablon CM, Henning PT, Kazmers IS, Urquhart A, Hallstrom B, Asheesh B, Aishwary P. Greater tronchanteric pain syndrome percutaneous tendon fenestration versus platelet-rich plasma injection for treatment of gluteal tendinosis. *Journal of Ultrasound in Medicine.* 2016; 35(11): 2413–2420.

Jia X, Peters PG, Schon L. The use of platelet-rich plasma in the management of foot and ankle conditions. *Operative Techniques in Sports Medicine.* 2011; 19(3): 177–184.

Jubert NJ, Rodríguez L, Reverté-Vinaixa MM, Navarro A. Platelet-rich plasma injections for advanced knee osteoarthritis: a prospective, randomized, double-blinded clinical trial. *Orthopaedic Journal of Sports Medicine.* 2017; 5(2): doi: 10.1177/2325967116689386.

Judson C, Wolf JM. Tennis elbow: blood and platelet-rich plasma (PRP) injections. In *Tennis Elbow* (pp. 73–83). New York, New York: Springer US; 2015.

Kadam R, Agrawal A, Chhallani A, Pandhare S, Gupta A, Sawant R. To assess the effects of platelet rich plasma application on pain in osteoarthritis knee. *International Journal of Research in Orthopaedics.* 2017 Apr 25; 3(3): 436–439.

Karli DC, Robinson BR. Platelet-rich plasma for hamstring tears. *Practical Pain Management.* 2010; 10(5): 10–14.

Kaux JF, Drion PV, Colige A, Pascon F, Libertiaux V, Hoffman A, Janssen L, Heyers A, Nusgens BV, LeGoff C, Gothot A, Cescotto S, Defraigne J-O, Rickert M, Crielaard J-M. Effects of platelet-rich plasma (PRP) on the healing of Achilles tendons of rats. *Wound Repair and Regeneration.* 2012; 20(5): 748–756.

Kazemi M, Azma K, Tavana B, Rezajee Moghaddam F, Panahi A. Autologous blood versus corticosteroid local injection in the short-term treatment of lateral elbow tendinopathy: a randomized clinical trial of efficacy. *American Journal of Physical Medicine & Rehabilitation.* 2010 Aug 1; 89(8): 660–667.

Kajikawa Y, Morihara T, Sakamoto H, Matsuda KI, Oshima Y, Yoshida A, Nagae M, Kawata M, Kubo T. Platelet-rich plasma enhances the initial mobilization of circulation-derived cells for tendon healing. *Journal of Cellular Physiology.* 2008; 215(3): 837–845.

Karaduman M, Okkaoglu MC, Sesen H, Taskesen A, Ozdemir M, Altay M. Platelet-rich plasma versus open surgical release in chronic tennis elbow: a retrospective comparative study. *Journal of Orthopaedics.* 2016; 13(1): 10–14.

Kesikburun S, Tan AK, Yılmaz B, Yaşar E, Yazıcıoğlu K. Platelet-rich plasma injections in the treatment of chronic rotator cuff tendinopathy: a randomized controlled trial with 1-year follow-up. The American journal of sports medicine. 2013 Nov; 41(11): Article ID 2609-16.

Kim E, Lee JH. Autologous platelet-rich plasma versus dextrose prolotherapy for the treatment of chronic recalcitrant plantar fasciitis. PM&R Journal. 2014; 6(2): 152–158.

Kim SA, Kim EH, Kim SY. The effects of hyperosmolar dextrose and autologous serum injection in the experimental articular defect of rabbit. Journal of Korean Academy of Rehabilitation Medicine. 2006; 30(2): 173–178.

Kirchner F, Anitua E. Intradiscal and intra-articular facet infiltrations with plasma rich in growth factors reduce pain in patients with chronic low back pain. Journal of Craniovertebral Junction & Spine. 2016; 7(4): 250.

Kiter E, Celikbas E, Akkaya S, Demirkan F, Kilic BA. Comparison of injection modalities in the treatment of plantar heel pain: a randomized controlled trial. Journal of the American Podiatric Medical Association. 2006; 96(4): 293–296.

Ko GD. Platelet-rich plasma prolotherapy for low back pain caused by sacroiliac joint laxity. Practical Pain Management. 2010: 10(7)55–67.

Ko GD. Mindra S, Lawson GE, Whitmore S, Arseneau L. Case series of ultrasound-guided platelet-rich plasma injections for sacroiliac joint dysfunction. Journal of Back and Musculoskeletal Rehabilitation. (2017): 1–8.

Kon E, Filardo G, Di Matteo B, Marcacci M. The role of platelet-rich plasma in cartilage repair. In Cartilage (pp. 127–138). Berlin, Heidelberg: Springer; 2017.

Kon E, Filardo G, Di Matteo B, Marcacci M. PRP for the treatment of cartilage pathology. The Open Orthopaedics Journal. 2013; 7: 120–128.

Kon E, Filardo G, Di Martino A, Marcacci M. Platelet-rich plasma (PRP) to treat sports injuries: evidence to support its use. Knee Surgery, Sports Traumatology, Arthroscopy. 2011; 19(4): 516–527.

Kon E, Mandelbaum B, Buda R, G Filardo, Delcogliano M, Timoncini A, Fornasari PM, Giannini S, Marcacci M. Platelet-rich plasma intra-articular injection versus hyaluronic acid viscosupplementation as treatments for cartilage pathology: from early degeneration to osteoarthritis. *Arthroscopy: The Journal of Arthroscopic & Related Surgery.* 2011; 27(11): 1490–1501.

Kon E, Buda R, Filardo G. Platelet-rich plasma: intra-articular knee injections produced favorable results on degenerative cartilage lesions. *Knee Surgery, Sports Traumatology, Arthroscopy.* 2010; 18(4): 472–479.

Kon E, Filardo G, Delcogliano M, Presti ML, Russo A, Bondi A, Martino AD, Cenacchi A, Fornasari PM, Marcacci M. Platelet-rich plasma: new clinical application: a pilot study for treatment of jumper's knee. *Injury.* 2009; 40(6): 598–603.

Krogh T, Ellingsen T, Christensen R, Jensen P, Fredberg U. Ultrasound-guided injection therapy of Achilles tendinopathy with platelet-rich plasma or saline: a randomized, blinded, placebo-controlled trial. *American Journal of Sports Medicine.* 2016; 44(8): 1990–1997.

Krogh T, Fredberg U, Stengaard-Pedersen K, Christensen R, Jensen P, Ellingsen T. Treatment of lateral epicondylitis with platelet-rich plasma, glucocorticoid, or saline: a randomized, double-blind, placebo-controlled trial. *American Journal of Sports Medicine.* 2013; 41(3): 625–635.

Krogh T, Bartels EM, Ellingsen T, Stengaard-Pedersen K, Buchbinder R, Fredberg U, Bliddal H, Christensen R. Comparative effectiveness of injection therapies in lateral epicondylitis: a systematic review and network meta-analysis of randomized controlled trials. *American Journal of Sports Medicine.* 2013; 41(6): 1435–1446.

Lana JFSD, Weglein A, Sampson SE, Vicente EF, Huber SC, Souza CV, Ambach MA, Vincent H, Urban-Paffaro A, Onodera CMK, Annichino-Bizzacchi JM, Santana MHA, Belangero WD. Randomized controlled trial comparing hyaluronic acid, platelet-rich plasma and the combination of both in the treatment of mild and moderate osteoarthritis of the knee. *Journal of Stem Cells and Regenerative Medicine.* 2016; 12(2): 69–78.

Lana JFSD, Santana MHA, Belangero WD, Malheiros Luzo AC. *Platelet-Rich Plasma*. Berlin, Heidelberg: Springer Publications; 2014.

Lana JFSD, Santana MHA, Belangero WD, Malheiros Luzo AC. *Platelet-Rich Plasma: Regenerative Medicine: Sports Medicine, Orthopedic, and Recovery of Musculoskeletal Injuries*. Berlin, Heidelberg: Springer Science & Business Media; 2013.

Lebiedziński R, Synder M, Buchcic P, Polguj M, Grzegorzewski A, Sibiński M. A randomized study of autologous conditioned plasma and steroid injections in the treatment of lateral epicondylitis. *International Orthopaedics*. 2015 Nov; 39(11): 2199–2203.

Lee KS, Wilson JJ, Rabago DP, Baer GS, Jacobson JA, Borrero CG. Musculoskeletal applications of platelet-rich plasma: fad or future? *American Journal of Roentgenology*. 2011; 196(3): 628–636.

Levi D, Horn S, Tyszko S, Levin J, Hecht-Leavitt C, Walko E. Intradiscal platelet-rich plasma injection for chronic discogenic low back pain: preliminary results from a prospective trial. *Pain Medicine*. 2016; 17(6): 1010–1022.

Levorova J, Machon V, Foltan R. Platelet-rich plasma in the therapy of osteoarthritis of temporomandibular joint. *International Journal of Oral and Maxillofacial Surgery*. 2017 Mar 1; 46(S1): 230.

Li Y, Cazilas K, Xue J, Tabor L, Luncsford C. Poster 275: Comprehensive Regenerative Therapies with Bone Marrow Stem Cell, PRP and Dextrose Prolotherapy to Treat Severe Degree of Osteoarthritis: A Case Report. *PM&R*. 2017 Sep 1; 9(9): S219.

Linetsky FS, Trescot AM, Wiederholz MH. Regenerative injection therapy. In *Pain Management and Palliative Care* (pp. 369–375). New York, New York: Springer US; 2015.

Lippross S, Moeller B, Haas H, Tohidnezhad M, Steubesand N, Wruck CJ, Kurz B, Seekamp A, Pufe T, Varoga D. Intraarticular injection of platelet-rich plasma reduces inflammation in a pig model of rheumatoid arthritis of the knee joint. *Arthritis & Rheumatology*. 2011; 63(11): 3344–3353.

López-Gavito E, Gómez-Carlín LA, Parra-Téllez P, Vázquez-Escamilla J. Platelet-rich plasma for managing calcaneus tendon tendinopathy and plantar fasciitis. *Acta Ortopedica Mexicana* 2011; 25(6): 380–385.

Lubowitz JH. Editorial commentary: the promise of platelet-rich plasma. *Arthroscopy: The Journal of Arthroscopic & Related Surgery.* 2016; 32(3): 506.

Lyras DN, Kazakos K, Verettas D, Polychronidis A, Tryfonidis M, Botaitis S, Agrogiannis G, Simopoulos C, Kokka A, Patsouris E. The influence of platelet-rich plasma on angiogenesis during the early phase of tendon healing. *Foot & Ankle International.* 2009 Nov; 30(11):1101–1106.

Mahindra P, Yamin M, Selhi HS, Singla S, Soni A. Chronic plantar fasciitis: effect of platelet-rich plasma, corticosteroid, and placebo. *Orthopedics.* 2016; 39(2): e285–289.

Malahias MA, Nikolaou VS, Johnson EO, Kaseta MK, Kazas ST, Babis GC. Platelet-rich plasma ultrasound-guided injection in the treatment of carpal tunnel syndrome: a placebo-controlled clinical study. *Journal of Tissue Engineering and Regenerative Medicine.* 2017 Sep 5 [cited 2017 December 9] https://doi.org/10.1002/term.2566.

Manoil L. Histologic effects of various sclerosing solutions. *Archives of Surgery.* 1938; 36(2): 171–189.

Martinelli N, Marinozzi A, Carnì S, Trovato U, Bianchi A, Denaro V. Platelet-rich plasma injections for chronic plantar fasciitis. *International Orthopaedics.* 2013; 37(5): 839–842.

Marx RE. Platelet-rich plasma: evidence to support its use. *Journal of Oral and Maxillofacial Surgery.* 2004; 62(4): 489–96.

Mautner K, Colberg RE, Malanga G, Borg-Stein JP, Harmon KG, Dharasmi AS, Chu S, Homer P. Outcomes after ultrasound-guided platelet-rich plasma injections for chronic tendinopathy: a multi-center, retrospective review. *PM&R Journal.* 2013; 5(3): 169–175.

Mayo Clinic Health Letter, Tendon Trouble: New treatment uses enhanced plasma. 2010 March, p.7 [cited 2017 February 12]. http://healthletter.mayoclinic.com/common/pdf/192/201003.PDF.

Meheux CJ, McCulloch PC, Lintner DM, Varner KE, Harris JD. Efficacy of intra-articular platelet-rich plasma injections in knee osteoarthritis: a systematic review. *Arthroscopy: The Journal of Arthroscopic & Related Surgery.* 2016; 32(3): 495–505.

Mei-Dan O, Carmont MR, Laver L, Mann G, Maffulli N, Nyska M. Platelet-rich plasma or hyaluronate in the management of osteochondral lesions of the talus. *American Journal of Sports Medicine.* 2012; 40(3): 534–541.

Mi B, Liu G, Zhou W, Lv H, Liu Y, Wu Q, Lui J. Platelet rich plasma versus steroid on lateral epicondylitis: meta-analysis of randomized clinical trials. *Physician and Sportsmedicine.* 2017; 97–104.

Mifune Y, Matsumoto T, Takayama K, Ota S, Li H, Meszaros LB, Usas A, Nagamune K, Gharaibeh B, Fu FH, Huard J. The effect of platelet-rich plasma on the regenerative therapy of muscle derived stem cells for articular cartilage repair. *Osteoarthritis and Cartilage.* 2013; 21(1): 175–185.

Miller LE, Parrish WR, Roides B, Bhattacharyya S. Efficacy of platelet-rich plasma injections for symptomatic tendinopathy: systematic review and meta-analysis of randomised injection-controlled trials. *BMJ Open Sport & Exercise Medicine.* 2017 Nov 1; 3(1): e000237.

Mishra AK, Skrepnik NV, Edwards SG, Jones GL, Sampson S, Vermillion DA, Ramsey ML, Karli DC, Rettig AC. Efficacy of platelet-rich plasma for chronic tennis elbow: a double-blind, prospective, multicenter, randomized controlled trial of 230 patients. *American Journal of Sports Medicine.* 2014; 42(2): 463–471.

Mishra A, Harmon K, Woodall J, Vieira A. Sports medicine applications of platelet rich plasma. *Current Pharmaceutical Biotechnology.* 2012; 13(7): 1185–1195.

Mishra A, Pavelko T. Treatment of chronic elbow tendinosis with buffered platelet-rich plasma. *American Journal of Sports Medicine.* 2006; 34(11): 1774–1778.

Mishra AK, Skrepnik NV, Edwards SG, Jones GL, Sampson S, Vermillion DA, Ramsey ML, Karli DC, Rettig AC. Efficacy of platelet-rich plasma for chronic tennis elbow: a double-blind, prospective, multicenter, randomized controlled trial of 230 patients. *American Journal of Sports Medicine.* 2014; 42(2): 463–471.

Mishra A, Woodall J, Vieira A. Treatment of tendon and muscle using platelet-rich plasma. *Clinical Sports Medicine.* 2009; 28(1): 113–125.

Mishra A, Pavelko T. Treatment of chronic elbow tendinosis with buffered platelet-rich plasma. *American Journal of Sports Medicine.* 2006; 34(11): 1774–1778.

Monfett M, Harrison J, Boachie-Adjei K, Lutz G. Intradiscal platelet-rich plasma (PRP) injections for discogenic low back pain: an update. *International Orthopaedics*. 2016; 40(6): 1321–1328.

Moon SY, Lee ST, Ryu JW. Ultrasound-guided platelet-rich plasma prolotherapy for temporomandibular disorders. *Journal of Oral Medicine & Pain*. 2014; 39(4): 140–145.

Monto RR. Platelet rich plasma treatment for chronic Achilles tendinosis. *Foot Ankle International*. 2012; 33(5): 379–385.

Moraes VY, Lenza M, Tamaoki MJ, Faloppa F, Belloti JC. Platelet-rich therapies for musculoskeletal soft tissue injuries. *Cochrane Database Systematic Reviews*. 2013; 12: CD010071.

Moussa M, Lajeunesse D, Hilal G, Atat OE, Haykal G, Serhal R, Chalhoub A, Khalil C, Alaaeddine N. Platelet rich plasma (PRP) induces chondroprotection via increasing autophagy, anti-inflammatory markers, and decreasing apoptosis in human osteoarthritic cartilage. *Experimental Cell Research*. 2017; 352(1): 146–156.

Munde SL, Jha V, Malik JS. Effectiveness of platelet-rich plasma in the treatment of moderate knee osteoarthritis. *Annals of International Medical and Dental Research*. 2017; 3(4): 42–47.

Murray DJ, Javed S, Jain N, Kemp S, Watts A. Platelet-rich-plasma injections in treating lateral epicondylosis: a review of the recent evidence. *Journal of Hand on Microsurgery*. 2015;7(2): 320–325.

Nasser MET, El Yasaki AZ, Mallah RM, Abdelazeem ASM. Treatment of lateral epicondylitis with platelet-rich plasma, glucocorticoid, or saline. A comparative study. *Egyptian Rheumatology and Rehabilitation*. 2017; 44(1): 1.

Nguyen RT, Borg-Stein J, McInnis K. Applications of platelet-rich plasma in musculoskeletal and sports medicine: an evidence-based approach. *PM&R Journal*. 2011; 3(3): 226–250.

Obata S, Akeda K, Imanishi T, Masuda K, Bae W, Morimoto R, Asanuma Y, Kasai Y, Uchida A, Sudo A. Effect of autologous platelet-rich plasma-releasate on intervertebral disc degeneration in the rabbit annular puncture model: a preclinical study. *Arthritis Research & Therapy*. 2012; 14(6): R241.

Özgürtaş T, Utku B, Yildiz C. Platelet-Rich Plasma. In *Musculoskeletal Research and Basic Science* (pp. 283–288). Berlin, Heidelberg: Springer; 2016.

Pandey V, Bandi A, Madi S, Agarwal L, Acharya KKV, Maddukuri S, Sambhaji C, Willem S. Does application of moderately concentrated platelet-rich plasma improve clinical and structural outcome after arthroscopic repair of medium-sized to large rotator cuff tear? A randomized controlled trial. *Journal of Shoulder and Elbow Surgery.* 2016; 25(8): 1312–1322.

Patel DN, Strauss EJ. Alternative therapeutic modalities in sports medicine. *Bulletin of the NYU Hospital for Joint Diseases.* 2015; 73(2): 122–127.

Patel S, Dhillon MS, Aggarwal S, Marwaha N, Jain A. Treatment with platelet-rich plasma is more effective than placebo for knee osteoarthritis a prospective, double-blind, randomized trial. *American Journal of Sports Medicine.* 2013; 41(2): 356–364.

Paterson KL, Nicholls M, Bennell KL, Bates D. Intra-articular injection of photo-activated platelet-rich plasma in patients with knee osteoarthritis: a double-blind, randomized controlled pilot study. *BMC Musculoskeletal Disorders.* 2016; 17(1): 1.

Paoloni J, De Vos RJ, Hamilton B, Murrell GA, Orchard J. Platelet-rich plasma treatment for ligament and tendon injuries. *Clinical Journal of Sports Medicine.* 2011; 21(1): 37–45.

Patel DN, Strauss EJ. Alternative therapeutic modalities in sports medicine. *Bulletin of the NYU Hospital for Joint Diseases.* 2015; 73(2): 122–122.

Patel M, Sheth C, Patel J, Tihoriwala P. Study of platelet rich plasma injections in patients of tendinopathy in south Gujarat population. *National Journal of Medical Research.* 2016; 6(2): 191–195.

Patel S, Dhillon MS, Aggarwal S, Marwaha N, Jain A. Treatment with platelet-rich plasma is more effective than placebo for knee osteoarthritis a prospective, double-blind, randomized trial. *American Journal of Sports Medicine.* 2013; 41(2): 356–364.

Paterson KL, Nicholls M, Bennell KL, Bates D. Intra-articular injection of photo-activated platelet-rich plasma in patients with knee osteoarthritis: a double-blind, randomized controlled pilot study. *BMC Musculoskeletal Disorders.* 2016; 17(1): 1.

Peerbooms JC, Sluimer J, Bruijn DJ, Gosens T. Positive effects of an autologous platelet concentrate in lateral epicondylitis in a double-blind randomized controlled trial: platelet-rich plasma versus corticosteroid injection with a 1-year follow-up. *American Journal of Sports Medicine*. 2010; 38(2): 255–262.

Piccin A, Di Pierro A, Canzian L, Primerano M, Corvetta D, Negri G, Mazzonleni G, Gastl G, Steurer M, Gentilini I, Eisendle K, Fontanella F. Platelet gel: a new therapeutic tool with great potential. *Blood Transfusion*. 2017; 15(4): 333.

Podesta L, Crow S, Volkmer D, Bert T, Yocum L. Treatment of partial ulnar collateral ligament tears in the elbow with platelet-rich plasma. *American Journal of Sports Medicine*. 2013; 41(7): 1689–1694.

Rabago D, Best TM, Zgierska AE, Zeisig E, Ryan M, Crane D. A systematic review of four injection therapies for lateral epicondylosis: prolotherapy, polidocanol, whole blood and platelet-rich plasma. *British Journal of Sports Medicine*. 2009; 43(7): 471–481.

Rabago D, Wilson J, Zgierska A. Platelet-rich plasma for treatment of Achilles tendinopathy. *Journal of the American Medical Association*. 2010; 303(17): 1696–1697.

Raeissadat SA, Rayegani SM, Hassanabadi H, Rahimi R, Sedighipour L, Rostami K. Plate-rich plasma superior to whole blood in the management of chronic tennis elbow: one year randomized clinical trial. *BMC Sports Science, Medicine, and Rehabilitation*. 2014; 6(12): 1–10.

Raeissadat SA, Sedighipour L, Rayegani SM, Bahrami MH, Bayat M, Rahimi R. Effect of platelet-rich plasma (PRP) versus autologous whole blood on pain and function improvement in tennis elbow: a randomized clinical trial. *Pain Research and Treatment*. 2014; 6(12): 8.

Randelli P, Arrigoni P, Ragone V, Aliprandi A, Cabitza P. Platelet rich plasma in arthroscopic rotator cuff repair: a prospective RCT study, 2-year follow-up. *Journal of Shoulder and Elbow Surgery*. 2011; 20(4): 518–528.

Randelli PS, Fossati C, Menon A, Ragone V, D'Ambrosi R, Cabitza P, de Girolamo L. Use of PRP in sports medicine. In *Arthroscopy and Sport Injuries* (pp. 439–443). Switzerland: Springer International Publishing; 2016.

Repetto I, Biti B, Cerruti P, Trentini R, Felli L. Conservative treatment of ankle osteoarthritis: can platelet-rich platelet rich plasma effectively postpone surgery. *Journal of Foot and Ankle Surgery.* 2017; 56(2): 362–365.

Reurink G, Goudswaard GJ, Moen MH, Weir A, Verhaar JAN, Bierma-Zeinstra SMA, Maas M, Tol JL. Platelet-rich plasma injections in acute muscle injury. *New England Journal of Medicine.* 2014; 370(26): 2546–2547.

Rha DW, Park GY, Kim YK, Kim MT, Lee SC. Comparison of the therapeutic effects of ultrasound-guided platelet-rich plasma injection and dry needling in rotator cuff disease: a randomized controlled trial. *Clinical Rehabilitation.* 2013; 27(2): 113–122.

Robins RJ. Platelet rich plasma: current indications and use in orthopaedic care. *Medical Research Archives.* 2017; 5(6): 1–17.

Sandrey MA. Autologous growth factor injections in chronic tendinopathy. *Journal of Athletic Training.* 2014; 49(3): 428–430.

Sampson S, Gerhardt M, Mandelbaum B. Platelet rich plasma injection grafts for musculoskeletal injuries: a review. *Current Reviews in Musculoskeletal Medicine.* 2008; 1(3): 165–174.

Sampson S, Reed M, Silvers H, Meng M, Mandelbaum B. Injection of platelet-rich plasma in patients with primary and secondary knee osteoarthritis: a pilot study. *Archives of Physical Medicine and Rehabilitation.* 2010; 89(12): 961–969.

Sampson S, Aufiero D, Meng M, Bledin A, Gillette T, Zall M. Platelet-rich plasma therapy as a first-line treatment for severe Achilles tendon tear: a case report. *International Journal of Therapy and Rehabilitation.* 2011; 18(2): 101.

Sánchez M, Anitua E, Diego D, Sanchez P, Prado R, Goiriena JJ, Prosper F, Orive G, Padilla S. A new strategy to tackle severe knee osteoarthritis: combination of intra-articular and intraosseous injections of platelet rich plasma. *Expert Opinion on Biological Therapy.* 2016; 627–643.

Sánchez M, Delgado D, Sánchez P, Anitua E, Padilla S. Plasma rich in growth factors for the treatment of skeletal muscle injury. In *Muscle Injuries in Sport Athletes* (pp. 451–464). Switzerland: Springer International Publishing; 2017.

Sánchez M, Anitua E, Orive G, Mujika I, Andia I. Platelet-rich therapies in the treatment of orthopaedic sport injuries. *Sports Medicine.* 2009; 39(5): 345–354.

Saucedo JM, Yaffe MA, Berschback JC, Hsu WK, Kalainov DM. Platelet-rich plasma. *Journal of Hand Surgery.* 2012; 37(3): 587–589.

Scarpone M, Rabago D, Snell E, DeMeo P, Ruppert K, Pritchard P, Arbogast G, Wilson JJ, Balzano JF. Effectiveness of platelet-rich plasma injection for rotator cuff tendinopathy: a prospective open-label study. *Global Advances in Health and Medicine.* 2013; 2(2): 26–31.

Schapiro A, Lee K, Rabago D, Wilson J. 2092355 Platelet-rich plasma and hyperosmolar dextrose (prolotherapy) for lateral epicondylosis: power Doppler sonographic assessment of tendon neovascularity as a measure of healing response. *Ultrasound in Medicine and Biology.* 2015; 41(4): S88–S89.

Schickendantz M, King D. Nonoperative management (including ultrasound-guided injections) of proximal biceps disorders. *Clinics in Sports Medicine.* 2016; 35(1): 57–73.

Scioli MW. Treatment of recalcitrant enthesopathy of the hip with platelet rich plasma—a report of three cases. *Clinical Orthopaedic Society News.* 2006: 6–7.

Scioli MW. Platelet-rich plasma injection for proximal plantar fasciitis. *Techniques in Foot & Ankle Surgery.* 2011; 10(1): 7–10.

Seppä H, Grotendorst G, Seppä S, Schiffmann E, Martin GR. Platelet-derived growth factor in chemotactic for fibroblasts. *Journal of Cell Biology.* 1982; 92(2): 584–588.

Shahid M, Kundra R. Platelet-rich plasma (PRP) for knee disorders. *EFORT Open Reviews.* 2017; 2(2): 28–34.

Shen L, Yuan T, Chen S, Xie X, Zhang C. The temporal effect of platelet-rich plasma on pain and physical function in the treatment of knee osteoarthritis: systematic review and meta-analysis of randomized controlled trials. *Journal of Orthopaedic Surgery and Research.* 2017; 12(1): 16.

Singla A, Jain M. Biological Regeneration of Tissues-Latest Therapeutic Approach Using Platelet Rich Plasma. *Blood Research and Transfusion Journal.* 2017;1(1):1-3.

Singla V, Batra YK, Bharti N, Goni VG, Marwaha N. Steroid vs. platelet-rich plasma in ultrasound-guided sacroiliac joint interjection for chronic low back pain. *Pain Practice*. 2017; 17(6): 782–791.

Soliman DM. Advantages of Dextrose, Platelet Rich Plasma and Stem Cells over the Traditional Conventional Methods in Treatment of Sports Injuries and Joint Osteoarthritis. *Journal of Sports Science*. 2017; 5: 113–118.

Sully KA, Sayeed YA, Patel BC. Poster 422: Successful Treatment of Cervical Facet Joint Pain using Platelet Rich Plasma—A Novel Case Report. *PM&R*. 2017 Sep 30; 9(9): S266.

Tan XX, Ju HY, Yan W, Jiang HJ, Su JP, Dong HJ, Wang L-S, Zou D-B. Autologous platelet lysate local injections for the treatment of refractory lateral epicondylitis. *Journal of Orthopaedic Surgery and Research*. 2016; 11(1): 17.

Tate KS, Crane D. Platelet rich plasma grafts in musculoskeletal medicine. *Journal of Prolotherapy*. 2010; 2: 371–376.

Taylor DW, Petrera M, Hendry M, Theodoropoulos JS. A systematic review of the use of plate-rich plasma in sports medicine as a new treatment for tendon and ligament injuries. *Clinical Journal of Sports Medicine*. 2011; 21(4): 344–352.

Tetschke E, Rudolf M, Lohmann CH, Stärke C. Autologous proliferative therapies in recalcitrant lateral epicondylitis. *American Journal of Physical Medicine & Rehabilitation*. 2015; 94(9): 696–706.

Thanasas C, Papadimitriou G, Charalambidis C, Paraskevopoulos I, Papanikolaou A. Platelet-rich plasma versus autologous whole blood for the treatment of chronic lateral elbow epicondylitis. *American Journal of Sports Medicine*. 2011; 39(10): 2130–2134.

Tiwari M, Bhargava R. Platelet rich plasma therapy: a comparative effective therapy with promising results in plantar fasciitis. *Journal of Clinical Orthopaedics and Trauma*. 2013; 4(1): 31–35.

Tolbert G. Poster 431: Ultrasound Guided Dextrose Prolotherapy with Platelet Rich Plasma for Sacroiliac Pain: A Case Report. *PM&R*. 2017 Sep 30; 9(9): S269.

Tolbert G, Roy D, Walker V. Ultrasound guided dextrose prolotherapy and platelet rich plasma therapy in chronic low back pain: three case reports. *International Journal of Physical Medicine and Rehabilitation.* 2013; 1(149): 2.

Tuakli-Wosornu YA, Terry A, Boachie-Adjei K, Harrison JR, Gribbin CK, LaSalle EE, Nguyen JT, Solomon JL, Lutz GE. Lumbar intradiskal platelet-rich plasma (PRP) injections: a prospective, double-blind, randomized controlled study. *PM&R Journal.* 2016; 8(1): 1–10.

Van Ark M, Zwerver J, Van den Akker-Scheek I. Injection treatments for patellar tendinopathy. *British Journal of Sports Medicine.* 2011; 45(13): 1068–1076.

Vannini F, Di Matteo B, Filardo G, Kon E, Marcacci M, Giannini S. Platelet-rich plasma for foot and ankle pathologies: a systematic review. *Foot & Ankle Surgery.* 2014; 20(1): 2–9.

Vetrano M, Castorina A, Vulpiani MC, Baldini R, Pavan A, Ferretti A. Platelet-rich plasma versus focused shock waves in the treatment of jumper's knee in athletes. *American Journal of Sports Medicine.* 2013; 41(4): 795–803.

Vora A, Borg-Stein J, Nguyen RT. Regenerative injection therapy for osteoarthritis: fundamental concepts and evidence-based review. *PM&R Journal.* 2012; 4: S104–S109.

Weglein A, Sampson S, Aufiero D. Platelet rich plasma practical use in non-surgical musculoskeletal pathology. In *Platelet-Rich Plasma* (pp. 187–201). Berlin, Heidelberg: Springer; 2014.

Wei LC, Gao SG, Xu M, Jiang W, Tian J, Lei GH. A novel hypothesis: the application of platelet-rich plasma can promote the clinical healing of white-white meniscal tears. *Medical Science Monitor.* 2012; 18(8): HY47.

Wesner M, Defreitas T, Bredy H, Pothier L, Qin Z, McKillop AB, Gross DP. A pilot study evaluating the effectiveness of platelet-rich plasma therapy for treating degenerative tendinopathies: a randomized control trial with synchronous observational cohort. *PLOS One.* 2016; 11(2): e0147842.

Wright-Carpenter T, Klein P, Schäferhoff P. Treatment of muscle injuries by local administration of autologous conditioned serum: animal experiments using a muscle contusion model. *International Journal of Sports Medicine.* 2004; 25(8): 588–593.

Wu J, Du Z, Lv Y, Zhang J, Xiong W, Wang R, Liu R, Zhang G, Liu Q. A new technique for the treatment of lumbar facet joint syndrome using intra-articular injection with autologous platelet rich plasma. *Pain Physician*. 2016; 19(8): 617–625.

Wu PI, Diaz R, Borg-Stein J. Platelet-rich plasma. *Physical Medicine & Rehabilitation Clinics of North America*. 2016; 27(4): 825–853.

Xie X, Chang C, Tuan R. Biology of platelet-rich plasma and its clinical application in cartilage repair. *Arthritis Research & Therapy*. 2014; 16(1): 204.

Yadav R, Kothari SY, Borah D. Comparison of local injection of platelet-rich plasma and corticosteroid in the treatment of lateral epicondylitis of humerus. *Journal of Clinical Diagnostic Research. JDCR*. 2015; 9(7): RC05.

Zhang JY, Fabricant PD, Ishmael CR, Wang JC, Petrigliano FA, Jones KJ. Utilization of platelet-rich plasma for musculoskeletal injuries: an analysis of current treatment trends in the United States. *Orthopaedic Journal of Sports Medicine*. 2016; 4(12): 2325967116676241.

Ziltener JL, Didisheim C, Borloz S. Injections of plate-rich plasma (PRP) for the treatment of sports injuries: a review. *Sportmedizin & Sporttraumatologie*. 2012; 60: 157–160.

Biocellular (Stem Cell–Rich) Prolotherapy

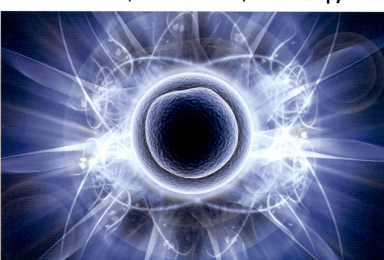

Adriani E, Moio M, Di Paola B, Salustri W, Alfieri A, Parisi P, Ruggiero M, Borab Z, Carlesimo B. Percutaneous Fat Transfer to Treat Knee Osteoarthritis Symptoms: Preliminary Results. *Joints*. 2017 Jun; 5(02): 89–92.

Albano JJ, Alexander RW. Autologous fat grafting as a mesenchymal stem cell source and living bioscaffold in a patellar tendon tear. *Clinical Journal of Sports Medicine*. 2011; 21(4): 359–361.

Alderman DD. State of the art: prolotherapy regenerative medicine. *Pain Week Journal*. 2016; 4(4): 44.

Alderman DD. Regenerative injection therapies for pain: traditional, rich platelet rich plasma and biocellular prolotherapy. In *Integrative Pain Management* (pp. 345–360). New York, New York: Oxford University Press; 2016.

Alderman DD. The new age of prolotherapy. *Practical Pain Management*. 2010; 10(4): 54–68.

Alderman DD, Alexander RW. Advances in regenerative medicine: high-density platelet-rich plasma and stem cell prolotherapy for musculoskeletal pain. *Practical Pain Management*. 2011; 11(8): 49–90.

Alderman DD, Alexander RW, Harris G, Astourian PC. Stem cell prolotherapy in regenerative medicine: background, theory and protocols. *Journal of Prolotherapy.* 2011; 3(3): 689–708.

Alexander RW. Biocellular regenerative medicine: use of adipose-derived stem/stromal cells and its native bioactive matrix. *Physical Medicine and Rehabilitation Clinics.* 2016 Nov 1; 27(4): 871–891.

Alexander RW. Understanding mechanical emulsification (nanofat) versus enzymatic isolation of tissue stromal vascular fraction (tSVF) cells from adipose tissue: potential uses in biocellular regenerative medicine. *Journal of Prolotherapy.* 2016; 8: e947–e960.

Alexander RW. Understanding adipose-derived stromal vascular fraction (AD-SVF) cell biology and use on the basis of cellular, chemical, structural and paracrine components: a concise review. *Journal of Prolotherapy.* 2012; 4: e855–e869.

Alexander RW. Autologous fat grafts as mesenchymal stromal stem cell source for use in prolotherapy: a simple technique to acquire lipoaspirants. *Journal of Prolotherapy.* 2011; 3(1): 680–688.

Andia I, Maffulli N. Biological therapies in regenerative sports medicine. *Sports Medicine.* 2017; 47(5): 807–828.

Behfar M, Sarrafzadeh-Rezaei F, Hobbenaghi R, Delirezh N, Dalir-Naghadeh B. Enhanced mechanical properties of rabbit flexor tendons in response to intratendinous injection of adipose derived stromal vascular fraction. *Current Stem Cell Research & Therapy.* 2012; 7(3): 173–178.

Brown MN, Shiple BJ, Scarpone M. Regenerative approaches to tendon and ligament conditions. *Physical Medicine and Rehabilitation Clinics of North America.* 2016; 27(4): 941–984.

Canapp DA, Sherman O, Ibrahim V, Carr BJ, Cox C, Barrett JG. The use of adipose-derived progenitor cells and platelet-rich plasma combination for the treatment of supraspinatus tendinopathy in 55 dogs: a retrospective study. *Frontiers in Veterinary Science.* 2016: 3.

Centeno CJ, Pitts J, Al-Sayegh H, Freeman M.D.. Anterior cruciate ligament tears treated with percutaneous injection of autologous bone marrow nucleated cells: a case series. *Journal of Pain Research.* 2015; 8: 437–447.

Correia SI, Pereira H, Silva-Correia J, Van Dijk CN, Espregueira-Mendes J, Oliveira JM. Current concepts: tissue engineering and regenerative medicine applications in the ankle joint. *Journal of the Royal Society Interface*. 2014; 11(92): 20130784.

Crane DM, Oliver KS, Bayes MC. Orthobiologics and knee osteoarthritis: a recent literature review, treatment algorithm, and pathophysiology discussion. *Physical Medicine and Rehabilitation Clinics of North America*. 2016; 27(4): 985–1002.

Davatchi F, Sadeghi Abdollahi B, Mohyeddin M, Nikbin B. Mesenchymal stem cell therapy for knee osteoarthritis: 5-years follow-up of three patients. *International Journal of Rheumatic Diseases*. 2015 [cited 2015 September 6] http://www.ncbi.nlm.nih.gov/pubmed/25990685.

DeChellis M.D., Cortazzo MH. Regenerative medicine in the field of pain medicine: prolotherapy, platelet-rich plasma therapy, and stem cell therapy—theory and evidence. *Techniques in Regional Anesthesia and Pain Management*. 2011; 15(2): 74–80.

De Girolamo L, Grassi M, Viganò M, Orfei CP, Montrasio UA, Usuelli F. Treatment of Achilles tendinopathy with autologous adipose-derived stromal vascular fraction results of a randomized prospective clinical trial. *Orthopaedic Journal of Sports Medicine*. 2016; 4(7): 232596711.

Eating HH. Osteoarthritis Pain Relief and Repair with Stem Cell Prolotherapy. PAIN. 2017 Nov 7. [cited 2017 Nov 7]. http://sflhealthandwellness.com/osteoarthritis-pain-relief-and-repair-with-stem-cell-prolotherapy/.

Emadedin M, Ghorbani Liastani M, Fazeli R, Mohseni F, Moghadasali R, Mardpour S, Hosseini SE, Niknejad M, Moeininia F, Fanni AA, Eslamine RB, Dizaji AV, Labibzadeh N, Bafghi AM, Baharvand H, Aghdam N. Long-term follow-up of intra-articular injection of autologous mesenchymal stem cells in patients with knee, ankle, or hip osteoarthritis. *Archives of Iranian Medicine*. 2015; 18(6): 336–344.

Garcia CJ. Treatment of lumbar degenerative disc disease with adipose derived stromal vascular fraction, point of care. Paper presented at the IFATS Quebec Conference; 2012.

Hauser RA, Speciale TL. Osteoarthritis pain relief and repair with stem cell prolotherapy. *Neuromodulation*; 2017 [cited 2017 June 5]. http://sflhealthandwellness.com/osteoarthritis-pain-relief-and-repair-with-stem-cell-prolotherapy/.

Hauser RA, Eteshola E. Rationale for using direct bone marrow aspirate as a proliferant for regenerative injection therapy (prolotherapy). *Open Stem Cell Journal*. 2013; 4(1): 7–14.

Hauser RA, Maddela HS, Alderman DD, Baehnisch G, Banner R, Blakemore PJ, Calderón JE, Clark GB, DeLaurentis M, Fauley S, Funck J, Gladstein B, Johnson ML, Kramer GH, Neustadt J, Resk J, Salazar JH, Swetlikoff G, Van Pelt RS, Wheaton MT. Journal of Prolotherapy international medical editorial board consensus statement on the use of prolotherapy for musculoskeletal pain. *Journal of Prolotherapy*. 2011; 3(4): 744–764.

Hauser RA, Orlofsky A. Regenerative injection therapy with whole bone marrow aspirate for degenerative joint disease: a case series. *Clinical Medicine Insights: Arthritis and Musculoskeletal Disorders*. 2013; 6: 65.

Hauser RA, Ostergaard S. Direct bone marrow injections for avascular necrosis of the talus. *Journal of Prolotherapy*. 2012; 4: e891–e894.

Hauser RA, Woldin B. Treating osteoarthritic joints using dextrose prolotherapy and direct bone marrow aspirate injection therapy. *Open Arthritis Journal*. 2014; 7(1): 1–9.

Herold C, Rennekampff HO, Groddeck R, Allert S. Autologous fat transfer for thumb carpometacarpal joint osteoarthritis: A prospective study. *Plastic and Reconstructive Surgery*. 2017 Aug 1; 140(2): 327-335.

Jo CH, Chai JW, Jeong EC, Oh S, Shin JS, Shim H, Yoon KS. Intra-articular Injection of Mesenchymal Stem Cells for the Treatment of Osteoarthritis of the Knee: A 2-Year Follow-up Study. *The American Journal of Sports Medicine*. 2017 Oct; 45(12): 2774–2783.

Jo CH, Lee YG, Shin WH, Kim H, Chai JW, Jeong EC, Kim JE, Shim H, Shin JS, Shin IS, Ra JC, Oh S, Yoon KS. Intra-articular injection of mesenchymal stem cells for the treatment of osteoarthritis of the knee: a proof-of-concept clinical trial. *Stem Cells*. 2014; 32(5): 1254–1266.

Kim YS, Kwon OR, Choi YJ, Suh DS, Heo DB, Koh YG. Comparative matched-pair analysis of the injection versus implantation of mesenchymal stem cells for knee osteoarthritis. *American Journal of Sports Medicine*. 2015; 43(11): 2738–2746.

Koh YG, Choi YJ. Infrapatellar fat pad-derived mesenchymal stem cell therapy for knee osteoarthritis. *Knee*. 2012; 19(6): 902–907.

Koh YG, Choi YJ, Kwon SK, Kim YS, Yeo JE. Clinical results and second-look arthroscopic findings after treatment with adipose-derived stem cells for knee osteoarthritis. *Knee Surgery, Sports Traumatology, Arthroscopy*. 2015; 23(5): 1308–1316.

Yokota N, Yamakawa M, Shirata T, Kimura T, Kaneshima H. Clinical results following intra-articular injection of adipose-derived stromal vascular fraction cells in patients with osteoarthritis of the knee. *Regenerative Therapy*. 2017; 6: 108–112.

Kristin C, Silbert R, Parlo M. Effects of the intradiscal implantation of stromal vascular fraction plus platelet rich plasma in patients with degenerative disc disease. *Journal of Translational Medicine*. 2017; 15(12): 12.

Lee JM, Kim BS, Lee H, Im GI. In vivo tracking of mesenchymal stem cells using fluorescent nanoparticles in an osteochondral repair model. *Molecular Therapy*. 2012; 20(7): 1434–1442.

Lee SY, Kim W, Lim C, Chung SG. Treatment of lateral epicondylosis by using allogeneic adipose-derived mesenchymal stem cells: a pilot study. *Stem Cells*. 2015; 33(10): 2995–3005.

Li Y, Cazilas K, Xue J, Tabor L, Luncsford C. Poster 275: Comprehensive Regenerative Therapies with Bone Marrow Stem Cell, PRP and Dextrose Prolotherapy to Treat Severe Degree of Osteoarthritis: A Case Report. *PM&R*. 2017 Sep 1; 9(9): S219.

Maffulli N. *Platelet Rich Plasma in Musculoskeletal Practice*. Berlin, Heidelberg: Springer; 2016.

Man Y, Wang P, Guo Y, Xiang L, Yang Y, Qu Y, Gong P, Deng L. Angiogenic and osteogenic potential of platelet-rich plasma and adipose-derived stem cell laden alginate microspheres. *Biomaterials*. 2012; 33(34): 8802–8811.

Mautner K, Blazuk J. Where do injectable stem cell treatments apply in treatment of muscle, tendon, and ligament injuries? *PM&R Journal*. 2015; 7(4): S33–S40.

Mitchell B, Bates D, Verrills P, Vivian D, Barnard A. Biological cell therapies for discogenic low back pain. *Journal of Science and Medicine in Sport*. 2017; 20: e43.

Oliver KS, Bayes M, Crane D, Pathikonda C. Clinical outcome of bone marrow concentrate in knee osteoarthritis. *Journal of Prolotherapy*. 2015; 7: e937–e946.

Oliver KS, Crane DM. A publication of regenerative medicine techniques. *Journal of Prolotherapy*. 2010; 2(2): 371–376.

Onishi K, Alderman DD, Alexander R. Autologous adipose-derived stromal/stem cells with platelet-rich plasma as biocellular regenerative therapy in the treatment of chronic proximal hamstring tendon tear. Poster presented in front of the Association of Academic Physiatrists; 2013.

Pak J, Lee JH, Park KS, Park M, Kang LW, Lee SH. Current use of autologous adipose tissue-derived stromal vascular fraction cells for orthopedic applications. *Journal of Biomedical Science*. 2017; 24(1): 9.

Pak J, Lee JH, Park KS, Lee SH. Efficacy of autologous adipose tissue-derived stem cells with extracellular matrix and hyaluronic acid on human hip osteoarthritis. *Biomedical Research*. 2017; 28(4).

Pak J, Lee JH, Kartolo WA, Lee SH. Cartilage regeneration in human with adipose tissue-derived stem cells: current status in clinical implications. *BioMedical Research International*. 2016; Article ID 4702674, 12 pages, doi:10.1155/2016/4702674.

Pak J, Lee JH, Lee SH. Regenerative repair of damaged meniscus with autologous adipose tissue-derived stem cells. *BioMedical Research International*. 2014; Article ID 436029, 10 pages, doi:10.1155/2014/436029.

Pascual-Garrido C, Rolón A, Makino A. Treatment of chronic patellar tendinopathy with autologous bone marrow stem cells: a 5-year-followup. *Stem Cells International*. 2012; Article ID 953510, 5 pages, doi:10.1155/2012/953510.

Perdisa F, GostyNska N, Roffi A, Filardo G, Marcacci M, Kon E. Adipose-derived mesenchymal stem cells for the treatment of articular cartilage: a systematic review on preclinical and clinical evidence. *Stem Cells International.* 2015; Article ID 597652, 13 pages, doi:10.1155/2015/597652.

Randelli P, Menon A, Ragone V, Carmont MR, Espregueira-Mendes J, Marcacci M, Neil J, Oliveira JM, Ortolani A, Azzalini E, Pereira H, Silva-Correia J, Reis RL, Ripóll P, Russo A, Cabitza P, Banfi G. Head, low-back and muscle injuries in athletes: PRP and stem cells in sports-related diseases. In *ESSKA Instructional Course Lecture Book* (pp. 273–311). Berlin, Heidelberg: Springer; 2014.

Sampson S, Botto-van-Bemden A, Aufiero D. Autologous bone marrow concentrate: review and application of a novel intra-articular orthobiologic for cartilage disease. *Physician and Sportsmedicine.* 2013; 41(3): 7–18.

Sampson S, Smith J, Vincent H, Aufiero D, Zall M, Botto-van-Bemden A. Intra-articular bone marrow concentrate injection protocol: short-term efficacy in osteoarthritis. *Regenerative Medicine.* 2016; 11(6): 511–520.

Singh A, Gangwar D, Singh S. Bone marrow injection: a novel treatment for tennis elbow. *Journal of Natural Science, Biology, and Medicine.* 2014; 5(2): 389–391.

Soliman DM. Advantages of dextrose, platelet rich plasma and stem cells over the traditional conventional methods in treatment of sports injuries and joint osteoarthritis. *Journal of Sports Science.* 2017; 5: 113–118.

Striano RD, Battista V, Bilboo N. Non-responding knee pain with osteoarthritis, meniscus and ligament tears treated with ultrasound guided autologous, micro-fragmented and minimally manipulated adipose tissue. *Open Journal of Regenerative Medicine.* 2017; 6(2): 17–26.

Tate-Oliver K, Alexander RW. Combination of autologous adipose-derived tissue stromal vascular fraction plus high density platelet-rich plasma or bone marrow concentrates in Achilles in tendon tears. *Journal of Prolotherapy.* 2013; 5: e895–e912.

Thompson C, Visco C. Lateral epicondylosis: emerging management options. *Current Sports Medicine Reports.* 2015; 14(3): 215–220.

Uysal CA, Tobita M, Hyakusoku H, Mizuno H. Adipose-derived stem cells enhance primary tendon repair: biomechanical and immunohistochemical evaluation. *Journal of Plastic, Reconstructive & Aesthetic Surgery.* 2012; 65(12): 1712–1719.

Vangsness CT, Farr J, Boyd J, Dellaero DT, Mills CR, Leroux-Williams M. Adult human mesenchymal stem cells delivered via intra-articular injection to the knee following partial medial meniscectomy: a randomized, double-blind, controlled study. *Journal of Bone and Joint Surgery.* 2014; 96(2): 90–98.

Vega A, Martín-Ferrero MA, Del Canto F, Alberca M, García V, Munar A, Orozco L, Soler R, Fuertes JJ, Huguet M, Sánchez A, García-Sancho J. Treatment of knee osteoarthritis with allogeneic bone marrow mesenchymal stem cells: a randomized controlled trial. *Transplant.* 2015; 99(8): 1681–1690.

Xia P, Wang X, Lin Q, Li X. Efficacy of mesenchymal stem cells injection for the management of knee osteoarthritis: a systematic review and meta-analysis. *International Orthopaedics.* 2015; 39(12): 2363–2372.

Yang X, Zhu TY, Wen LC. Intraarticular injection of allogenic mesenchymal stem cells has a protective role for the osteoarthritis. *Chinese Medical Journal.* 2015; 128(18): 2516–2523.

Yu H, Adesida AB, Jomha NM. Meniscus repair using mesenchymal stem cells—a comprehensive review. *Stem Cell Research & Therapy.* 2015; 6(1): 86.

Zeckser J, Wolff M, Tucker J, Goodwin J. Multipotent mesenchymal stem cell treatment for discogenic low back pain and disc degeneration. *Stem Cells International.* 2016; Article ID 3908389, 13 pages, doi:10.1155/2016/3908389.

References Cited

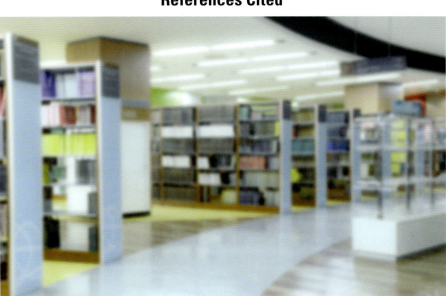

Preface

[1] Uhl RL, Roberts TT, Papaliodis DN, Mulligan MT, Dubin AH. Management of chronic musculoskeletal pain. *Journal of the American Academy of Orthopaedic Surgeons.* 2014; 22(2): 101–110.

[2] American Academy of Orthopaedic Surgeons. One in two Americans have a musculoskeletal condition: New report outlines the prevalence, scope, cost and projected growth of musculoskeletal disorders in the U.S. ScienceDaily. 2016 March 1 [cited 2017 August 24] www.sciencedaily.com/releases/2016/03/160301114116.htm.

[3] Kay MC, Register-Mihalik JK, Gray AD, Djoko A, Dompier TP, Kerr ZY. The epidemiology of severe injuries sustained by national collegiate athletic association student-athletes, 2009–2010 through 2014–2015. *Journal of Athletic Training.* 2017; 52(2): 117–128; Åman M, Forssblad M, Henriksson-Larsén K. Incidence and severity of reported acute sports injuries in 35 sports using insurance registry data. *Scandinavian Journal of Medicine & Science in Sports.* 2016; 26(4): 451–462.

[4] Center for Disease Control and Prevention, Osteoarthritis Fact Sheet, last update 2017 Feb [cited 2017 May 17] https://www.cdc.gov/arthritis/basics/osteoarthritis.htm.

[5] Wehling P, Moser C, Maixner W. How does surgery compare with advanced intra-articular therapies in knee osteoarthritis: Current thoughts. *Therapeutic Advances in Musculoskeletal Disease.* 2016; 8(3): 72–85.

[6] Tyson P. The Hippocratic oath today. PBS/KQED. 2001 Mar 27 [cited 2016 March 27] http://www.pbs.org/wgbh/nova/body/hippocratic-oath-today.html.

Chapter 1: The Exciting Possibilities of Regenerative Medicine

[1] Alexander RW. Biocellular regenerative medicine: Use of adipose-derived stem/stromal cells and its native bioactive matrix. *Physical Medicine & Rehabilitation Clinics of North America.* 2016; 27(4): 871–891; Liu S, Jiang L, Li H, Shi H, Luo H, Zhang Y, Yu C, Jin Y. Mesenchymal stem cells prevent hypertrophic scar formation via inflammatory regulation when undergoing apoptosis. *Journal of Investigative Dermatology.* 2014 Oct 31; 134(10): 2648-2657; Zhang Q, Liu LN, Yong Q, Deng JC, Cao WG. Intralesional injection of adipose-derived stem cells reduces hypertrophic scarring in a rabbit ear model. *Stem Cell Research & Therapy.* 2015 Aug 18; 6(1): 145.

Chapter 2: Osteopathic Medicine and What is a D.O.?

[1] The Business and Professions Code for of California (where I live) notes, "It is the policy of this state that holders of M.D. degrees and D.O. degrees shall be accorded equal professional status and privileges as licensed physicians and surgeons." *State of California, Business and Professions Code.* Section 2453(a). [cited 2016 March 17] http://www.leginfo.ca.gov/cgi-bin/displaycode?section=bpc&group=02001-03000&file=2450-2459.7.

[2] Still AT. Philosophy of Osteopathy. Kirksville, Missouri: Still AT, 1899. As cited in Stark, Jane Eliza. Quoting A. T. Still with rigor: An historical and academic review. *Journal of the American Osteopathic Association.* 2012; 112(6): 366–373.

[3] *Journal of Osteopathy.* Kirksville, MO. 1895 October; II (7) from Still National Osteopathic Museum. [cited 2016 March 17] https://www.atsu.edu/museum/subscription/pdfs/JournalofOsteopathyVol2No71895October.pdf.

[4] Gevitz N. The 'Little M.D.' or the 'Big D.O.': The path to the California merger. *Journal of the American Osteopathic Association.* 2014; 114(5): 390–402.

Chapter 3: The History of Prolotherapy Regenerative Medicine

[1] Gedney E. Special technic: hypermobile joint: A preliminary report. *Osteopathic Profession.* 1937; 4(9): 30–31.

[2] Shuman D. Sclerotherapy–injections may be best way to restrengthen ligaments in case of slipped knee cartilage. *The Osteopathic Profession.* 1949 March; 16(6): 18–19.

[3] Pomeroy KL. Schlerotherapy, prolotherapy and orthopedic medicine: A historical review. Presented at the American College of Osteopathic Schlerotherapeutic Pain Management seminar, 2002.

[4] Hauser RA, Hauser MA. *Prolo Your Pain Away, 3rd Edition,* Caring Medical and Rehabilitation, Oak Park, Illinois, 2004.

[5] Schultz LW. A treatment for subluxation of the temporomandibular joint. *Journal of the American Medical Association.* 1937 September 25; 109(13): 1032–1035.

[6] C. Everett Koop, Preface. In *Hauser, Prolo Your Pain Away, 1st Edition.* Oak Park, Illinois: Beulah Land Press, 1998.

Chapter 5: Prolotherapy Basics

[1] Andriacchi T, Sabiston P, DeHaven K, Dahners L, Woo S, Frank C, Oakes B, Brand R, Lewis J. Ligament: Injury and repair. In *Injury and Repair of the Musculoskeletal Soft Tissues* (pp. 103–128). Park Ridge, Illinois: American Academy of Orthopedic Surgeons, 1988.

[2] Benjamin M, Ralphs JR. Tendons and ligaments-an overview. *Histology and Histopathology.* 1997; 12(4): 1135–1144.

[3] Medical definition of "chronic." *Medicine Net.com* [cited 2017 August 13] http://www.medicinenet.com/script/main/art.asp?articlekey=2728.

[4] Hackett GS, Henderson DG. Joint stabilization: An experimental, histologic study with comments on the clinical application in ligament proliferation. *American Journal of Surgery.* 1955; 80: 968–973; Alpers B.J. The problem of sciatica. *Medical Clinics of North America.* 1953; 37: 503.

[5] Hackett GS, Hemwall GA, Montgomery GA. In *Ligament and Tendon Relaxation Treated by Prolotherapy*, 5th ed. (p. 9). Commenting on work of Newman PH. Oak Brook, Illinois: Institute in Basic Life Principles, 1991.

[6] Reeves KD. Prolotherapy: Basic science, clinical studies and technique. In *Pain Procedures in Clinical Practice, 2nd Edition* (pp. 172–190). Philadelphia, Pennsylvania: Hanley and Belfus, 2000.

[7] Reeves KD, Fullerton BD, Topol G. Evidence-based regenerative injection therapy (prolotherapy) in sports medicine. In *The Sports Medicine Resource Manual* (p. 611–619). Philadelphia, Pennsylvania: Saunders (Elsevier), 2008.

[8] Liu Y. An in situ study of the influence of a sclerosing solution in rabbit medial collateral ligaments and its junction strength. *Connective Tissue Research*. 1983; 2: 95–102; Maynard J. Morphological and biomechanical effects of sodium Morrhuate on tendons. *Journal of Orthopaedic Research*. 1985; 3: 236–248; Klein R. Proliferant injections for low back pain: Histologic changes of injected ligaments and objective measures of lumbar spine mobility before and after treatment. *Journal of Neurology, Orthopedic Medicine and Surgery*. 1989; 10: 141–144; Reeves KD, Hassanein K. Randomized prospective double-blind placebo-controlled study of dextrose prolotherapy for knee osteoarthritis with or without ACL laxity. *Alternative Therapies*. 2000; 6(2): 68–80.

[9] Reeves KD, Hassanein K. Randomized prospective double-blind placebo-controlled study of dextrose prolotherapy for knee osteoarthritis with or without ACL laxity. *Alternative Therapies in Health and Medicine*. 2000 Mar 1; 6(2): 68.

[10] Otsuka Y, Mizuta H, Takagi K, Iyama K, Yoshitake Y, Nishikawa K, Suzuki F, Hiraki Y. Requirement of fibroblast growth factor signaling for regeneration of epiphyseal morphology in rabbit full-thickness defects of articular cartilage. *Development, Growth & Differentiation*. 1997; 39: 143–156; Van Beuningen H, Glansbeek HL, van der Kraan PM, van den Berg WB. Differential effects of local application of BMP-2 or TGF-beta 1 on both articular cartilage composition and osteophyte formation. *Osteoarthritis Cartilage*.1998; 6: 306–317; Madry H, Gao L, Eichler H, Orth P, Cucchiarini M. Bone marrow aspirate concentrate-enhanced marrow stimulation of chondral defects. *Stem Cells International*. 2017 May 18; 2017.

[11] Dagenais S, Haldeman S, Wooley JR. Intraligamentous injection of sclerosing solutions (prolotherapy) for spinal pain: A critical review of the literature. *Spine Journal*. 2005; 5: 310–328.

[12] Reeves KD. Prolotherapy: Basic science, clinical studies and technique. In *Pain Procedures in Clinical Practice, 2nd Edition* (pp. 172–190). Philadelphia, Pennsylvania: Hanley and Belfus, 2000.

[13] Reeves KD. Prolotherapy: Present and future applications in soft-tissue pain and disability. Injection techniques: principles and practice. *Physical Medicine and Rehabilitation Clinics of North America*. 1995; 6(4): 917–923.

[14] Hackett GS. *Ligament and Tendon Relaxation Treated by Prolotherapy*, 1st ed. Charles C. Thomas Publishers, Springfield, Illinois, 1956.

Chapter 6: Causes of Chronic Musculoskeletal Pain and Why Prolotherapy Works

[1] Andriacchi T, Sabiston P, DeHaven K, Dahners L, Woo S, Frank C, Oakes B, Brand R, Lewis J. Ligament: Injury and repair. In *Injury and Repair of the Musculoskeletal Soft Tissues* (pp. 103–128). Park Ridge, Illinois: American Academy of Orthopedic Surgeons, 1988.

[2] Khan KM, Cook JL, Bonar F, Hardcourt P. Histopathology of common overuse tendon conditions: Update and implications for clinical management. *Sports Medicine*. 1999; 27: 393–408.

[3] Taber's Cyclopedic Medical Dictionary, 18th ed. s.v. Definition of Collagen (p. 411). Philadelphia, Pennsylvania: F.A. Davis Company, 1997.

[4] Finan PH, Goodin BR, Smith MT. The association of sleep and pain: an update and a path forward. *Journal of Pain*. 2013 Dec 31; 14(12): 1539–1552.

[5] Jorgensen LN, Kallehave F, Christensen E, Siana JE, Gottrup F. Less collagen production in smokers. *Surgery*. 1998 Apr 30; 123(4): 450–455.

[6] Silverstein P. Smoking and wound healing. *American Journal of Medicine*. 1992 Jul 15; 93(1): S22–S24.

[7] Jam, B. Questioning the use of NSAIDs given inflammation is a perfectly healthy response following acute musculoskeletal injuries. 2014 Jul 14 [cited 2017 March 30] https://www.researchgate.net/profile/Bahram_Jam/publication/306372948_Questioning_the_use_of_NSAIDs_Given_Inflammation_is_a_Perfectly_Healthy_Response_Following_Acute_Musculoskeletal_Injuries/links/57bb12f708ae9fdf82ef016e.pdf; Banks AR. A rationale for prolotherapy. *Journal of Orthopaedic Medicine.* 1991; 13(3): 55–59.

[8] Stovitz SD, Johnson RJ. NSAIDs and musculoskeletal treatment: What is the clinical evidence? *The Physician and Sportsmedicine.* 2003; 31(1): 35–52.

[9] Cervoni TD, Martire JR, Curl LA, McFarland EG. Recognizing upper-extremity stress lesions. *Physician and Sportsmedicine.* 1997 Aug 1; 25(8): 69–86.

[10] Blalock D, Miller A, Tilley M, Wang J. Joint instability and osteoarthritis. *Clinical Medical Insights Arthritis Musculoskeletal Disorder.* 2015 Feb 19; 8: 15–23; Farrow CD, Newton CD. Ligamentous injury (sprain). In *Textbook of Small Animal Orthopaedics.* Ithaca, New York: International Veterinary Information Service, 1985.

[11] Morehead K, Sack KE. Osteoarthritis: What therapies for this disease of many causes? *Postgraduate Medicine.* 2003 Nov 1; 114(5): 11–17; Radin EL, Paul IL, Rose RM. Role of mechanical factors in pathogenesis of primary osteoarthritis. *The Lancet.* 1972 March 4; 299(7749): 519–522.

[12] Lohmander LS, Ostenberg A, Englund M, Roos H. High prevalence of knee osteoarthritis, pain and functional limitations in female soccer players twelve years after anterior cruciate ligament injury. *Arthritis & Rheumatism.* 2004 Oct; 50(10): 3142–3152.

[13] Panush R. Recreational activities and degenerative joint disease. *Sports Medicine.* 1994 Jan; 17(1): 1–5.

[14] Hauser RA, Blakemore PJ, Wang J, Steilen D. Structural basis of joint instability as cause for chronic musculoskeletal pain and its successful treatment with regenerative injection therapy (prolotherapy). *Open Pain Journal.* 2014; 7:9–22 [cited 2017

March 15] https://benthamopen.com/contents/pdf/TOPAINJ/ TOPAINJ-7-9.pdf.

[15] Li Y, Peng B. Pathogenesis, Diagnosis, and Treatment of Cervical Vertigo. *Pain Physician.* 2014 Dec; 18(4): E583–E595.

[16] Hauser RA, Steilen D, Sprague IS. Cervical instability as a cause of Barré-Liéou Syndrome and definitive treatment with pro-lotherapy: A case series. *European Journal of Preventive Medicine.* 2015; 3(5): 155–166.

[17] Soliman DMI, Sherif NM, Omar OH, El Zohiery AK. Healing effects of prolotherapy in treatment of knee osteoarthritis healing effects of prolotherapy in treatment of knee osteoarthritis. *Egyptian Rheumatology Rehabilitation.* 2016; 43(2): 47.

[18] Linetsky FS, Botwin K, Gorfine L, Jay GW, McComb B, Miguel R, Mikulinksky A, Parris W, Pollak S, Ray A, Saberski L, Taraschi P, Torres F, Trescot A. Position paper: Regenerative injection therapy (RIT) effectiveness and appropriate usage. *Pain Clinic Magazine.* 2002 June; 4(3): 38–45; Reeves KD, Hassanein K. Randomized prospective double-blind placebo-controlled study of dextrose prolotherapy for knee osteoarthritis with or without ACL laxity. *Alternative Therapies.* 2000; 6(2): 68–79; Reeves KD, Hassanein K. Randomized prospective placebo controlled double blind study of dextrose prolotherapy for osteoarthritic thumbs and finger (DIP, PIP and Trapeziometacarpal) joints: Evidence of clinical efficacy. *Journal of Alternative and Complementary Medicine.* 2000; 6(4): 311–320.

[19] Hassan F, Trebinjac S, Murrell WD, Maffulli N. The effectiveness of prolotherapy in treating knee osteoarthritis in adults: a systematic review. *British Medical Bulletin.* 2017 Mar 4; 122(1): 91–108.

Chapter 7: The Importance of a Correct Diagnosis

[1] Ombregt L, Bisschop P, Ter Veer HJ. *A System of Orthopaedic Medicine,* 2nd ed. (p. 59). London, England: Churchill Livingstone, 2003; MacRae DL. Asymptomatic intervertebral disc protrusion. *Acta Radiologica.* 1956; 46–49; Hitselberger WE, Whitten RM. Abnormal myelograms in asymptomatic patients. *Journal of Neurosurgery.* 1968; 28: 204; Wiesel SW, Tsourmas N, Feffer HL, Citrin CM, Patronas N. A study of computer-assisted tomography: 1. The incidence of positive CAT scans in an asymptomatic

group of patients. *Spine.* 1984; 9: 549–551; Powell MC, Wilson M, Szypryt P, Symonds EM, Worthington BS. Prevalence of lumbar disc degeneration observed by magnetic resonance in symptomless woman. *The Lancet.* 1986; 13: 1366–1367; Boden SD, Davis D.O., Dina TS, Patronas NJ, Wiesel SW. Abnormal magnetic resonance scans of the lumbar spine in asymptomatic subjects. *Journal of Bone and Joint Surgery.* 1990; 72A: 503–408; Kaplan PA. MR imaging of the normal shoulder: Variants and pitfalls. *Radiology.* 1992; 184: 519–524; Baker AD. Abnormal magnetic-resonance scans of the lumbar spine in asymptomatic subjects. A prospective investigation. In *Classic Papers in Orthopaedics* (pp. 245–247). London, England: Springer, 2014; Brinjikji W, Luetmer PH, Comstock B, Bresnahan BW, Chen LE, Deyo RA, Halabi S, Turner JA, Avins AL, James K, Wald JT. Systematic literature review of imaging features of spinal degeneration in asymptomatic populations. *American Journal of Neuroradiology.* 2015 Apr 1; 36(4): 811–816; Jensen MC, Brant-Zawadzki MN, Obuchowski N, Modic MT, Malkasian D, Ross JS. Magnetic resonance imaging of the lumbar spine in people without back pain. *New England Journal of Medicine.* 1994 July 14; 331: 69–73.

[2] Deyo R. Magnetic resonance imaging of the lumbar spine—terrific test or tar baby? *New England Journal of Medicine.* 1994; 331: 115–116.

[3] Chandnani V, Ho C, Gerharter J, Neumann C, Kursunoglu-Brahme S, Sartoris DJ, Resnick D. MR findings in asymptomatic shoulders: A blind analysis using symptomatic shoulders as controls. *Clinical Imaging.* 1992; 16: 25–30; Sher JS, Uribe JW, Posada A, Murphy BJ, Zlatkin MB. Abnormal findings on magnetic resonance images of asymptomatic shoulders. *Journal of Bone and Joint Surgery.* 1995; 75A: 10–15; Miniaci A, Dowdy PA, Willits KR, Vellet AD. Magnetic resonance imaging evaluation of the rotator cuff tendons in the asymptomatic shoulder. *American Journal of Sports Medicine.* 1995; 23: 142–145; Thompson WO, Debski RE, Boardman ND 3rd, Taskiran E, Warner JJ, Fu FH, Woo SY. A biomechanical analysis of rotator cuff deficiency in a cadaveric model. *American Journal of Sports Medicine.* 1996; 24(3): 286–292.

[4] Miniaci A, Mascia AT, Salonen DC, Becker EJ. Magnetic imaging of the shoulder in asymptomatic professional baseball pitchers. *American Journal of Sports Medicine.* 2002; 20: 66–73.

[5] Matsumoto M, Fujimura Y, Suzuki N, Nishi Y, Nakamura M, Yabe Y, Shiga H. MRI of the cervical intervertebral discs in asymptomatic subjects. *Journal of Bone and Joint Surgery (Br).* 1998; 80(1): 19–24; Humphreys SC, Hodges SD, Fisher DL, Eck JC, Covington LA. Reliability of magnetic resonance imaging in predicting disc material posterior to the posterior longitudinal ligament in the cervical spine, a prospective study. *Spine.* 1998; 23(22): 2468–2471; Kaiser JA, Holland BA. Imaging of the cervical spine. *Spine.* 1998; 23(24): 2701–2712.

[6] Deshpande BR, Losina E, Smith SR, Martin SD, Wright RJ, Katz JN. Association of MRI findings and expert diagnosis of symptomatic meniscal tear among middle-aged and older adults with knee pain. *BMC Musculoskeletal Disorders.* 2016 Apr 11; 17(1):154; Jerosch J, Castro WH, Assheuer J. Age related magnetic resonance imaging morphology of the menisci in asymptomatic individuals. *Archives of Orthopedic Trauma Surgery.* 1996; 115(3–4): 199–202; LaPrade RF, Burnett QM, Veenstra MA, Hodgman CG. The prevalence of abnormal magnetic resonance imaging findings in asymptomatic knees: with correlation of magnetic resonance imaging to arthroscopic findings in symptomatic knees. *American Journal of Sports Medicine.* 1994; 22(6): 739–745.

[7] Boeth H, MacMahon A, Eckstein F, Diederichs G, Schlausch A, Wirth W, Duda GN. MRI findings of knee abnormalities in adolescent and adult volleyball players. *Journal of Experimental Orthopaedics.* 2017: 4(1): 6; Major NM, Helms CA. MR imaging of the knee: findings in asymptomatic collegiate basketball players. *American Journal of Roentgenology.* 2002; 179(3): 641–644.

[8] Stanitski CL. Correlation of arthroscopic and clinical examinations with magnetic resonance imaging findings of injured knees in children and adolescents. *American Journal of Sports Medicine.* 1998; 26: 2–6.

[9] Connor PM, Banks DM, Tyson AB, Coumas JS, D'Alessandro DF. Magnetic resonance imaging of the asymptomatic shoulder of overhead athletes: A 5-year follow-up study. *American Journal of Sports Medicine.* 2003; 31: 724–727.

[10] Primack SJ. Past, present, and future considerations for musculoskeletal ultrasound. *Physical Medicine & Rehabilitation Clinics of North America.* 2016; 27(3): 749–752; Fullerton BD, Reeves KD.

Ultrasonography in regenerative injection (prolotherapy) using dextrose, platelet-rich plasma, and other injectants. *Physical Medicine & Rehabilitation Clinics of North America.* 2010; 21(3): 585–605.

[11] Özçakar L, Kara M, Chang KV, Carl AB, Akkaya N, Tok F, Chen WS, Wang TG, Tekin L, Ulasl AM, Chen CP, Capkn E, De Muynck M. Nineteen reasons why physiatrists should do musculoskeletal ultrasound: EURO-MUSCULUS/USPRM recommendations. *American Journal of Physical Medicine & Rehabilitation.* 2015; 94(6): e45–e49.

[12] Finnoff JT. The evolution of diagnostic and interventional ultrasound in sports medicine. *PM&R.* 2016; 8(3): S133–S138.

[13] Donegan RJ, Stauffer A, Heaslet M, Poliskie M. Comparing magnetic resonance imaging and high-resolution dynamic ultrasonography for diagnosis of plantar plate pathology: A case series. *Journal of Foot and Ankle Surgery.* 2017; 56(2): 371–374; de Jesus JO, Parker L, Frangos AJ, Nazarian LN. Accuracy of MRI, MR arthrography, and ultrasound in the diagnosis of rotator cuff tears: A meta-analysis. *American Journal of Roentgenology.* 2009; 192(6): 1701–1707; Delzell PB, Tritle BA, Bullen JA, Chiunda S, Forney MC. Clinical utility of high-frequency musculoskeletal ultrasonography in foot and ankle pathology: How ultrasound imaging influences diagnosis and management. *Journal of Foot and Ankle Surgery.* 2017; 2017; 56(4): 735–739; Stone M, Eyler W, Rhodenizer J, van Holsbeeck M. Accuracy of sonography in plantar plate in tears in cadavers. *Journal of Ultrasound in Medicine.* 2017; 36(7): 1355–1361; Podlipská J, Guermazi A, Lehenkari P, Niinimäki J, Roemer FW, Arokoski JP, Kaukinen P, Liukkonen E, Lammentausta E, Nieminen MT, Tervonen O, Koski JM, Saarakkala S. Comparison of diagnostic performance of semi-quantitative knee ultrasound and knee radiography with MRI: Oulu knee osteoarthritis study. *Scientific Reports.* 2016; 6: 22365; Fischer CA, Weber MA, Neubecker C, Bruckner T, Tanner M, Zeifang F. Ultrasound vs. MRI in the assessment of rotator cuff structure prior to shoulder arthroplasty. *Journal of Orthopaedics.* 2015; 12(1): 23–30.

[14] Szkudlarek M, Klarlund M, Narvestad E, Strandberg C, Jensen KE, Thomsen HS, Østergaard M. Ultrasonography of the metacarpophalangeal and proximal interphalangeal joints in rheumatoid arthritis: A comparison with magnetic resonance imaging,

conventional radiography and clinical examination. *Arthritis Research & Therapy*. 2006; 8(2): R52; Dinnes J, Loveman E, McIntyre L, Waugh N. The effectiveness of diagnostic tests for the assessment of shoulder pain due to soft tissue disorders: a systematic review. *NIHR Health Technology Assessment Programme: Executive Summaries, 7(29)*. Southampton (UK): NIHR Journals Library, 2003. [cited 2017 July 7] https://www.ncbi.nlm.nih.gov/books/NBK62241.

[15] Lento PH, Primack S. Advances and utility of diagnostic ultrasound in musculoskeletal medicine. *Current Reviews in Musculoskeletal Medicine*. 2008; 1(1): 24–31.

[16] Kane D, Grassi W, Sturrock R, Balint PV. A brief history of musculoskeletal ultrasound: "From bats and ships to babies and hips." *Rheumatology*. 2004; 43(7): 931–933; Tsung J. History of ultrasound and technological advances. Presentation at Mount Sinai School of Medicine [cited 2017 April 17] http://www.wcume.org/wp-content/uploads/2011/05/Tsung.pdf.

[17] McDonald DG. Leopold GR. Ultrasound B-scanning in the differentiation of Baker's cyst and thrombophlebitis. *British Journal of Radiology*. 1972; 45(538): 729–732.

[18] Drakonaki EE, Allen GM, Wilson DJ. Ultrasound elastography for musculoskeletal applications. *British Journal of Radiology*. 2012 Nov; 85(1019):1435–1445.

[19] Galletti S, Oliva F, Masiero S, Frizziero A, Galletti R, Schiavone C, Salini V, Abate M. Sonoelastography in the diagnosis of tendinopathies: an added value. *Muscles, Ligaments and Tendons Journal*. 2015; 5(4): 325–330.

[20] Cyriax System of Orthopedic Medicine. [Cited December 26, 2017]. http://www.aaomed.org/Cyriax-System-of-Orthopaedic-Medicine.

Chapter 8: Prolotherapy Regenerative Medicine is Evidence Based

[1] Alternative treatments: Dealing with chronic pain. *Mayo Clinic Health Letter*. 2005 April; 23(4) [cited 2016 March 7] http://www.prolotherapy.com/Mayo-Clinic-Prolo%202005.pdf.

[2] Tendon Trouble: New treatment uses enhanced plasma. *Mayo Clinic Health Letter*, 2010 March, p.7 [cited 2017 October 24] http://healthletter.mayoclinic.com/common/pdf/192/201003.PDF.

[3] Mayo Clinic Health System. Physical Medicine & Rehabilitation Department information page [cited 2017 August 1] http://mayoclinichealthsystem.org/locations/la-crosse/medical-services/physical-medicine-and-rehabilitation.

[4] Mayo Clinic Center for Regenerative Medicine [Internet]. Musculoskeletal Regeneration. [cited 2017 March 6] http://www.mayo.edu/research/centers-programs/center-regenerative-medicine/focus-areas/musculoskeletal-regeneration.

[5] Liu YK, Tipton CM, Matches RD, Bedford TG, Maynard JA, Walmer HC. An in situ study of a sclerosing solution in rabbit medical collateral ligaments and its junction strength. *Connective Tissue Research*, 1983; 11(2–3): 95–102.

[6] Maynard JA, Pedrini VA, Pedrini-Mille A, Romanus B, Ohlerking F. Morphological and biochemical effects of sodium morrhuate on tendons. *Journal of Orthopaedic Research*. 1985; 3(2): 236–248.

[7] Klein RG, Dorman TA, Johnson CE. Proliferant injections for low back pain: Histologic changes of injected ligaments and objective measures of lumbar spine mobility before and after treatment. *Journal of Neurological and Orthopaedics Medicine and Surgery*. 1989; 10: 141–144.

[8] Reeves KD, Hassanein K. Randomized, prospective, placebo-controlled double-blind study of dextrose prolotherapy for osteoarthritic thumb and finger (DIP, PIP, and trapeziometacarpal) joints: Evidence of clinical efficacy. *Journal of Alternative & Complementary Medicine*. 2000 Aug; 6(4): 311–320.

[9] Dechow E, Davies RK, Carr AJ, Thompson PW. A randomized, double-blind, placebo-controlled trial of sclerosing injections in patients with chronic low back pain. *Rheumatology*. 1999; 38(12): 1255–1259; Klein RG, Eek BC, DeLong WB, Mooney V. A randomized double-blind trial of dextrose-glycerine-phenol injections for chronic, low back pain. *Journal of Spinal Disorders & Techniques*. 1993; 6(1): 23–33.

[10] Rabago D, Patterson JJ, Mundt M, Kijowski R, Grettie J, Segal NA, Zgierska A. Dextrose prolotherapy for knee osteoarthritis: A randomized controlled trial. *Annals of Family Medicine*. 2013; 11(3): 229–237.

[11] Reeves KD, Hassanein K. Randomized prospective double-blind placebo-controlled study of dextrose prolotherapy for knee osteoarthritis with or without ACL laxity. *Alternative Therapies in Health and Medicine.* 2000; 6(2): 68–80.

[12] Reeves KD, Hassanein K. Randomized, prospective, placebo-controlled double-blind study of dextrose prolotherapy for osteoarthritic thumb and finger (DIP, PIP, and trapeziometacarpal) joints: Evidence of clinical efficacy. *Journal of Alternative & Complementary Medicine.* 2000; 6(4): 311–320.

[13] Refai H, Altahhan O, Elsharkawy R. The efficacy of dextrose prolotherapy for temporomandibular joint hypermobility: A preliminary prospective, randomized, double-blind, placebo-controlled clinical trial. *Journal of Oral and Maxillofacial Surgery.* 2011; 69(12): 2962–2970.

[14] Bertrand H, Reeves KD, Bennett CJ, Bicknell S, Cheng AL. Dextrose prolotherapy versus control injections in painful rotator cuff tendinopathy. *Archives of Physical Medicine and Rehabilitation.* 2016; 97(1): 17–25.

[15] Reeves KD, Hassanein KM. Long term effects of dextrose prolotherapy for anterior cruciate ligament laxity. *Alternative Therapies in Health and Medicine,* 2003; 9(3): 58–62.

[16] Topol GA, Reeves KD, Hassanein KM. Efficacy of dextrose prolotherapy in elite male kicking-sport athletes with chronic groin pain. *Archives of Physical Medicine and Rehabilitation.* 2005; 86(4): 697–702.

[17] Hauser RA, Hauser MA, Page RD. Dextrose prolotherapy for unresolved neck pain. *Practical Pain Management.* 2007; 7(8): 56–60; Hooper RA, Ding M. Retrospective case series on patients with chronic spinal pain treated with dextrose prolotherapy. *Journal of Alternative & Complementary Medicine.* 2004; 10(4): 670–674.

[18] Steilen D, Hauser R, Woldin B, Sawyer S. Chronic neck pain: Making the connection between capsular ligament laxity and cervical instability. *Open Orthopaedics Journal.* 2014; 8: 326; Hooper RA, Frizzell JB, Faris P. Case series on chronic whiplash-related neck pain treated with intraarticular zygapophysial joint regeneration injection therapy. *Pain Physician.* 2007; 10(2): 313–318.

[19] Kim WM, Lee HG, Jeong CW, Kim CM, Yoon MH. A randomized controlled trial of intra-articular prolotherapy versus steroid injection for sacroiliac joint pain. *Journal of Alternative and Complementary Medicine*. 2010; 16(12): 1285–129.

[20] Ryan MB, Wong AD, Gillies JH, Wong J, Taunton JE. Sonographically guided intratendinous injections of hyperosmolar dextrose/lidocaine: a pilot study for the treatment of chronic plantar fasciitis. British journal of sports medicine. 2009 Apr 1; 43(4): 303–306.

[21] Rabago D, Lee KS, Ryan M, Chourasia AO, Sesto ME, Zgierska A, Kijowski R, Grettie J, Wilson J, Miller D. Hypertonic dextrose and morrhuate sodium injections (prolotherapy) for lateral epicondylosis (tennis elbow): Results of a single-blind, pilot-level randomized controlled trial. *American Journal of Physical Medicine & Rehabilitation/Association of Academic Physiatrists*. 2013; 92(7): 587.

[22] Hackett GS, Henderson DG. Joint stabilization: An experimental, histologic study with comments on the clinical application in ligament proliferation. *American Journal of Surgery*. 1955; 89(5): 968–973.

[23] Caring Medical Regenerative Medicine Clinics. Hackett Hemwall Prolotherapy. [cited 2016 March 7] https://www.caring-medical.com/prolotherapy/hackett-hemwall-prolotherapy/.

[24] Kiliç CS, Güngörmüş M. Is dextrose prolotherapy superior to placebo for the treatment of temporomandibular joint hypermobility? A randomized clinical trial. *International Journal of Oral and Maxillofacial Surgery*. 2016; 45(7): 813–819.

[25] University of Alberta. Platelet-rich plasma injections may lead to improvements in tissue healing. *Science Daily*; 2016 March 2 [cited 2016 March 6] www.sciencedaily.com/releases/2016/03/160302132531.htm.

[26] Paterson KL, Nicholls M, Bennell KL, Bates D. Intra-articular injection of photo-activated platelet-rich plasma in patients with knee osteoarthritis: A double-blind, randomized controlled pilot study. *BMC Musculoskeletal Disorders*. 2016; 17(1): Görmeli G, Görmeli CA, Ataoglu B, Çolak C, Aslantürk O, Ertem K. Multiple PRP injections are more effective than single injections and hyaluronic acid in knees with early osteoarthritis: A

randomized, double-blind, placebo-controlled trial. *Knee Surgery, Sports Traumatology, Arthroscopy.* 2015: 1–8; Sandeep P, Dhillon MS, Aggarwal S, Marwaha N, Jain A. Treatment with platelet-rich plasma is more effective than placebo for knee osteoarthritis a prospective, double-blind, randomized trial. *American Journal of Sports Medicine.* 2013; 41(2): 356–364; Smith PA. Intra-articular autologous conditioned plasma injections proved safe and efficacious treatment for knee osteoarthritis: An FDA-sanctioned, randomized, double-blind, placebo-controlled clinical trial. *American Journal of Sports Medicine.* 2016; 44(4): 884–891.

[27] Tuakli-Wosornu YA, Terry A, Boachie-Adjei K, Harrison JR, Gribbin CK, LaSalle EE, Nguyen JT, Solomon JL, Lutz GE. Lumbar intradiskal platelet-rich plasma (PRP) injections: A prospective, double-blind, randomized controlled study. *PM&R.* 2016; 8(1): 1–10.

[28] Dragoo JL, Wasterlain AS, Braun HJ, Nead KT. Platelet-rich plasma as a treatment for patellar tendinopathy: a double-blind, randomized controlled trial. *American Journal of Sports Medicine.* 2014; 42(3): 610–618.

[29] Hauser RA, Phillips HJ, Maddela H. Platelet rich plasma Prolotherapy as first-line treatment for meniscal pathology. *Practical Pain Management.* 2010 Jul; 10(6): 53–64.

[30] de Jonge S, de Vos RJ, Weir A, van Schie HTM, Bierma-Zeinstra SMA, Verhaar JAN, Weinans H, Tol JL. One-year follow-up of platelet-rich plasma treatment in chronic Achilles tendinopathy a double-blind randomized placebo-controlled trial. *American Journal of Sports Medicine.* 2011; 39(8): 1623–1629.

[31] Ko GD, Mindra S, Lawson GE, Whitmore S, Arseneau L. Case series of ultrasound-guided platelet-rich plasma injections for sacroiliac joint dysfunction. *Journal of Back and Musculoskeletal Rehabilitation.* 2016; 30(2): 363–370.

[32] Mishra AK, Skrepnik NV, Edwards SG, Jones GL, Sampson S, Vermillion DA, Ramsey ML, Karli DC, Rettig AC. Platelet-rich plasma significantly improves clinically outcomes in patients with chronic tennis elbow: A double-blind, prospective, multicenter, controlled trial of 230 patients. *American Journal of Sports Medicine.* 2013; (42)2: 463–471; Peerbooms JC, Sluimer J, Bruijn DJ, Gosens T. Positive effect of an autologous platelet concentrate in lateral epicondylitis in a double-blind randomized controlled trial

platelet-rich plasma versus corticosteroid injection with a 1-year follow-up. *American Journal of Sports Medicine.* 2010; 38(2): 255–262.

[33] Deal JB, Smith E, Heard W, O'Brien MJ, Savoie III FH. Platelet-Rich Plasma for Primary Treatment of partial ulnar collateral ligament tears: MRI correlation with results. *Orthopaedic Journal of Sports Medicine.* 2017 Nov 8; 5(11) [cited December 26, 2017]. http://journals.sagepub.com/doi/full/10.1177/2325967117738238.

[34] Gosens T, Peerbooms JC, van Laar W, den Oudsten BL. Ongoing positive effect of platelet-rich plasma versus corticosteroid injection in lateral epicondylitis: A double-blind, randomized controlled trial with 2-year follow up. *American Journal of Sports Medicine.* 2011; 39(6): 1200–1208.

[35] Singh A, Goel SC, Gupta KK, Kumar M, Arun GR, Patil H, Kumaraswamy V, Jha S. The role of stem cells in osteoarthritis. *Bone & Joint Research.* 2014; 3: 32–37.

[36] Perdisa F, Gostyńska N, Roffi A, Filardo G, Marcacci M, Kon E. Adipose-derived mesenchymal stem cells for the treatment of articular cartilage: A systematic review on preclinical and clinical evidence. *Stem Cells International.* 2015; Article ID 597652,13 pages.

[37] Bui, KHT, Duong TD, Nguyen NT, Nguyen TD, Le VT, Mai VT, Phan N, Le DM, Phan NK, Pham PV. "Symptomatic knee osteoarthritis treatment using autologous adipose derived stem cells and platelet-rich plasma: A clinical study." *Biomedical Research and Therapy.* 2014; 1(1): 2–8.

[38] Koh, YG, Choi YJ, Kwon SK, Kim YS, Yeo JE. Clinical results and second-look arthroscopic findings after treatment with adipose-derived stem cells for knee osteoarthritis. *Knee Surgery, Sports Traumatology, Arthroscopy.* May 2015; 23(5): 1308–1316.

[39] Oe K, Kushida T, Okamoto N, Umeda M, Nakamura T, Ikehara S, Iida H. New strategies for anterior cruciate ligament partial rupture using bone marrow transplantation in rats. *Stem Cells and Development.* 2011; 20(4): 671–679; Soon MY, Hassan A, Hui JHJ, Goh JC, Lee EH. An analysis of soft tissue allograft anterior cruciate ligament reconstruction in a rabbit model: a short-term study of the use of mesenchymal stem cells to enhance tendon osteointegration. *The American Journal of Sports Medicine.* 2007; 35(6): 962–971.

[40] Albano JJ, Alexander RW. Autologous fat grafting as a mesenchymal stem cell source and living bioscaffold in a patellar tendon tear. *Clinical Journal of Sport Medicine*. 2011; 21(4): 359–361.

[41] Alexander RW. Biocellular regenerative medicine: Use of adipose-derived stem/stromal cells and its native bioactive matrix. *Physical Medicine & Rehabilitation Clinics of North America*. 2012; 27: 871–891.

[42] Oliver KS, Alexander RW. Combination of autologous adipose-derived tissue stromal vascular fraction plus high density platelet-rich plasma or bone marrow concentrates in Achilles tendon tears. *Journal of Prolotherapy*. 2013; 5: e895–e912.

[43] Journal of Prolotherapy [cited 2017 March 26] http://www.journalofprolotherapy.com.

[44] Solomon DJ. The role of peer review for scholarly journals in the information age. *The Journal of Electronic Publishing*. 2007; 10(1) [cited 2017 March 4] http://quod.lib.umich.edu/j/jep/3336451.0010.107?view=text;rgn=main.

[45] Hauser RA, Maddela HS, Alderman DD, Baehnisch G, Banner R, Blakemore PJ, Calderón JE, Clark GB, DeLaurentis M, Fauley S, Funck J, Gladstein B, Johnson ML, Kramer GH, Neustadt J, Resk J, Salazar JH, Swetlikoff G, Van Pelt RS, Wheaton MT. Journal of Prolotherapy international medical editorial board consensus statement on the use of prolotherapy for musculoskeletal pain. *Journal of Prolotherapy*. 2011; 3(4): 744–764.

[46] Aims & Scope. *PM&R*. [cited 2017 March 4] http://www.pmr-journal.org/content/aims.

[47] The American Osteopathic Association of Prolotherapy Regenerative Medicine. Teaching physicians since 1938. Committed to the long term education of Prolotherapy [cited 2016 February 28] http://www.prolotherapycollege.org/.

[48] Department of Family Medicine and Community Health, University of Wisconsin School of Medicine and Public Health. The UW Prolotherapy and Research Lab (UWPRL): Advancing a promising treatment in chronic pain [cited 2016 February 28] http://www.fammed.wisc.edu/prolotherapy/.

[49] Rabago D, Slattengren A, Zgierska A. Prolotherapy in primary care practice. *Primary Care: Clinics in Office Practice*. 2010; 37(1):

65–80; Rabago D, Best TM, Zgierska AE, Zeisig E, Ryan M, Crane D. A systematic review of four injection therapies for lateral epicondylosis: Prolotherapy, polidocanol, whole blood and platelet-rich plasma. *British Journal of Sports Medicine.* 2009; 43(7): 471–481; Scarpone M, Rabago D, Zgierska A, Arbogest J, Snell E. The efficacy of prolotherapy for lateral epicondylosis: A pilot study. *Clinical Journal of Sport Medicine: Official Journal of the Canadian Academy of Sport Medicine.* 2008; 18(3): 248; Rabago D, Best TM, Beamsley M, Patterson J. A systematic review of prolotherapy for chronic musculoskeletal pain. *Clinical Journal of Sport Medicine.* 2005; 15(5): E376; Rabago D, Patterson JJ, Mundt M, Kijowski R, Grettie J, Segal NA, Zgierska A. Dextrose prolotherapy for knee osteoarthritis: A randomized controlled trial. *Annals of Family Medicine.* 2013; 11(3): 229–237; Rabago D, Zgierska A, Fortney L, Kijowski R, Mundt M, Ryan M, Grettie J, Patterson JJ. Hypertonic dextrose injections (prolotherapy) for knee osteoarthritis: results of a single-arm uncontrolled study with 1-year follow-up. *Journal of Alternative and Complementary Medicine.* 2012; 18(4): 408–414; Rabago D, Lee KS, Ryan M, Chourasia AO, Sesto ME, Zgierska A, Kijowski R, Grettie J, Wilson J, Miller D. Hypertonic dextrose and morrhuate sodium injections (prolotherapy) for lateral epicondylosis (tennis elbow): Results of a single-blind, pilot-level randomized controlled trial. *American Journal of Physical Medicine & Rehabilitation/ Association of Academic Physiatrists.* 2013; 92(7): 587–596.

[50] American Association of Orthopaedic Medicine. Orthopedic Problems, Innovative Solutions. Since 1983. About Us [2016 Mar 6] http://www.aaomed.org/About-AAOM.

[51] The Hackett Hemwall Foundation. About Us [2016 March 6] http://www.hacketthemwall.org/About_Us.html.

[52] TOBI: The Orthobiological Institute. About Us [cited 2016 March 6] http://www.prpseminar.com/about/.

[53] Prolotherapy is Not Experimental. [cited 2017 September 30] http://www.neurofascial.com/sites/default/files/Prolotherapy% 20is%20Not%20Experimental,%20February%202014.pdf.

[54] Strongside Solutions. Press Release: Emerging therapies act of 2017. 2017 April 10 [cited 1 August 2017] http://strongsidesolutions.com/press-release-emerging-therapies-act-of-2017/ [press release].

Chapter 9: Platelet Rich Plasma (PRP) Prolotherapy

[1] Kazakos K, Lyras DN, Verettas D, Tilkeridis K, Tryfonidis M. The use of autologous PRP gel as an aid in the management of acute trauma wounds. *Injury*. 2009; 40(8): 801–805; Sánchez M, Delgado D, Sánchez P, Anitua E, Padilla S. Plasma rich in growth factors for the treatment of skeletal muscle injury. In *Muscle Injuries in Sport Athletes* (pp. 451–464). Switzerland: Springer International Publishing, 2017; A Hamid MS, Mohamede Ali MR, Yusof A, George J, Lee LP. Platelet-rich plasma injections for the treatment of hamstring injuries: A randomized controlled trial. *American Journal of Sports Medicine*. 2014 Oct; 42(10): 2410–2418.

[2] Kon E, Filardo G, Di Matteo B, Marcacci M. The role of platelet-rich plasma in cartilage repair. In *Cartilage* (pp. 127–138). Switzerland: Springer International Publishing, 2017.

[3] Marx R, Kevy S, Jacobson M. Platelet rich plasma (PRP): A primer. *Practical Pain Management*. 2008; 8(2); Foster TE, Puskas BL, Mandelbaum BR, Gerhardt MB, Rodeo SA. Platelet-rich plasma: From basic science to clinical applications. *American Journal of Sports Medicine*. 2009; 37(11): 2259–2272.

[4] Hall M, Bank P, Meislin R, Jazrawi L, Cardone D. Platelet-rich plasma: current concepts and application in sports medicine. *Journal of the American Academy of Orthopaedic Surgeons*. 2009; 27: 602–608.

[5] US National Library of Medicine, National Institute of Health, search for "PRP" [cited 2017 July 29] https://www.ncbi.nlm.nih.gov/pubmed/?term=PRP.

[6] Google Scholar, search for "platelet rich plasma" [cited 2017 July 29] https://scholar.google.com/scholar?q=Platelet+rich+plasma&btnG=&hl=en&as_sdt=0%2C5.

[7] Yuan T, Zhang CQ, Wang JHC. Augmenting tendon and ligament repair with platelet-rich plasma (PRP). *Muscles, Ligaments and Tendons Journal*. 2013; 3(3): 139–149; Hall M, Band P, Meislin R, Jazrawi L, Cardone D. Platelet-rich plasma: Current concepts and application in sports medicine. *Journal of the American Academy of Orthopaedic Surgeons*. 2009; 17: 602–608; Deal JB, Smith E, Heard W, O'Brien MJ, Savoie III FH. Platelet-rich plasma for primary treatment of partial ulnar collateral ligament tears: MRI correlation

with results. *Orthopaedic Journal of Sports Medicine.* 2017 Nov 8; 5(11) [cited December 26, 2017]. http://journals.sagepub.com/doi/full/10.1177/2325967117738238.

[8] Fitzpatrick J, Bulsara M, Zheng MH. 2017. The effectiveness of platelet-rich plasma in the treatment of tendinopathy: A meta-analysis of randomized controlled clinical trials. *American Journal of Sports Medicine.* 2017; 45(1): 226–233; Balasubramaniam U, Dissanayake R, Annabell L. Efficacy of platelet-rich plasma injections in pain associated with chronic tendinopathy: a systematic review. *Physician and Sportsmedicine.* 2015; 43(3): 253–261.

[9] Sanchez M, Anitua E, Azofra J, Aguirre JJ, Andia I. Intra-articular injection of an autologous preparation rich in growth factors for the treatment of knee OA: A retrospective cohort study. *Clinical and Experimental Rheumatology.* 2008; 26(5): 910–913; Raeissadat SA, Rayegani SM, Hassanabadi H, Fathi M, Ghorbani E, Babaee M, Azma K. Knee osteoarthritis injection choices: Platelet-rich plasma (PRP) versus hyaluronic acid (a one-year randomized clinical trial). *Clinical Medicine Insights: Arthritis and Musculoskeletal Disorders.* 2015; 8: 1–8; Andia I, Maffulli N. Platelet-rich plasma for managing pain and inflammation in osteoarthritis. *Nature Reviews Rheumatology.* 2013; 9(12): 721–730; Sanchez M, Guadilla J, Fiz N, Andia I. Ultrasound-guided platelet-rich plasma injections for the treatment of osteoarthritis of the hip. *Rheumatology.* 2012; 41: 144–150.

[10] Blanke F, Vavken P, Haenle M, von Wehren L, Pagenstert G, Majewski M. Percutaneous injections of platelet rich plasma for treatment of intrasubstance meniscal lesions. *Muscles, Ligaments and Tendons Journal.* 2015; 5(3): 162; Wei LC, Gao SG, Xu M, Jiang W, Tian J, Lei GH. A novel hypothesis: The application of platelet-rich plasma can promote the clinical healing of white-white meniscal tears. *Medical Science Monitor.* 2012; 18(8): HY47–HY50; Hauser RA, Phillips HJ, Maddela H. PRP prolotherapy as first line treatment for meniscal pathology. *Practical Pain Management.* 2010; 53–63; Braun HJ, Wasterlain AS, Dragoo JL. The use of PRP in ligament and meniscal healing. *Sports Medicine and Arthroscopy Review.* 2013; 21(4): 206–212.

[11] Moussa M, Lajeunesse D, Hilal G, Atat OE, Haykal G, Serhal R, Chalhoub A, Khalil C, Alaaeddine N. Platelet rich plasma (PRP) induces chondroprotection via increasing autophagy,

anti-inflammatory markers, and decreasing apoptosis in human osteoarthritic cartilage. *Experimental Cell Research.* 2017; 352(1): 146–156; Kon E, Buda R, Filardo G, Di Martino A, Timoncicni A, Cenacchi A, Fornasari PM, Giannini S, Marcacco M. Platelet-rich plasma: Intra-articular knee injections produced favorable results on degenerative cartilage lesions. *Knee Surgery, Sports Traumatology, Arthroscopy.* 2010; 18(4): 472–479; Vannini F, Di Matteo B, Filardo G. Platelet-rich plasma to treat ankle cartilage pathology-from translational potential to clinical evidence: A systematic review. *Journal of Experimental Orthopaedics.* 2015 Dec 14; 2(1): 2.

[12] Gosens T, Peerbooms JC, Van Laar W, den Oudsten BL. Ongoing positive effect of platelet-rich plasma versus corticosteroid injection in lateral epicondylitis: A double-blind randomized controlled trial with 2-year follow-up. *American Journal of Sports Medicine.* 2011; 39(6): 1200–1208.

[13] Mishra A, Harmon K, Woodall J, Vieira A. Sports medicine applications of platelet rich plasma. *Current Pharmaceutical Biotechnology.* 2012; 13: 1185–1195.

[14] Hammond J, Hinton R, Curl LA, Muriel JM, Lovering RM. Use of autologous platelet-rich plasma to treat muscle strain injuries. *American Journal of Sports Medicine.* 2009; 37(6): 1135–1142.

[15] Sanchez M, Anitua E, Andia I. Application of autologous growth factors on skeletal muscle healing. *Poster Presentation at the 2nd World Conference on Regenerative Medicine.* Leipzig, Germany; May 18–20, 2005.

[16] Filardo G, Kon E, Della Villa S, Vincentelli F, Maria Fornasari P, Marcacci M. Use of platelet-rich plasma for the treatment of refractory jumper's knee. *International Orthopaedics.* 2010; 34(6): 909–915.

[17] Boesen AP, Hansen R, Boesen MI, Malliaras P, Langberg H. Effect of high-volume injection, platelet-rich plasma, and sham treatment in chronic midportion Achilles tendinopathy: A randomized double-blind prospective study. *American Journal of Sports Medicine* (2017): Di Matteo B, Filardo G, Kon E, Marcacci M. Platelet-rich plasma: Evidence for the treatment of patellar and Achilles tendinopathy—a systematic review. *Musculoskeletal Surgery.* 2015; 99(1): 1–9.

[18]Muralidharagopalan NR, Loganathan D, Iyer KMJ, Boopathikumar KK. Functional outcomes of platelet rich plasma injections in plantar fasciitis. *International Journal of Research in Orthopaedics*; 2017 Jul 3; (4): 734–737; Barrett S, Erredge S. Growth factors for chronic plantar fasciitis? *Podiatry Today*. 2004; 17(11): 35–42; Kumar V, Millar T, Murphy PN, Clough T. The treatment of intractable plantar fasciitis with platelet-rich plasma injection. *The Foot*. 2013 Sep 30; 23(2): 74–77.

[19] Hanci M, Karamese M, Tosun Z, Aktan TM, Suman S, Savaci N. Intra-articular platelet-rich plasma injection for the treatment of temporomandibular disorders and a comparison with arthro-centesis. *Journal of Cranio-Maxillofacial Surgery*. 2015; 43(1): 162–166; Hegab AF, Ali HE, Elmasry M, Khallaf MG. Platelet-rich plasma injection as an effective treatment for temporomandibular joint osteoarthritis. *Journal of Oral and Maxillofacial Surgery*. 2015; 73(9): 1706–1713.

[20] Cameron JA, Thielen KM. Autologous platelet rich plasma for neck and lower back pain secondary to spinal disc herniation: Midterm results. *Spine Research*. 2017 Aug 30; 3(2): Article ID 100030: 5 pages; Lutz GE. Increased nuclear T2 signal intensity and improved function and pain in a patient one year after an intradiscal platelet–rich plasma injection. *Pain Medicine*. 2017; 18 (6), 1197–1199; Wang SZ, Chang Q, Lu J, Wang C. Growth factors and platelet-rich plasma: Promising biological strategies for early intervertebral disc degeneration. *International Orthopaedics*. 2015; 39(5): 927–934; Bhatia R, Chopra G. Efficacy of Platelet Rich Plasma via Lumbar Epidural Route in Chronic Prolapsed Intervertebral Disc Patients-A Pilot Study. *Journal of Clinical and Diagnostic Research*. 2016 Sep; 10(9): UC05–UC07.

[21] Ko GD, Mindra S, Lawson GE, Whitmore S, Arseneau L. Case series of ultrasound-guided platelet-rich plasma injections for sacroiliac joint dysfunction. *Journal of Back and Musculoskeletal Rehabilitation*. 2017 Mar 2: 30(2): 363–370.

[22] Sánchez M, Guadilla J, Fiz N, Andia I. Ultrasound-guided plate-let-rich plasma injections for the treatment of osteoarthritis of the hip. *Rheumatology*. 2011 Nov 9; 51(1): 144–150; Dallari D, Stagni C, Rani N, Sabbioni G, Pelotti P, Torricelli P, Tschon M, Giavaresi G. Ultrasound-guided injection of platelet-rich plasma and hyal-uronic acid, separately and in combination, for hip osteoarthritis:

a randomized controlled study. *The American Journal of Sports Medicine*. 2016 Mar; 44(3): 664–671.

[23] Wu J, Zhou J, Liu C, Zhang J, Xiong W, Lv Y, Liu R, Wang R, Du Z, Zhang G, Liu Q. A prospective study comparing platelet-rich plasma and local anesthetic (LA)/corticosteroid in intra-artic-ular injection for the treatment of lumbar facet joint syndrome. *Pain Practice*. 2017; 17(7): 914–924; Ko GD, Mindra S, Lawson GE, Whitmore S, Arseneau L. Case series of ultrasound-guided plate-let-rich plasma injections for sacroiliac joint dysfunction. *Journal of Back and Musculoskeletal Rehabilitation*. 2017; 30(2): 363–370; Aufiero D. Vincent H, Sampson S, Bodor M. Regenerative injec-tion treatment in the spine: review and case series with platelet rich plasma. *Journal of Stem Cell Research, Reviews and Reports*. 2015; 2(1): 1019.

[24] Tolbert G. Roy D, Walker V. Ultrasound guided dextrose pro-lotherapy and platelet rich plasma therapy in chronic low back pain: three case reports. *International Journal of Physical Medicine & Rehabilitation*; 2013; 1: 149 [cited 2017 September 30] https://www.omicsonline.org/ultrasound-guided-dextrose-prolother-apy-2329-9096.1000149.php?aid=17937.

[25] Gumina S. PRP in rotator cuff healing. In *Rotator Cuff Tear* (pp. 357–360). Switzerland: Springer International Publishing, 2017; Barker SL, Bell SN, Connell D, Coghlan JA. Ultrasound-guided platelet-rich plasma injection for distal biceps tendinopathy. *Shoulder & Elbow*. 2015; 7(2): 110–114; Scarpone M, Rabago D, Snell E, DeMeo P, Ruppert K, Pritchard P, Arbogast G, Wilson JJ, Balzono JF. PRP as a treatment alternative for symptomatic rota-tor cuff tendinopathy for patients failing conservative treatments. *Techniques in Orthopaedics*. 2007; 22(1): 26–33; Alderman DD. Platelet rich plasma for rotator cuff tears. *Practical Pain Management*. 2012 September: 21–23.

[26] Papalia R, Zampogna B, Vadala G, Di Martino A, Nobile C. Are platelet rich plasma injections more effective in tendinopathy or enthesopathy. *Journal of Pain & Relief*. 2017; 6(3): Article ID 1000288, 5 pages; Cohn CS, Lockhart E, McCullough JJ. The use of autolo-gous platelet-rich plasma in the orthopedic setting. *Transfusion*. 2015; 55(7): 1812–1820; Kovacevic D, Bedi A, Dines JS, Athwal GS. Upper extremity: biologics in treating shoulder disease. *Current Orthopaedic Practice*. 2015; 26(2): 90–98.

[27] Salamanna F, Veronesi F, Maglio M, Della Bella E, Sartori M, Fini M. New and emerging strategies in platelet-rich plasma application in musculoskeletal regenerative procedures: general overview on still open questions and outlook. *BioMed Research International*. 2015: Article ID 846045, 24 pages.

[28] Jo CH, Shin JS, Shin WH, Lee SY, Yoon KS, Shin S. Platelet-rich plasma for arthroscopic repair of medium to large rotator cuff tears: a randomized controlled trial. *American Journal of Sports Medicine*. 2015; 43(9): 2102–2110; Sanchez M, Anuita E, Azofra J, Andia I, Padilla S, Mujika I. Comparison of surgically repaired Achilles tendon tears using platelet-rich fibrin matrices. *The American Journal of Sports Medicine*. 2007; 25(2): 245–251.

[29] Foster T, Puskas B, Mandelbaum BR, Gerhardt MB, Rodeao SA. Platelet-rich plasma: From basic science to clinical applications. *American Journal of Sports Medicine*. 2009; 37(11): 2259–2272.

[30] Garg, A. "The use of platelet rich plasma to enhance the success of bone grafts around dental implants." *Dental Implantology Update*. 2000; 11(3):17–21.

[31] Alexander R, Abuzeni P. Enhancement of autologous fat transplantation with platelet rich plasma. *American Journal of Cosmetic Surgery*. 2001; 18: 59–70.

[32] Kazakos K, Lyras DN, Verettas D, Tilkeridis K, Tryfonidis M. The use of autologous PRP gel as an aid in the management of acute trauma wounds. *Injury*. 2009; 40(8): 801–805.

[33] Mishra A, Pavelko T. Treatment of chronic elbow tendinosis with buffered platelet-rich plasma. *American Journal of Sports Medicine*. 2006; 34(11): 1774–1778.

[34] Dines J, Positano R. Plasma helps Hines Ward be super. *New York Daily News, Sports*. 2009 Feb 8 [cited 2017 August 26] http://www.nydailynews.com/sports/2009/02/07/2009-02-07_plasma_helps_hines_ward_be_super-2.html#ixzz0ivc1qaXu.

[35] Tendon Trouble: New treatment uses enhanced plasma. *Mayo Clinic Health Letter*. 2010 March, p. 7. [cited 2017 April 24] http://healthletter.mayoclinic.com/common/pdf/192/201003.PDF.

[36] NBA Warriors' Stephen Curry has platelet-rich plasma treatment on knee. *Sports Illustrated*. 2016 May 4 [cited 2016 May 29]

http://www.si.com/nba/2016/05/04/stephen-curry-golden-state -warriors-knee-injury-platelet-rich-plasma-treatment.

[37] Marx R, Garg A. *Dental and Craniofacial Applications of Platelet-Rich Plasma*. Hanover, Illinois: Quintessence Publishing Co., Inc. 2005.

[38] Langer HE, Stellos K, Steingen C, Froihofer A, Schonberger T, Kramer B, Bigalke B, May AE, Seizer P, Muller I, Gieseke F, Siegel-Axel D, Meuth SG, Schmidt A, Wendel HP, Bloch W, Gawaz M, Muller I. Platelet derived bFGF mediates vascular integrative mechanisms of mesenchymal stem cells in vitro. *Journal of Molecular and Cellular Cardiology*. 2009; 47(2): 315–325; Lyras D, Kazakos K, Verettas D, Botaitis S, Agrogiannis G, Kokka A, Pitiakoudis M, Kotzakaris A. The effect of platelet-rich plasma gel in the early phase of patellar tendon healing. *Archives of Orthopaedic and Trauma Surgery*. 2009; 129: 1577–1582.

[39] Kakudo N, Morimoto N, Kushida S, Ogawa T, Kusumoto K. Platelet-rich plasma releasate promotes angiogenesis in vitro and in vivo. *Medical Molecular Morphology*. 2014; 47(2): 83–89; Lyras DN, Kazakos K, Verettas D, Polychronidis A, Tryfonidis M, Botaitis S, Agrogiannis G, Simopoulos C, Kokka A, Patsouris E. The influence of platelet-rich plasma on angiogenesis during the early phase of tendon healing. *Foot & Ankle International*. 2009 Nov; 30(11): 1101–1106.

[40] Haynesworth SF, Kadiyala S, Liang LN, Thomas T, Bruder SP. Chemotactic and mitogenic stimulation of human mesenchymal stem cells by platelet rich plasma suggests a mechanism for enhancement of bone repair. Presented at the 48th Annual Meeting of the Orthopaedic Research Society, Dallas, Texas; February 10–13, 2002 www.perstat.com/ortho1.pdf; Haynesworth SE, Bruder SP. Mitogenic stimulation of human mesenchymal stem cells by platelet releasate. Poster Presentation, *American Academy of Orthopedic Surgery*. 2001 March.

[11] Fitzpatrick J, Bulsara MK, McCrory PR, Richardson M.D., Zheng MH. Analysis of platelet-rich plasma extraction: Variations in platelet and blood components between 4 common commercial kits. *Orthopaedic Journal of Sports Medicine*. 2017; 5(1).

[42] Marx R. Platelet-rich plasma: Evidence to support its use. *Journal of Oral and Maxillofacial Surgery*. 2004; 62: 489–496; Haynesworth

SE, Kadiyala S, Liang LN, Thomas T, Bruder SP. Chemotactic and mitogenic stimulation of human mesenchymal stem cells by platelet rich plasma suggests a mechanism for enhancement of bone repair. Presented at the 48th Annual Meeting of the Orthopaedic Research Society, Dallas, Texas; February 10–13, 2002. www.perstat.com/ortho1.pdf; Lansdown DA, Fortier LA. Platelet-rich plasma: formulations, preparations, constituents, and their effects. *Operative Techniques in Sports Medicine.* 2017; 25(1): 7–12.

[43] Weibrich G, Hansen T, Kleis W, Buch R, Hitzler WE. Effect of platelet concentration in platelet-rich plasma on peri-implant bone regeneration. *Bone.* 2004; 34(3): 665–671.

[44] Boswell SG, Schnabel LV, Mohammed HO, Sundman EA, Minas T, Fortier LA. Increasing platelet concentrations in leukocyte-reduced platelet-rich plasma decrease collagen gene synthesis in tendons. *American Journal of Sports Medicine.* 2014 Jan; 42(1): 42–49; Giusti I, Rughetti A, D'ascenzo S, Millimaggi D, Pavan A, Dell'Orso L, Dolo V. Identification of an optimal concentration of platelet gel for promoting angiogenesis in human endothelial cells. *Transfusion.* 2009 Apr 1; 49(4): 771–778.

[45] Dhillon MS, Patel S, John R. PRP in OA knee–update, current confusions and future options. *SICOT-J.* 2017; 3: 27.

[46] Filardo G, Kon E, Di Matteo B, Di Martino A, Sessa A, Letizia Merli M, Marcacci M. Leukocyte-poor PRP application for the treatment of knee osteoarthritis. *Joints.* 2013; 1(3): 112–120.

[47] Kawazoe T, Kim HH. Tissue augmentation by white blood cell-containing platelet-rich plasma. *Cell Transplantation.* 2012; 21(2–3): 601–607; Bielecki T, Dohan-Ehrenfest DM, Everts PA, Wiczkowski A. The role of leukocytes from L-PRP/L-PRF in wound healing and immune defense: New perspectives. *Current Pharmaceutical Biotechnology.* 2012; 13(7): 1153–1162.

[48] Weglein A, Sampson S, Aufiero D. Platelet rich plasma practical use in non-surgical musculoskeletal pathology. In *Platelet Rich Plasma: Lecture Notes in Bioengineering* (pp. 187–201). Berlin, Germany: Springer-Verlag, 2014.

[49] Alsousou J, Thompson M, Hulley P, Noble A, Willett K. The biology of platelet-rich plasma and its application in trauma

and orthopaedic surgery. *Journal of Bone and Joint Surgery (British Volume)*. 2009; 91(8): 987–996.

[50] Fufa D, Shealy B, Jacobson M, Kevy S, Murray MM. Activation of platelet-rich plasma using soluble type I collagen. *Journal of Oral and Maxillofacial Surgery*. 2008; 66(4): 684–690; Hall M. Band P, Meislin R, Jazrawi L, Cardone D. Platelet-rich plasma: Current concepts and application in sports medicine. *Journal of the American Academy of Orthopaedic Surgeons*. 2009; 17(10): 602–608.

[51] Wu J, Zhou J, Liu C, Zhang J, Xiong W, Lv Y, Liu R, Wang R, Du Z, Zhang G, Liu Q. A prospective study comparing platelet-rich plasma and local anesthetic(LA)/corticosteroid in intra-articular injection for the treatment of lumbar facet joint. *Pain Practice*. 2017; 17(7): 914–924; Mundla GKR, Venkataramana PK, Koduru MKR, Ravindran B. Study comparing the efficacy of platelet rich plasma versus steroid versus placebo in lateral epicondylitis. *International Journal of Research in Orthopaedics*. 2017; 3(2): 207–212; Nasser MET, El Yasaki AZ, El Mallah RME, Abdelazeem ASM. Treatment of lateral epicondylitis with platelet-rich plasma, glucocorticoid, or saline. A comparative study. *Egyptian Rheumatology and Rehabilitation*. 2017; 44(1): 1.

[52] Gosens T, Peerbooms JC, van Laar W, den Oudsten BL. Ongoing positive effect of platelet-rich plasma versus corticosteroid injection in lateral epicondylitis: A double-blind randomized controlled trial with 2-year follow-up. *The American Journal of Sports Medicine*. 2011; 39(6): 1200–1208.

[53] Mi B, Liu G, Zhou W, Lv H, Liu Y, Wu Q, Liu J. Platelet rich plasma versus steroid on lateral epicondylitis: meta-analysis of randomized clinical trials. *The Physician and Sportsmedicine*. 2017; 45(2): 97–104.

[54] Monto RR. Platelet-rich plasma efficacy versus corticosteroid injection treatment for chronic severe plantar fasciitis. *Foot & Ankle International*. 2014; 35(4): 313–318.

[55] Wu J, Zhou J, Liu C, Zhang J, Xiong W, Lv Y, Liu R, Wang R, Du Z, Zhang G, Liu Q. A prospective study comparing platelet-rich plasma and local anesthetic(LA)/corticosteroid in intra-articular injection for the treatment of lumbar facet joint. *Pain Practice*. 2017; 17(7): 914–924.

[56] Moussa M, Lajeunesse D, Hilal G, El Atat O, Haykal G, Serhal R, Chalhoub A, Khalil C, and Alaaeddine N. Platelet rich plasma (PRP) induces chondroprotection via increasing autophagy, anti-inflammatory markers, and decreasing apoptosis in human osteoarthritic cartilage. *Experimental Cell Research.* 2017; 352(1): 146–156; Xie, X, Ulici V, Alexander P, Jiang Y, Zhang C, Tuan RS. Platelet-rich plasma inhibits mechanically induced injury in chondrocytes. *Arthroscopy: The Journal of Arthroscopic and Related Surgery.* 2015 Jun; 31(6): 1142–1150; Gato-Calvo L, Vela-Anero A, Loures-Fraga E, Ruiz Romero C, Blanco FJ, Burguera EF. Proliferative and anti-inflammatory effect of platelet-rich plasma on osteoarthritic chondrocytes. *Osteoarthritis and Cartilage.* 2017; 25: S270–S271.

[57] Creaney L, Hamilton B. Growth factor delivery methods in the management of sports injuries: The state of play. *British Journal of Sports Medicine.* 2008; 42(5): 314–320.

[58] Marx R. The biology of platelet-rich plasma (reply to letter to the editor). *Journal of Oral and Maxillofacial Surgery.* 2001; 59: 1120.

[59] Schmitz JP, Hollinger J. The biology of platelet-rich plasma (letter to the editor). *Journal of Oral and Maxillofacial Surgery.* 2001 Sept 30; 59(9): 1119–1120.

[60] Sanchez A, Sheridan P, Kupp L. Is platelet-rich plasma the perfect enhancement factor? A current review. *International Journal of Oral & Maxillofacial Implants.* 2002; 18: 93–103.

[61] Bielecki T, Gazdik T, Arendt J, Szxzepanski T, Kroi W, Wielkoszynski T. Antibacterial effect of autologous platelet gel enriched with growth factors and other active substances. *Journal of Bone and Joint Surgery (British Volume).* 2007; 89(3): 417–420.

[62] Clark G. Platelet rich plasma (PRP) therapy literature reviews. *Journal of Prolotherapy.* August 2009; 1(3): 185–191.

Chapter 10: Biocellular (Stem Cell–Rich) Prolotherapy

[1] Jackson WM, Nesti LJ, Tuan RS. Mesenchymal stem cell therapy for attenuation of scar formation during wound healing. *Stem Cell Research & Therapy.* 2012; 3: 20.

[2] National Institutes of Heatlh, US Department of Health and Human Services, Stem Cell Information, Basics [cited 2017 January 22] https://stemcells.nih.gov/info/basics/1.htm.

[3] Boregowda S, Phinney D. Reconciling the stem cell and paracrine paradigms of mesenchymal stem cell function. In *The Biology and Therapeutic Application of Mesenchymal Cells*. Hoboken, New Jersey: John Wiley & Sons; published online 2016 Nov 26 [cited 2017 February 15] http://onlinelibrary.wiley.com/doi/10.1002/9781118907474.ch64 /summary.

[4] Izadpanah R, Trygg C, Patel B, Kriedt C, Dufour J, Gimble JM, Bunnell BA. Biologic properties of mesenchymal stem cells derived from bone marrow and adipose tissue. *Journal of Cellular Biochemistry*. 2006; 99(5): 1285–1297; Kern S, Eichler H, Stoeve J, Kluter H, Bieback K. Comparative analysis of mesenchymal stem cells from bone marrow, umbilical cord blood, or adipose tissue. *Stem Cells*. 2006; 24(5): 1294–1301; Jang Y, Koh YG, Choi YJ, Kim SH, Yoon DS, Lee M, Lee JW. Characterization of adipose tissue-derived stromal vascular fraction for clinical application to cartilage regeneration. *Vitro Cellular & Developmental Biology-Animal*. 2015 Feb 1; 51(2): 142–150; Zuk PA, Zhu M, Ashijan P, De Ugarte DA, Huang JI, Mizuno H, Alfonso ZC, Fraser JK, Benhaim P, Hedrick MH. Human adipose tissue is a source of multipotent stem cells. *Molecular Biology of the Cell*. 2002; 13(12): 4279–4295.

[5] Fraser JK, Wulur I, Alfonso Z, Hedrick MH. Fat tissue: An underappreciated source of stem cells for biotechnology. *Trends in Biotechnology*. 2006; 24(4): 150–154; Prockop DJ, Phinney DG, Bunnell BA. *Mesenchymal Stem Cells: Methods and Protocols*. Totowa, New Jersey: Humana Press, 2008.

[6] Beane OS, Fonseca VC, Cooper LL, Koren G, Darling EM. Impact of aging on the regenerative properties of bone marrow-, muscle-, and adipose-derived mesenchymal stem/stromal cells. *PLOS ONE*. 2014; 26(12) [cited 2017 October 1] http://journals.plos.org/plosone/article?id=10.1371/journal.pone.0115963.

[7] Kim WS, Park BS, Sung JH, Yang JM, Park SB, Kwak SJ, Park SJ. Wound healing effect of adipose-derived stem cells: A critical role of secretory factors on human dermal fibroblasts." *Journal of Dermatological Science*. 2007; 48(1): 15–24; Ebrahimian TG, Pouzoulet F, Squiban C, Buard V, Andre M, Cousin B, Gourmelon P, Benderitter M, Casteilla L, Tamarat R. Cell therapy based on adipose tissue-derived stromal cells promotes physiological and pathological wound healing. *Arteriosclerosis, Thrombosis, and Vascular Biology*. 2009; 29(4): 503–510.

[8] Little D, Guilak F, Ruch D. Ligament-derived matrix stimulates a ligamentous phenotype in human adipose-derived stem cells. *Tissue Engineering Part A.* 2010; 16(7): 2307–2319; Figueroa D, Espinosa M, Calvo R, Scheu M, Vaisman A, Gallegos M, Conget P. Anterior cruciate ligament regeneration using mesenchymal stem cells and collagen type I scaffold in a rabbit model. *Knee Surgery, Sports Traumatology, Arthroscopy.* 2014; 22(5): 1196–1202.

[9] Chen X, Zou X, Yin G, Ouyang H. Tendon tissue engineering with mesenchymal stem cells and biografts: An option for large tendon defects? *Frontiers in Bioscience (Scholar Edition).* 2009 Jun; 1: 23–32; Uysal AC, Mizuno H. Tendon regeneration and repair with adipose derived stem cells. *Current Stem Cell Research & Therapy.* 2010; 5(2): 161–167; Uysal, AC, Mizuno H. Differentiation of adipose-derived stem cells for tendon repair. *Methods in Molecular Biology.* 2011; 702: 443–451; Uysal AC, Mizuno H. Tendon regeneration and repair with adipose derived stem cells. *Current Stem Cell Research & Therapy.* 2010; 5(2): 161–167.

[10] Jung M, Kaszap B, Redöhl A, Steck E, Breusch S, Richter W, Gotterbarn T. Enhanced early tissue regeneration after matrix-assisted autologous mesenchymal stem cell transplantation in full thickness chondral defects in a minipig model. *Cell Transplantation.* 2009; 18(8): 923–932; Lee KB, Hui JH, Song IC, Ardany L, Lee EH. Injectable mesenchymal stem cell therapy for large cartilage defects: A porcine model. *Stem Cells.* 2007; 25(11): 2964–2971; Dragoo JL, Samimi B, Zhu M, Hame SL, Thomas BJ, Lieberman JR. Tissue-engineered cartilage and bone using stem cells from human infrapatellar fat pads. *Journal of Bone & Joint Surgery (British volume).* 2003; 85(5): 740–747; Gobbi A, Karnatzikos G, Sankineani SR. One-step surgery with multipotent stem cells for the treatment of large full-thickness chondral defects of the knee. *American Journal of Sports Medicine.* 2014; 42(3): 648–657.

[11] Hoogendoom RJW, Lu ZF, Kroeze RJ, Bank RA, Wuisman PI, Helder MN. Adipose stem cells for intervertebral disc regeneration: Current status and concepts for the future. *Journal of Cellular and Molecular Medicine.* 2008; 12(6A): 2205–2216; Richardson SM, Kalamegam G, Pushparaj PN, Matta C, Memic A, Khademhosseini A, Mobasheri R, Poletti FL, Hoyland JA, Mobasheri A. Mesenchymal stem cells in regenerative medicine:

Focus on articular cartilage and intervertebral disc regeneration. *Methods*. 2016; 99(April): 69–80.

[12] Bacou F, El Andalousi RB, Daussin PA, Micallef JP, Levin JM, Chammas M, Casteilla L, Reyne Y, Nougues J. Transplantation of adipose tissue-derived stromal cells increases mass and functional capacity of damaged skeletal muscle. *Cell Transplantation*. 2004; 13(2): 103–111; Rodriguez LV, Alfonso Z, Zhang R, Leung J, Wu B, Ignarro LJ. Clonogenic multipotent stem cells in human adipose tissue differentiate into functional smooth muscle cells. *Proceedings of the National Academy of Sciences of the United States of America*. 2006; 103(32): 12167–12172; Goudenege S, Pisani DF, Wdziekonski B, Di Santo JP, Bagnis C, Dani C, Dechesne CA. Enhancement of myogenic and muscle repair capacities of human adipose-derived stem cells with forced expression of MyoD. *Molecular Therapy*. 2009; 17(6): 1064–1072.

[13] Murphy JM, Dixon K, Beck S, Fabian D, Feldman A, Barry F. Reduced chondrogenic and adipogenic activity of mesenchymal stem cells from patients with advanced osteoarthritis. *Arthritis & Rheumatism*. 2002; 46(3): 704–713; Luyten FP. Mesenchymal stem cells in osteoarthritis. *Current Opinion in Rheumatology*. 2004; 16(5): 599–603; Haynesworth SE, Kadiyala S, Liang LN, Thomas T, Bruder SP. Chemotactic and Mitogenic Stimulation of Human Mesenchymal Stem Cells by Platelet Rich Plasma Suggests a Mechanism for Enhancement of Bone Repair. Presented at the 48th Annual Meeting of the Orthopaedic Research Society, Dallas, Texas; February 10–13, 2002 www.perstat.com/ortho1.pdf.

[14] Wakitani S, Goto T, Pineda SJ, Young RG, Mansour JM, Caplan AI, Goldberg VM. Mesenchymal cell-based repair of large, full-thickness defects of articular cartilage. *Journal of Bone & Joint Surgery (American volume)*. 1994; 76(4): 579–592; Wakitani S, Imoto K, Yamamoto T, Saito M, Murata N, Yoneda M. Human autologous culture expanded bone marrow mesenchymal cell transplantation for repair of cartilage defects in osteoarthritic knees. *Osteoarthritis and Cartilage*. 2002; 10(3): 199–206; Bui KHT, Pham PV, Duong TD, Nguyen NT, Nguyen TD, Le VT, Mai VT, Phan NLC, Le DM, Ngoc NK. Symptomatic knee osteoarthritis treatment using autologous adipose derived stem cells and platelet-rich plasma: A clinical study. *Biomedical Research and Therapy*. 2014; 1(1): 2–8.

[15] Filardo G, Perdisa F, Roffi A, Marcacci M, Kon E. Stem cells in articular cartilage regeneration. *Journal of Orthopaedic Surgery and Research.* 2016; 11(1): 1; Koh YG, Choi YJ, Kwon SK, Kim YS, Yeo JE. Clinical results and second-look arthroscopic findings after treatment with adipose-derived stem cells for knee osteoarthritis. *Knee Surgery, Sports Traumatology, Arthroscopy.* 2015; 23(5): 1308–1316.

[16] International Federation for Adipose Therapeutics and Science [cited 2016 January 24] http://www.ifats.org.

[17] Crisan M, Corselli M, Chen WC, Péault B. Perivascular cells for regenerative medicine. *Journal of Cellular and Molecular Medicine.* 2012; 16(12): 2851–2860.

[18] Malan T. Adipose-derived regenerative cells. In *Stem Cells in Aesthetic Procedures* (pp. 299–302). Berlin, Germany: Springer, 2014.

[19] Van Pham P, Bui KH, Ngo DQ, Vu NB, Truong NH, Phan NL, Le DM, Duong TD, Nguyen TD, Le VT, Phan NK. Activated platelet-rich plasma improves adipose-derived stem cell transplantation efficiency in injured articular cartilage. *Stem Cell Research & Therapy.* 2013; 4: 91.

[20] Blanton MW, Hadad I, Johnstone BH, Mund JA, Rogers PI, Eppley BL, March KL. Adipose stromal cells and platelet-rich plasma therapies synergistically increase revascularization during wound healing. *Plastic and Reconstructive Surgery.* 2009; 123(2 Suppl): 56S–64S; 91; Fukaya Y, Kuroda M, Aoyagi Y, Asada S, Kubota Y, Okamoto Y, Nakayama T, Saito Y, Satoh K, Bujo H. Platelet-rich plasma inhibits the apoptosis of highly adipogenic homogeneous preadipocytes in an in vitro culture system. *Experimental & Molecular Medicine.* 2012; 44(5): 330–339; Uysal CA, Tobita M, Hyakusoku H, Mizuno H. Adipose-derived stem cells enhance primary tendon repair: Biomechanical and immunohistochemical evaluation. *Journal of Plastic, Reconstructive & Aesthetic Surgery.* 2012; 65(12): 1712–1719.

[21] Uysal CA, Tobita M, Hyakusoku H, Mizuno H. Adipose-derived stem cells enhance primary tendon repair: Biomechanical and immunohistochemical evaluation. *Journal of Plastic, Reconstructive & Aesthetic Surgery.* 2012; 65(12): 1712–1719.

[22] Wyles CC, Houdek MT, Behfar A, Sierra, RJ. Mesenchymal stem cell therapy for osteoarthritis: current perspectives. *Stem Cells and Cloning: Advances and Applications.* 2015; 8: 117–124.

[23] van Lent, PL, van den Berg, WB. Mesenchymal stem cell therapy in osteoarthritis: Advanced tissue repair or intervention with smouldering synovial activation? *Arthritis Research & Therapy.* 2013 Mar 20; 15(2): 112.

[24] Wolfstadt JI, Cole BJ, Ogilvie-Harris DJ, Viswanathan S, Chahal J. Current concepts: The role of mesenchymal stem cells in the management of knee osteoarthritis. *Sports Health.* 2015; 7(1): 38–44.

[25] Buckwalter, JA, Saltzman C, Brown T. The impact of osteoarthritis: Implications for research. *Clinical Orthopaedics and Related Research.* 2004; 427: S6–S15.

[26] Ruetze M, Richter W. Adipose-derived stromal cells for osteoarticular repair: Trophic function versus stem cell activity. *Expert Reviews in Molecular Medicine.* 2014 May [cited 2017 October 1] https://www.ncbi.nlm.nih.gov/pmc/articles/PMC4017835/; Reich CM, Raabe O, Wenisch S, Bridger PS, Kramer M, Arnhold S. Isolation, culture and chondrogenic differentiation of canine adipose tissue- and bone marrow-derived mesenchymal stem cells: A comparative study. *Veterinary Research Communications.* 2012; 36(2): 139–148; Afizah H, Yang Z, Hui JH, Ouyang HW, Lee EH. A comparison between the chondrogenic potential of human bone marrow stem cells (BMSCs) and adipose-derived stem cells (ADSCs) taken from the same donors. *Tissue Engineering.* 2007 April; 13(4): 659–666.

[27] Dragoo JL, Carlson G, McCormick F, Khan-Farooqi H, Zhu M, Zuk PA, Benhaim P. Healing full-thickness cartilage defects using adipose-derived stem cells. *Tissue Engineering.* 2007; 13(7): 1615–1621.

[28] Im GI, Shin YW, Lee KB. Do adipose tissue-derived mesenchymal stem cells have the same osteogenic and chondrogenic potential as bone marrow-derived cells? *Osteoarthritis and Cartilage.* 2005; 13: 845–53.

[29] Freitag J, Shah K, Wickham J, Boyd R, Tenen A. The effect of autologous adipose derived mesenchymal stem cell therapy in the treatment of a large osteochondral defect of the knee following unsuccessful surgical intervention of osteochondritis dissecans–a case study. *BMC Musculoskeletal Disorders.* 2017 Jul 14; 18(1): 298.

[30] Melief SM, Zwaginga JJ, Fibbe WE, Roelofs H. Adipose tissue-derived multipotent stromal cells have a higher immunomodulatory capacity than their bone marrow-derived counterparts. *Stem Cells Translational Medicine*. 2013; 2(6): 455–463.

[31] Oshita T, Tobita M, Tajima S, Mizuno H. Adipose-derived stem cells improve collagenase-induced tendinopathy in a rat model. *American Journal of Sports Medicine*. 2016 Aug; 44(8): 1983–1989: Choi YS, Vincent LG, Lee AR, Dobke MK, Engler AJ. Mechanical derivation of functional myotubes from adipose-derived stem cells. *Biomaterials*. 2012 Mar; 33(8): 2482–2491; De Francesco F, Ricci G, D'Andrea F, Nicoletti GF, Ferraro GA. Human adipose stem cells: from bench to bedside. *Tissue Engineering Part B: Reviews*. 2015; 21(6): 572–584; Obaid, H, Connell D. Cell therapy in tendon disorders: What is the current evidence? *American Journal of Sports Medicine*. 2010; 38(10): 2123–2132.

[32] Adriani E, Moio M, Di Paola B, Salustri W, Alfieri A, Parisi P, Ruggiero M, Borab Z, Carlesimo B. Percutaneous Fat Transfer to Treat Knee Osteoarthritis Symptoms: Preliminary Results. *Joints*. 2017 Jun; 5(2): 89–92.

[33] Tangchitphisut P, Srikaew N, Numhom S, Tangprasittipap A, Woratanarat P, Wongsak S, Kijkunasathian C, Hongeng S, Murray IR, Tawonsawatruk T. Infrapatellar Fat Pad: An alternative source of adipose-derived mesenchymal stem cells. *Arthritis*. 2016 Apr 26 [cited 2017 October 1] https://www.hindawi.com/journals/arthritis/2016/4019873/abs; English A, Jones EA, Corscadden D, Henshaw K, Chapman T, Emery P, McGonagle D. A comparative assessment of cartilage and joint fat pad as a potential source of cells for autologous therapy development in knee osteoarthritis. *Rheumatology*. 2007 Sep 26; 46(11): 1676–1683.

[34] Hindle P, Khan N, Biant L, Péault B. The Infrapatellar fat pad as a source of perivascular stem cells with increased chondrogenic potential for regenerative medicine. *Stem Cells Translational Medicine*. 2017; 6(1): 77–87.

[35] Teichtahl AJ, Wulidasari E, Brady SRE, Wang Y, Wluka AE, Ding C, Giles GG, Cicuttini FM. A large infrapatellar fat pad protects against knee pain and lateral tibial cartilage volume loss. *Arthritis Research & Therapy*. 2015; 17(1): 318.

[36] Adriani E, Moio M, Di Paola B, Salustri W, Alfieri A, Parisi P, Ruggiero M, Borab Z, Carlesimo B. Percutaneous Fat Transfer to Treat Knee Osteoarthritis Symptoms: Preliminary Results. *Joints.* 2017 Jun; 5(2): 89–92.

[37] Ruhdorfer A, Haniel F, Petersohn T, Dörrenberg J, Wirth W, Dannhauer T, Hunter DJ, Eckstein F. Between-group differences in infra-patellar fat pad size and signal in symptomatic and radiographic progression of knee osteoarthritis vs non-progressive controls and healthy knees–data from the FNIH Biomarkers Consortium Study and the Osteoarthritis Initiative. *Osteoarthritis and Cartilage.* 2017; 25(7): 1114–1121.

[38] Cowan, S.M., H.F. Hart, S.J. Warden, and K.M. Crossley. Infrapatellar fat pad volume is greater in individuals with patellofemoral joint osteoarthritis and associated with pain. *Rheumatology International.* August 2015; 35(8): 1439–1442; Clockaerts S, Bastiaansen-Jenniskens YM, Runhaar J, Van Osch GJ, Van Offel JF, Verhaar JA, De Clerck LS, Somville J. The infrapatellar fat pad should be considered as an active osteoarthritic joint tissue: A narrative review. *Osteoarthritis and Cartilage.* 2010 Jul 31; 18(7): 876–882.

[39] Antony BSE, Jin X, Wang X, Han W, Cicuttini F, Ding C, Jones G. OP0144 Infra patellar fat pad signal intensity alterations and effusion-synovitis predict knee pain, cartilage volume loss and total knee replacement over 10.7 years in older adults. *Annals of the Rheumatic Diseases.* 2016; 75(2): 110–111.

[40] Gwyn R, Kotwal RS, Holt M.D., Davies AP. Complete excision of the infrapatellar fat pad is associated with patellar tendon shortening after primary total knee arthroplasty. *European Journal of Orthopaedic Surgery & Traumatology.* 2016 Jul 1; 26(5): 545–549.

[41] Hernigou P, Homma Y, Flouzat-Lachaniette CH, Poignard A, Chevallier N, Rouard H. Cancer risk is not increased in patients treated for orthopaedic diseases with autologous bone marrow cell concentrate. *Journal of Bone & Joint Surgery (American Volume).* 2013 Dec; 95(24): 2215–2221.

[42] Pak J, Chang JJ, Lee JH, Lee SH. Safety reporting on implantation of autologous adipose tissue-derived stem cells with platelet-rich plasma into human articular joints. *BMC Musculoskeletal Disorders.* 2013; 14: 337.

[43] Hatzistergos KE, Blum A, Ince T, Grichnik JM, Hare JM. What is the oncologic risk of stem cell treatment for heart disease? *Circulation Research*. 2011; 108(11): 1300–1303; Heldman AW, DiFede DL, Fishman JE, Zambrano JP, Trachtenberg BH, Karantalis V, Mushtaq M, Williams AR, Suncion VY, McNiece IK, Ghersin E. Transendocardial mesenchymal stem cells and mononuclear bone marrow cells for ischemic cardiomyopathy: The TAC-HFT randomized trial. *JAMA*. 2014; 311(1): 62–73.

[44] Filardo G, Perdisa F, Roffi A, Marcacci M, Kon E. Stem cells in articular cartilage regeneration. *Journal of Orthopaedic Surgery and Research*. 2016 Apr 12; 11:42, 15 pages.

[45] Chirba MA, Sweetapple B, Hannon CP, Anderson JA. FDA regulation of adult stem cell therapies as used in sports medicine. *The Journal of Knee Surgery*. 2015; 28(1): 55–62.

[46] Alderman DD. Regenerative injection therapies for pain: Traditional, platelet rich plasma and biocellular prolotherapy. In *Integrative Pain Management* (pp. 346–360). New York, New York: Oxford University Press, 2016; Shapiro E, Grande D, Drakos M. Biologics in Achilles tendon healing and repair: A review. *Current Reviews in Musculoskeletal Medicine*. 2015; 8(1): 9–17.

Chapter 11: Pain Medication: A Double-Edged Sword

[1] Eligon J, Kovaleski SF, Cosecarilli J. Prince's addiction and an intervention too late. *New York Times*. 2016 May 4 [cited 2017 March 27] https://www.nytimes.com/2016/05/05/arts/music/friends-sou ght-help-for-princes-addiction-lawyer-says.html?_r=0.

[2] Frieden TR, Houry D. Reducing the risks of relief—the CDC opioid-prescribing guideline. *New England Journal of Medicine*. 2016 Apr 21; 2016(374): 1501–1504; Opioid Addiction 2016 Facts & Figures. American Society of Addiction Medicine [cited 31 October 2017] https://www.asam.org/docs/default-source/advocacy/opioid-addiction-disease-facts-figures.pdf; Moghe S. Opioid history: From "wonder drug" to abuse epidemic. 2016 Oct 14 [cited 2017 August 10] http://www.cnn.com/2016/05/12/health/opioid-addiction-history/index.html.

[3] Loh RS. Effects of opioids on the immune system. *Neurochemical Research*. 1996; 21(11): 1375–1386; Stovitz SD, Johnson RJ. NSAIDs and musculoskeletal treatment: What is the clinical evidence?

Physician and Sportsmedicine. 2003 Jan (31)1: 35–52; Juni P, Nartey L, Reichenbach S, Sterchi R, Dieppe PA. Risk of cardiovascular events and Rofecoxib [Vioox]: Cumulative meta-analysis. *The Lancet.* 2004 Dec 10; 364(9450): 2021–2029.

[4] Welters I. Opioids and immunosuppression. Clinical relevance? *Anaesthesist.* 2003; 52(5): 442–452; Plein LM, Rittner HL. Opioids and the immune system-friend or foe. *British Journal of Pharmacology.* 2017 Mar [cited 2017 March 27] http://onlinelibrary.wiley.com/doi/10.1111/bph.13750/full.

[5] Scopsi L, Balslev E, Brunner N, Poulsen HS, Andersen J, Rank F, Larsson LI. Immunoreactive opioid peptides in human breast cancer. *American Journal of Pathology.* 1989; 134(2): 473–479; Simon RH, Arbo TE. Morphine increases metastatic tumor growth. *Brain Research Bulletin.* 1986; 16(3): 363–367; Ishikawa M, Tanno K, Kamo A, Takayanagi Y, Sasaki Y. Enhancement of tumor growth by morphine and its possible mechanism in mice. *Biological and Pharmaceutical Bulletin.* 1993; 16(3): 762–766; Bryant HU, Bernton EW, Holaday JW. Immunosuppressive effects of chronic morphine treatment in mice. *Life Science.* 1987; 41(14): 1731–1738.

[6] Zhang N, Hodge D, Rogers TJ, Oppenheim JJ. Ca+2- independent protein kinase C's mediate heterologous desensitization of leukocyte chemokine receptors by opioid receptors. *Journal of Biological Chemistry.* 2003; 278(15): 12729–12736.

[7] Ninkovic' J, Roy S. Role of the mu-opioid receptor in opioid modulation of immune function. *Amino Acids.* 2013; 45(1): 9–24.

[8] Wiegand TJ, Vernetti CM. Nonsteroidal anti-inflammatory drug (NSAID) toxicity. Medscape [cited 2017 March 27] http://emedicine.medscape.com/article/816117-overview.

[9] Guo S, DiPietro LA. Factors affecting wound healing. *Journal of Dental Research.* 2010; 89(3): 219–229.

[10] Kotsiou OS, Zarogiannis SG, Gourgoulianis KI. Prehospital NSAIDs use prolong hospitalization in patients with pleuro-pulmonary infection. *Respiratory Medicine.* 2017; 123: 28–33.

[11] Stovitz SD, Johnson RJ. NSAIDs and musculoskeletal treatment. What is the clinical evidence? *Physician and Sportsmedicine.* 2003 Jan; (31)1: 35–52; Golden BD, Abramson SD. Selective

cyclooxygenase-2 inhibitors. *Rheumatology Clinics of North America.* 1999; 25(2): 359–278.

[12] Manjuran RJ, History of Aspirin. *Kerala Heart Journal.* 2015; 5 (2): 28–29.

[13] History of Aspirin. *Wikipedia.* [cited 2017 March 27] https://en.wikipedia.org/wiki/History_of_aspirin.

[14] Segev G, Katz R. Selective COX-2 inhibitors and risk of cardiovascular events. *Hospital Physician.* 2004 Feb: 39–46.

[15] US Food and Drug Administration. Information for Health care Professionals: Valdecoxib (marketed as Bextra). 2005 [cited 2017 March 27] https://www.fda.gov/Drugs/DrugSafety/Postmarket DrugSafetyInformationforPatientsandProviders/ucm124649.htm.

[16] Harvard Health Publications, Harvard Medical School. Heart-safer NSAID alternatives. 2015 Nov [cited 2017 March 27] http://www.health.harvard.edu/heart-health/heart-safer-nsaid-alternatives; Trelle S, Reichenbach S, Wandel S, Hildebrand P, Tschannen B, Villiger PM, Egger M, Jüni P. Cardiovascular safety of non-steroidal anti-inflammatory drugs: network meta-analysis. *British Medical Journal.* 2011 Jan 11; 342: c7086.

[17] Chang DS, Hsu E, Hottinger DG, Cohen SP. Anti-nerve growth factor in pain management: current evidence. *Journal of Pain Research.* 2016; 9: 373–383.

[18] Stovitz SD, Johnson RJ. NSAIDs and musculoskeletal treatment. What is the clinical evidence? *Physician and Sportsmedicine.* 2003 Jan (31)1: 35–52.

[19] Almekinders LC. Anti-inflammatory treatment of muscular injuries in sports. *Sports Medicine.* 1993; 15: 139–145.

[20] Andriacchi T, Sabiston P, DeHaven K, Dahners L, Woo S, Frank C, Oakes B, Brand R, Lewis J. Ligament: Injury and repair. In *Injury and Repair of the Musculoskeletal Soft Tissues* (pp. 103–128). Park Ridge, Illinois: American Academy of Orthopedic Surgeons, 1988.

[21] Jam, B. Questioning the use of NSAIDs given inflammation is a perfectly healthy response following acute musculoskeletal injuries. 2014 Jul 14 [cited 2017 March 30] https://www.researchgate.net/profile/Bahram_Jam/publication/306372948_Questioning_

the_use_of_NSAIDs_Given_Inflammation_is_a_Perfectly_
Healthy_Response_Following_Acute_Musculoskeletal_Injuries/
links/57bb12f708ae9fdf82ef016e.pdf.

[22] Orchard J, Best T. The management of muscle strain injuries:
An early return versus the risk of recurrence. *Clinical Journal
of Sports Medicine.* 2002; 12(1): 3–5; Almekinders LC, Gilbert JA.
Healing of experimental muscle strains and the effects of non-
steroidal anti-inflammatory medication. *American Journal of Sports
Medicine.* 1986; 14: 303–308; Mishra DK, Friden J, Schmitz MC,
Lieber RL. Anti-inflammatory medication after muscle injury.
Journal of Bone and Joint Surgery. 1995; 77(10): 1510–1519; Obremsky
WY, Seaber AV, Ribbeck BM, Garrett WE Jr. Biomechanical and
histologic assessment of a controlled muscle strain injury treated
with piroxicam. *American Journal of Sports Medicine.* 1994; 22(4):
558–561.

[23] Hauser RA. The acceleration of articular cartilage degeneration
in osteoarthritis by nonsteroidal anti-inflammatory drugs. *Journal
of Prolotherapy.* 2010; 2(1): 305–322.

[24] Walker LA, Zambraski EJ, Williams RF. Widespread use of prescription nonsteroidal anti-inflammatory drugs among US army
active duty soldiers. *Military Medicine.* 2017; 182(3): e1709.

[25] Ziltener JL, Leal S, Fournier PE. Non-steroidal anti-inflammatory drugs for athletes: An update. *Annals of Physical and
Rehabilitation Medicine.* 2010; 53(4): 278–288.

[26] Morelli KM, Brown LB, Warren GL. Effect of NSAIDs on
recovery from acute skeletal muscle injury: a systematic review
and meta-analysis. *American Journal of Sports Medicine.* March
2017 [cited 2017 October 1] http://journals.sagepub.com/doi/
abs/10.1177/0363546517697957.

[27] Almekinders LC. Anti-inflammatory treatment of muscular
injuries in sports: An update of recent studies. *Sports Medicine.*
1999; 28(6): 383–388.

[28] Mishra DK, Fridén J, Schmitz MC, Lieber RL. Anti-inflammatory
medication after muscle injury. A treatment resulting in short-
term improvement but subsequent loss of muscle function. *Journal
of Bone and Joint Surgery* 1995 Oct 1; 77(10): 1510–1519.

[29] Ziltener JL, Leal S, Fournier PE. Non-steroidal anti-inflammatory drugs for athletes: an update. *Annals of Physical and Rehabilitation Medicine.* 2010; 53(4): 278–288.

[30] Mackey AL, Mikkelsen UR, Magnusson SP, Kjaer M. Rehabilitation of muscle after injury–the role of anti-inflammatory drugs. *Scandinavian Journal of Medicine & Science in Sports.* 2012; 22(4): e8–e14.

[31] Stanley KL, Weaver JE. Pharmacologic management of pain and inflammation in athletes. *Clinics in Sports Medicine.* 1998; 17(2): 374–392.

[32] Bissinger O, Kreutzer K, Götz C, Hapfelmeier A, Pautke C, Vogt S, Wexel G, Wolff KD, Tischer T, Prodinger PM. A biomechanical, micro-computer tomographic and histological analysis of the influence of diclofenac and prednisolone on fracture healing in vivo. *BMC Musculoskeletal Disorders.* 2016; 17(1): 383.

[33] Dahners LE, Mullis BH. Effects of nonsteroidal anti-inflammatory drugs on bone formation and soft-tissue healing. *Journal of the American Academy of Orthopaedic Surgeons.* 2004; 12(3): 139–143.

[34] O'Connor JP, Lysz T. Celecoxib, NSAIDs and the skeleton. *Drugs of Today.* 2008; 9: 693.

[35] Giannoudis PV. Nonunion of the femoral diaphysis: The influence of reaming and non-steroidal anti-inflammatory drugs. *Journal of Bone and Joint (British).* 2001; 83(2): 308.

[36] Van Esch RW. Kool MM, van As S. NSAIDs can have adverse effects on bone healing. *Medical Hypotheses.* 2013; 81(2): 343–346.

[37] Pountos I, Georgouli T, Calori GM, Giannoudis PV. Do nonsteroidal anti-inflammatory drugs affect bone healing? A critical analysis. *The Scientific World Journal.* 2012: Article ID 606404, 14 pages.

[38] Glassman SD, Rose SM, Dimar JR, Puno RM, Campbell MJ, Johnson JR. The Effect of Postoperative Nonsteroidal Anti-inflammatory Drug Administration on Spinal Fusion. *Spine.* 1998 Apr 1; 23(7): 834–838. Glassman DS. The effect of postoperative nonsteroidal anti-inflammatory drug administration on spinal fusion. *Spine.* 1998; 23(7): 834–838.

[39] Tscholl PM, Gard S, Schindler M. A sensible approach to the use of NSAIDs in sports medicine. *Schweizerische Zeitschrift für Sportmedizin & Sporttraumatologie.* 2017; 65(2): 15–20.

[40] Elder C, Dahners L, Weinhold P. Cox-2 inhibitor impairs ligament healing in the rat. *American Journal of Sports Medicine.* 2001; 29(6): 801–805.

[41] Packer JD, Varthi A, Zhu D, Javier FG, Garver JV, Tommasini SM, Blaine TA. Ibuprofen impairs capsulolabral healing in a rat model of anterior glenohumeral instability. *Journal of Shoulder and Elbow Surgery.* 2016; 25(10): e315.

[42] Hauser RA, Dolan EE, Phillips HJ, Newlin AC, Moore RE, Woldin BA. Ligament injury and healing: A review of current clinical diagnostics and therapeutics. *Open Rehabilitation Journal.* 2013; 6: 1–20.

[43] Brandt KD, Palmoski MJ. Effects of salicylates and other nonsteroidal anti-inflammatory drugs on articular cartilage. *American Journal of Medicine.* 1984; 77(1): 65–69.

[44] Newman NM, Ling RSM. Acetabular bone destruction related to non-steroidal anti-inflammatory drugs. *The Lancet.* 1985; 326(8445): 11–14.

[45] Ronningen H, Langeland N. Indomethacin treatment in osteoarthritis of the hip joint – Does the treatment interfere with the natural course of the disease? *Acta Orthopaedica Scandinavica.* 1979; 50(2): 169–174.

[46] Huskisson EC, Berry H, Gishen P, Jubb RW, Whitehead J. Effects of antiinflammatory drugs on the progression of osteoarthritis of the knee. LINK Study Group. Longitudinal Investigation of Nonsteroidal Antiinflammatory Drugs in Knee Osteoarthritis. *Journal of Rheumatology.* 1995; 22(10): 1941–1946.

[47] Kahn KM, Cook LJ, Kannus P, Maffulli N, Bonar SF. Time to abandon the "tendinitis" myth. Painful, overuse tendon conditions have noninflammatory pathology. *British Medical Journal.* 2002; 324(7338): 626–627; Khan KM, Cook JL, Taunton JE, Bonar F. Overuse tendinosis, not tendonitis. Part 1: A new paradigm for a difficult clinical problem. *The Physician and Sportsmedicine.* 2000; 28(5): 38–48.

[48] Connizzo BK, Yannascoli SM, Tucker JJ, Caro AC, Riggin CN, Mauck RL, Soslowsky LJ, Steinberg DR, Bernstein J. The detrimental effects of systemic Ibuprofen delivery on tendon healing are time-dependent. *Clinical Orthopaedics and Related Research®.* 2014; 472(8): 2433–2439.

[49] Ferry ST, Dahners LE, Afshari HM, Weinhold PS. The effects of common anti-inflammatory drugs on the healing rat patellar tendon. *American Journal of Sports Medicine.* 2007; 35(8): 1326–1333.

[50] Dimmen S, Engebretsen L, Nordsletten L, Madsen JE. Negative effects of parecoxib and indomethacin on tendon healing: An experimental study in rats. *Knee Surgery, Sports Traumatology, Arthroscopy.* 2009; 17(7): 835–839.

[51] Magra M, Maffulli N. Nonsteroidal anti-inflammatory drugs in tendinopathy: Friend or foe. *Clinical Journal of Sports Medicine.* 2006; 16(1): 1–3.

[52] Landefeld K, Gonzales H, Sander GE. Hypertensive crisis: the causative effects of nonsteroidal anti-inflammatory drugs. *Journal of Clinical Case Reports.* 2016; 6(838): 2; MacFarlane LL, Orak DJ, Simpson WM. NSAIDs, antihypertensive agents and loss of blood pressure control. *American Family Physician.* 1995; 51(4): 849–856.

[53] Vitting KE, Nichols NJ, Seligson GR. Naproxen and acute renal failure in a runner, letter. *Annals of Internal Medicine.* 1986; 105(1): 144; Walker RJ, Fawcett JP, Flannery EM, Gerrard DF. Indomethacin potentiates exercise-induced reduction in renal hemodynamics in athletes. *Medicine and Science in Sports and Exercise.* 1994; 26(11): 1302–1306.

[54] Nessa A, Fakir MAH. Nonsteroidal anti-inflammatory drugs (NSAIDS) induced acute kidney injury (AKI): patient profile outcome in Bangladesh armed forces. *Journal of Armed Forces Medical College, Bangladesh.* 2015; 10(2): 39–43.

[55] Perneger TV, Whelton PK, Klag MJ. Risk of kidney failure associated with the use of acetaminophen, aspirin and nonsteroidal anti-inflammatory drugs. *New England Journal of Medicine.* 1994; 331(25): 1675–1679.

[56] Wolfe MM, Lichtenstein DR, Singh G. Gastrointestinal toxicity of nonsteroidal anti-inflammatory drugs. *New England Journal*

of Medicine. 1999; 340(24): 1888–1899 [Published erratum, *New England Journal of Medicine* 1999; 341(7): 548)].

[57] ACR 68th Annual Scientific Meeting regarding the Adenomatous Polyp Prevention on Vioxx (APPROVe) trial, presented October 18, 2004.

[58] Segev G, Katz R. Selective COX-2 inhibitors and risk of cardiovascular events. *Hospital Physician.* February 2004: 39–46.

[59] Public Health Advisory—FDA announces important changes and additional warnings for COX-2 selective and non-selective non-steroidal anti-inflammatory drugs (NSAIDs). *US Food and Drug Administration.* [Internet] 2005 Apr 7 [cited 2017 July 26] https://www.fda.gov/Drugs/DrugSafety/ucm150314.htm.

[60] FDA drug safety communication: FDA strengthens warning that non-aspirin nonsteroidal anti-inflammatory drugs (NSAIDs) can cause heart attacks or strokes. US Food and Drug Administration. 2005 Jul 9 [cited 2017 March 27] https://www.fda.gov/Drugs/DrugSafety/ucm451800.htm.

[61] FDA strengthens warning of heart attack and stroke risk for non-steroidal anti-inflammatory drugs. 2016 Sept 28 [cited 2017 March 30] https://www.fda.gov/ForConsumers/ConsumerUpdates/ucm453610.htm#1.

[62] FDA recommendations on NSAID use: what you need to know. *NSAID Dilemma* [cited 2017 Mar 30] https://www.nsaidilemma.com/wp-content/uploads/2016/10/FDA_Recommendations.pdf; FDA strengthens warning that non-aspirin nonsteroidal anti-inflammatory drugs (NSAIDs) can cause heart attacks or strokes. *US Food and Drug Administration.* 2005 Jul 9 [cited 2017 July 26] https://www.fda.gov/downloads/Drugs/DrugSafety/UCM453941.pdf.

[63] Anderson JL, Adams CD, Antman EM, Bridges CR, Califf RM, Casey DE Jr, Chavey WE 2nd, Fesmire FM, Hochman JS, Levin TN, Lincoff AM, Peterson ED, Theroux P, Wenger NK, Wright RS, Smitch SC Jr, Jacobs AK, Halperin JL, Hunt SA, Krumholz HM, Kushner FG, Lytle BW, Nishimura R, Ornato JP. Page RL. Riegel B. ACC/AHA 2007 guidelines for the management of patients with unstable angina/ non-ST-Elevation myocardial infarction: A report of the American College of Cardiology/American Heart Association Task Force on Practice

Guidelines (Writing Committee to Revise the 2002 Guidelines for the Management of Patients With Unstable Angina/Non-ST-Elevation Myocardial Infarction) Developed in collaboration with the American College of Emergency Physicians, the Society for Cardiovascular Angiography and Interventions, and the Society of Thoracic Surgeons endorsed by the American Association of Cardiovascular and Pulmonary Rehabilitation and the Society for Academic Emergency Medicine. *Journal of the American College of Cardiology.* 2007; 50(7): e1–e157.

[64] American College of Rheumatology Ad Hoc Group on use of Selective and Nonselective Nonsteroidal Antiinflammatory Drugs. Recommendations for use of selective and nonselective nonsteroidal antiinflammatory drugs: An American College of Rheumatology white paper. Arthritis Rheum. 2008; 59(8):1058–1073.

[65] National Kidney Foundation. Pain medicines (analgesics) [cited 2017 March 30] www.kidney.org/atoz/content/painMeds_Analgesics.

[66] Alliance for Rational Use of NSAIDs – NSAID Alliance HCP Brochure. Western Pain. 2014 [cited 2016 June 29] http://www.nsaidalliance.com/wp-content/uploads/2014/09/NSAID-Alliance-HCP-Brochure-Web.pdf.

[67] Stovitz SD, Johnson RJ. NSAIDs and musculoskeletal treatment. What is the clinical evidence? *Physician and Sportsmedicine.* 2003; (31)1: 35–52.

[68] Su B, O'Connor JP. NSAID therapy effects on healing of bone, tendon, and the enthesis. *Journal of Applied Physiology.* 2013 Sep 15; 115(6): 892–899.

Chapter 12: Prolotherapy Regenerative Medicine for Tendinopathy, Ligament Sprains, Muscle, and Meniscal Tears

[1] Liou, J, Landhans, M, Gottardi, R and Tuan, R. Chapter 6: Injury and repair of tendon, ligament and meniscus. Meniscus. In *Translating Regenerative Medicine to the Clinic* (pp.75–86). Los Angeles, California: Academic Press Elsevier. 2016.

[2] Docheva D, Müller SA, Majewski M, Evans CH. Biologics for tendon repair. *Advanced Drug Delivery Reviews*. 2015 Apr 30; 84: 222–239.

[3] Chahla J, Gannon J, Moatshe G, LaPrade RF. Outside-in Meniscal Repair: Technique and Outcomes. In *The Menisci* (pp. 129–135). Heidelberg, Germany: Springer. 2017.

[4] Khan KM, Cook JL, Bonar F, Hardcourt P. Histopathology of common overuse tendon conditions: Update and implications for clinical management. *Sports Medicine*. 1999; 27: 393–408; Almekinders L, Temple J. Etiology, diagnosis, and treatment of tendonitis: An analysis of the literature. *Medicine & Science in Sports & Exercise*. 1998 Aug; 30(8): 1183–1190.

[5] Liu Y. An in situ study of the influence of a sclerosing solution in rabbit medial collateral ligaments and its junction strength. *Connective Tissue Research*. 1983 Jan 1; 11(2–3): 95–102; Maynard J. Morphological and biomechanical effects of sodium morrhuate on tendons. *Journal of Orthopaedic Research*. 1985; 3(2): 236–248.

[6] Reeves KD, Hassanein K. Randomized prospective double-blind placebo-controlled study of dextrose Prolotherapy for knee osteoarthritis with or without ACL laxity. *Alternative Therapies*. March 2000; 6(2): 68–80.

[7] Seven MM, Ersen O, Akpancar S, Ozkan H, Turkkan S, Yıldız Y, Koca K. Effectiveness of prolotherapy in the treatment of chronic rotator cuff lesions. Orthopaedics & Traumatology: Surgery & Research. 2017 May 31; 103(3): 427–433; Chan O, Havard B, Morton S, Pritchard M, Maffulli N, Crisp T, Padhiar, N, Perry, JD, King, J, Morrissey, D. Outcomes of prolotherapy for intra-tendinous Achilles tears: a case series. *Muscles, Ligaments and Tendons Journals*. 2017; 7(1): 78–87; Morath O, Kubosch EJ, Taeymans J, Zwingmann J, Kostantinidis L, Südkamp NP, Hirschmüller A. The effect of sclerotherapy and prolotherapy on chronic painful Achilles tendinopathy–a systematic review including meta-analysis. *Scandinavian Journal of Medicine & Science in Sports*. 2017; 1–12; Hauser RA, Lackner JB, Steilen-Matias D, Harris DK. A systematic review of dextrose prolotherapy for chronic musculoskeletal pain. *Clinical Medicine Insights. Arthritis and Musculoskeletal Disorders*. 2016; 9: 139–159; Lee DH, Kawck KS, Rah UW, Yoon SH. Prolotherapy for refractory rotator cuff disease: retrospective

case-control study of 1-year follow up. *Archives of Physical Medicine and Rehabilitation*. 2015; 96(11): 2027–2032; Bertrand H, Reeves KD, Bennett CJ, Bicknell S, Cheng A. Dextrose prolotherapy versus control injections in painful rotator cuff tendinopathy. *Archives of Physical Medicine and Rehabilitation*. 2016; 97(1): 17–25; Rabago D, Yelland M, Patterson JJ, Zgierska A. Prolotherapy for chronic musculoskeletal pain. *American Family Physician*. 2011; 84(11): 1208–1210.

[8] Filardo G, Kon E, Di Matteo B, Pelotti P, Di Martino A, Marcacci M. Platelet-rich plasma for the treatment of patellar tendinopathy: clinical and imaging findings at medium-term follow-up. *International Orthopaedics*. 2013 Aug 1; 37(8): 1583–1589.

[9] Kadam R, Vijay S, Chhallani A, Pandhare S, Gupta A, Singh RS. Efficacy of platelet rich plasma injection in treatment of plantar fasciitis. *International Journal of Research in Orthopaedics*. 2017 Apr 25;3(3): 451–455; Baz AA, Gad AM, Waly MR. Ultrasound guided injection of platelet rich plasma in cases of chronic plantar fasciitis. *The Egyptian Journal of Radiology and Nuclear Medicine*. 2017 Mar 31; 48(1): 125–132; Papalia R, Zampogna B, Vadala G, Di Martino A, Nobile C, Del Buono A, Torre G, Tirindelli, C, Maffulli, N, Denaro, V. Are Platelet Rich Plasma Injections More Effective in Tendinopathy or Enthesopathy? *Journal of Pain & Relief*. 2017; 6(288): ISSN 2167-0846.

[10] Mautner K, Colberg RE, Malanga G, Borg-Stein JP, Harmon KG, Dharamsi AS, Chu S, Homer P. Outcomes after ultrasound-guided platelet-rich plasma injections for chronic tendinopathy: a multicenter, retrospective review. *PM&R*. 2013; 5(3): 169–175; Fitzpatrick J, Bulsara M, Zheng MH. The effectiveness of platelet-rich plasma in the treatment of tendinopathy: a meta-analysis of randomized controlled clinical trials. *American Journal of Sports Medicine*. 2017 Jan; 45(1): 226–233; Sahu A, Singh PK, Khan S, Singhania S, Gudhe M, Mundada G, Gawande V. Ultrasound-guided platelet-rich plasma infiltration: A stupendous treatment for chronic tendinopathy. *Saudi Journal of Sports Medicine*. 2016 Sep 1; 16(3): 185.

[11] Pascual-Garrido C, Rolón A, Makino A. Treatment of chronic patellar tendinopathy with autologous bone marrow stem cells: a 5-year-followup. *Stem Cells International*. 2012: Article ID 953510, 5 pages.

[12] de Girolamo L, Grassi M, Viganò M, Orfei CP, Montrasio UA, Usuelli F. Treatment of achilles tendinopathy with autologous adipose-derived stromal vascular fraction: Results of a randomized prospective clinical trial. *Orthopaedic Journal of Sports Medicine.* 2016 Jul 18; 4(7) Suppl 4.

[13] Oliver KS, Alexander RW. Combination of autologous adipose-derived tissue stromal vascular fraction plus high density platelet-rich plasma or bone marrow concentrates in Achilles tendon tears. *Journal of Prolotherapy.* 2013; 5: e89–e912.

[14] Hauser R, Hauser M, Cukla J. Dextrose prolotherapy injection for chronic ankle pain. *Practical Pain Management.* 2010; 10(1): 7–76; Van Pelt RS. Ankle and foot treatment with prolotherapy. *Journal of Prolotherapy.* 2011; 3(1): 576–581; Fullerton BD. High-resolution ultrasound and magnetic resonance imaging to document tissue repair after prolotherapy: A report of 3 cases. *Archives of Physical Medicine and Rehabilitation.* 2008 Feb 29; 89(2): 377–385.

[15] Sinoff C. Prolotherapy for 20 year old ankle injury. *Journal of Prolotherapy.* 2010; 2(4): 497–488.

[16] Reeves KD, Hassanein KM. Fullerton BD, Reeves KD. Ultrasonography in regenerative injection (prolotherapy) using dextrose, platelet-rich plasma, and other injectants. *Physical Medicine and Rehabilitation Clinics of North America.* 2010 Aug 31; 21(3): 585–605; Hauser RA, Dolan EE, Phillips HJ, Newlin AC, Moore RE, Woldin BA. Ligament injury and healing: a review of current clinical diagnostics and therapeutics. *Open Rehabilitation Journal.* 2013 Jan 23; 6: 1–20; Ahmet Mustafa ADA M.D., Yavuz F. Treatment of a medial collateral ligament sprain using prolotherapy: a case study. *Alternative Therapies in Health and Medicine.* 2015 Jul 1; 21(4): 68.

[17] Whyte GP, Gobbi A, Szwedowski D. Partial Anterior Cruciate Ligament Lesions: A Biological Approach to Repair. In *Bio-Orthopaedics* (pp. 665–670). Heidelberg, Germany: Springer. 2017; Chellis DM, Cortazzo MH. Regenerative medicine in the field of pain medicine: Prolotherapy, platelet-rich plasma therapy, and stem cell therapy—Theory and evidence. *Techniques in Regional Anesthesia and Pain Management.* 2011 Apr 30; 15(2): 74–80; Long term effects of dextrose prolotherapy for anterior cruciate ligament laxity. *Alternative Therapies in Health and Medicine.* 2003 May

1; 9(3): 58–62; Grote W, Delucia R, Waxman R, Zgierska A, Wilson J, Rabago D. Repair of a complete anterior cruciate tear using prolotherapy: a case report. *International Musculoskeletal Medicine.* 2009 Dec 1; 31(4): 159–165.

[18] Oe K, Kushida T, Okamoto N, Umeda M, Nakamura T, Ikehara S, Iida H. New strategies for anterior cruciate ligament partial rupture using bone marrow transplantation in rats. *Stem Cells and Development.* 2011; 20(4): 671–679; Soon MY, Hassan A, Hui JH, Goh JC, Lee EH. An analysis of soft tissue allograft anterior cruciate ligament reconstruction in a rabbit model: A short-term study of the use of mesenchymal stem cells to enhance tendon osteointegration. *American Journal of Sports Medicine.* 2007; 35(6): 962–971.

[19] Lazzara MA. The non-surgical repair of a complete Achilles tendon rupture by prolotherapy: biological reconstruction. A case report. *Journal of Orthopaedic Medicine.* 2005 Jan 1; 27(3): 128–132; Grote W, Delucia R, Waxman R, Zgierska A, Wilson J, Rabago D. Repair of a complete anterior cruciate tear using prolotherapy: a case report. *International Musculoskeletal Medicine.* 2009 Dec 1; 31(4): 159–165.

[20] Pihlajamäki H, Hietaniemi K, Paavola M, Visuri T, Mattila VM. Surgical versus functional treatment for acute ruptures of the lateral ligament complex of the ankle in young men: a randomized controlled trial. *The Journal of Bone & Joint Surgery.* 2010 Oct 20; 92(14): 2367–2374.

[21] Petersen W, Rembitzki IV, Koppenburg AG, Ellermann A, Liebau C, Brüggemann GP, Best R. Treatment of acute ankle ligament injuries: a systematic review. *Archives of Orthopaedic and Trauma Surgery.* 2013 Aug 1; 133(8): 1129–1141.

[22] Sánchez M, Delgado D, Sánchez P, Anitua E, Padilla S. Plasma Rich in Growth Factors for the Treatment of Skeletal Muscle Injury. In *Muscle Injuries in Sport Athletes,* Chapter 28 (pp. 451–464). Switzerland: Springer International Publishing. 2017.

[23] Alexander RW. Biocellular regenerative medicine: Use of adipose-derived stem/stromal cells and its native bioactive matrix. *Physical Medicine & Rehabilitation Clinics of North America.* 2016; 27(4): 871–891.

[24] Kimura M, Shirakura K, Hasegawa A et al. Second look arthroscopy after meniscal repair. Factors affecting the healing rate. *Clinical Orthopedics and Related Research* 1995; 314: 185–191.

[25] Cengiz IF, Silva-Correia J, Pereira H, Espregueira-Mendes J, Oliveira JM, Reis RL. Basics of the Meniscus. In *Regenerative Strategies for the Treatment of Knee Joint Disabilities* (pp. 237–247). Switzerland: Springer International Publishing. 2017.

[26] Bhattacharyya T, Gale D, Dewire P, Totterman S, Gale ME, McLaughlin S, Einhorn TA, Felson DT. The clinical importance of meniscal tears demonstrated by magnetic resonance imaging in osteoarthritis of the knee. *The Journal of Bone & Joint Surgery.* 2003 Jan 1; 85(1): 4–9; Kornick J, Trefelner E, McCarthy S, Lange R, Lynch K, Jokl P. Meniscal abnormalities in the asymptomatic population at MR imaging. *Radiology.* 1990 Nov; 177(2): 463–465; Beattie KA, Boulos P, Pui M, O'Neill J, Inglis D, Webber CE, Adachi JD. Abnormalities identified in the knees of asymptomatic volunteers using peripheral magnetic resonance imaging. *Osteoarthritis and Cartilage.* 2005 Mar 31; 13(3): 181–186.

[27] Kaplan LD, Schurhoff MR, Selesnick H, Thorpe M, Uribe JW. Magnetic resonance imaging of the knee in asymptomatic professional basketball players. *Arthroscopy: The Journal of Arthroscopic & Related Surgery.* 2005 May 31; 21(5): 557–561.

[28] Chahla J, Gannon J, Moatshe G, LaPrade RF. Outside-in Meniscal Repair: Technique and Outcomes. In *The Menisci* (pp. 129–135). Heidelberg, Germany: Springer. 2017; Rongen JJ, Rovers MM, van Tienen TG, Buma P, Hannink G. Increased risk for knee replacement surgery after arthroscopic surgery for degenerative meniscal tears: a multi-center longitudinal observational study using data from the osteoarthritis initiative. *Osteoarthritis and Cartilage.* 2017 Jan 31; 25(1): 23–29.

[29] Hauser RA, Phillips HJ, Maddela HS. The Case for Utilizing Prolotherapy as First-Line Treatment for Meniscal Pathology. *Journal of Prolotherapy.* 2010; 2(3): 416–437; Braun HJ, Wasterlain AS, Dragoo JL. The use of PRP in ligament and meniscal healing. *Sports Medicine and Arthroscopy Review.* 2013 Dec 1; 21(4): 206–201; Hauser RA, Phillips HJ, Maddela H. Platelet rich plasma Prolotherapy as first-line treatment for meniscal pathology. *Practical Pain Management.* 2010 Jul; 10(6): 53–64

[30] Blanke F, Vavken P, Haenle M, von Wehren L, Pagenstert G, Majewski M. Percutaneous injections of platelet rich plasma for treatment of intrasubstance meniscal lesions. *Muscles, Ligaments and Tendons Journal.* 2015 Jul; 5(3): 162–166.

[31] Yu H, Adesida AB, Jomha NM. Meniscus repair using mesenchymal stem cells–a comprehensive review. *Stem Cell Research & Therapy.* 2015 Apr 30; 6(1): 86.

[32] Pak J, Lee JH, Lee SH. Regenerative repair of damaged meniscus with autologous adipose tissue-derived stem cells. *BioMed Research International.* 2014 Jan 30; 2014: Article ID 436029, 10 pages.

[33] Pak J, Lee JH, Park KS, Jeon JH, Lee SH. Potential use of mesenchymal stem cells in human meniscal repair: current insights. *Open Access Journal of Sports Medicine.* 2017; 8: 33; Striano RD, Battista V, Bilboo N. Non-responding knee pain with osteoarthritis, meniscus and ligament tears treated with ultrasound guided autologous, micro-fragmented and minimally manipulated adipose tissue. *Open Journal of Regenerative Medicine.* 2017 Jun 27; 6(02): 17; Whitehouse MR, Howells NR, Parry MC, Austin E, Kafienah W. Brady K, Goodship AE, Eldridge JD, Blom AW and Hollander AP, 2017. Repair of torn avascular meniscal cartilage using undifferentiated autologous mesenchymal stem cells: From in vitro optimization to a first-in-human study. *Stem Cells Translational Medicine;* 6(4): 1237–1248.

Chapter 13: Prolotherapy Regenerative Medicine for Osteoarthritis

[1] Felson DT, Lawrence RC, Dieppe PA, Hirsch R, Helmick CG, Jordan JM, Kington RS, Lane NE, Nevitt MC, Zhang Y, Sowers M, McAlindon T, Spector TD, Poole AR, Yanovski SZ, Ateshian G, Sharma L, Buckwalter JA, Brandt KD, Fries JF. Osteoarthritis: New insights. Part 1: The disease and its risk factors. *Annals of Internal Medicine.* 2000; 133(8): 635–646; Blalock D, Miller A, Tilley M, Wang J. Joint instability and osteoarthritis. *Clinical Medicine Insights. Arthritis and Musculoskeletal Disorders.* 2015; 8: 15.

[2] Fleming BC, Hulstyn MJ, Oksendahl HL, Fadale PD. Ligament injury, reconstruction and osteoarthritis. *Current Opinion in Orthopaedics.* 2005; 16(5): 354–362.

[3] Carbone A, Rodeo S. Review of current understanding of post-traumatic osteoarthritis resulting from sports injuries. *Journal of Orthopaedic Research*. 2017; 35(3): 397–405; Lohmander LS, Ostenberg A, Englund M, Roos H. High prevalence of knee osteoarthritis, pain and functional limitations in female soccer players twelve years after anterior cruciate ligament injury. *Arthritis & Rheumatism*. 2004; 50(10): 3145–3152.

[4] Blalock D, Miller A, Tilley M, Wang J. Joint instability and osteoarthritis. *Clinical Medicine Insights. Arthritis and Musculoskeletal Disorders*. 2015; 8: 15; Lowman E. Osteoarthritis. *Journal of the American Medical Association*. 1955; 157: 487–488.

[5] Radin E, Paul I, Rose R. Role of mechanical factors in pathogenesis of primary osteoarthritis. *The Lancet*. 1972 Mar 4; 299(7749): 519–522.

[6] Hunter DJ, Zhang Y, Sokolove J, Niu J, Aliabadi P, Felson DT. Trapeziometacarpal subluxation predisposes to incident trapeziometacarpal osteoarthritis (OA): The Framingham Study. *Osteoarthritis and Cartilage*. 2005 Nov 30; 13(11): 953–957.

[7] Tan AL, Toumi H, Benjamin M, Grainger AJ, Tanner SF, Emery P, McGonagle D. Combined high-resolution magnetic resonance imaging and histological examination to explore the role of ligaments and tendons in the phenotypic expression of early hand osteoarthritis. *Annals of the Rheumatic Diseases*. 2006; 65(10): 1267–1272; Brandt KD, Radin EL, Dieppe PA, Van De Putte L. Yet more evidence that osteoarthritis is not a cartilage disease. *Annals of the Rheumatic Diseases*. 2006; 65: 1261–1264; Hunter DJ, Zhang Y, Sokolove J, Niu J, Aliabadi P, Felson DT. Trapeziometacarpal subluxation predisposes to incident trapeziometacarpal osteoarthritis (OA): The Framingham study. *Osteoarthritis and Cartilage*. 2005 Nov 30; 13(11): 953–957.

[8] Kamekura S, Hoshi K, Shimoaka T, Chung U, Chikuda H, Yamada T, Uchida M, Ogata N, Seichi A, Nakamura K, Kawaguchi H. Osteoarthritis development in novel experimental mouse models induced by knee joint instability. *Osteoarthritis and Cartilage*. 2005; 13(7): 632–641; Van Osch GJ, van der Kraan PM, Blankevoort L, Huiskes R, van den Berg WB. Relation of ligament damage with site specific cartilage loss and osteophyte formation in collagenase induced osteoarthrthritis in mice. *Journal of Rheumatology*.

1996; 23(7): 1227–1232; Farrow CS, Newton CD. Ligamentous injury (sprain). In *Textbook of Small Animal Orthopaedics*. Ithaca, New York: International Veterinary Information Service, 1985.

[9] Beattie KA, Boulos P, Pui M, O'Neill J, Inglis D, Webber CE, Adachi JD. Abnormalities identified in the knees of asymptomatic volunteers using peripheral magnetic resonance imaging. *Osteoarthritis and Cartilage*. 2005; 13(3): 181–186.

[10] High incidence of pain common one year following TKA. *Orthopedics Today*. 2016 May [cited 2017 May 17] https://www.hss.edu/newsroom_thomas-sculco-study-on-pain-after-total-knee-arthroplasty.asp.

[11] Fleeton G, Harmer AR, Nairn L, Crosbie J, March L, Crawford R, Van der Esch M, Fransen M. Self-reported knee instability before and after total knee replacement surgery. *Arthritis Care & Research*. 2016; 68(4): 463–471.

[12] Wehling P, Moser C, Maixner W. How does surgery compare with advanced intra-articular therapies in knee osteoarthritis: Current thoughts. *Therapeutic Advances in Musculoskeletal Disease*. 2016; 8(3): 72–85.

[13] McGrory B, Weber K, Lynott JA, Richmond JC, Davis CM, Yates A, Kamath AF, Dasa V, Brown GA, Gerlinger TL, Villanueva T, Piva S, Hebl J, Jevsevar D, Shea KG, Bozic KJ, Shaffer W, Cummins D, Murray JN, Donnelly P, Patel N, Brenton B, Shores P, Woznica A, Linskey E, Servarino K. The American Academy of Orthopaedic Surgeons evidence-based clinical practice guideline on surgical management of osteoarthritis of the knee. *Journal of Bone and Joint Surgery. American Volume*. 2016; 98(8): 688–692.

[14] Moseley JB, O'Malley K, Petersen NJ, Menke TJ, Brody BA, Kuykendall DH, Hollingsworth JC, Ashton CM, Wray NP. A controlled trial of arthroscopic surgery for osteoarthritis of the knee for osteoarthritis of the knee. *New England Journal of Medicine*. 2002; 347(2): 81–88.

[15] Kirkley A, Birmingham TB, Litchfield RB, Giffin JR, Willits KR, Wong CJ, Feagan BG, Donner A, Griffin SH, D'Ascanio LM, Pope JE, Fowler PJ. A randomized trial of arthroscopic surgery for osteoarthritis of the knee. *New England Journal of Medicine*. 2008; 359(11): 1097–1107.

[16] Rongen JJ, Rovers MM, van Tienen TG, Buma P, Hannink G. Increased risk for knee replacement surgery after arthroscopic surgery for degenerative meniscal tears: A multi-center longitudinal observational study using data from the osteoarthritis initiative. *Osteoarthritis and Cartilage*. 2017; 25(1): 23–29.

[17] Brunk D. Meniscectomy associated with knee osteoarthritis. *Family Practice News*. 2006 Feb 15: 50 [cited 2017 May 19] https://www.highbeam.com/doc/1G1-142922562.html.

[18] Soliman DM, Sherif INM, Omar OH, El Zohiery AK. Healing effects of prolotherapy in treatment of knee osteoarthritis healing effects of prolotherapy in treatment of knee osteoarthritis. *Egyptian Rheumatology and Rehabilitation*. 2016; 43(2): 47; Nourani B, Rabago D. Prolotherapy for knee osteoarthritis: A descriptive review. *Current Physical Medicine and Rehabilitation Reports*. 2016; 4(1): 42–49; Ekinci S, Tatar O, Akpancar S, Turgut H, Seven MM. A new treatment option in osteoarthritis: prolotherapy injections. *Journal of Orthopaedic Research*. 2016; 26: 816–823; Reeves KD, Hassanein K. Randomized prospective double-blind placebo-controlled study of dextrose prolotherapy for knee osteoarthritis with or without ACL laxity. *Alternative Therapies*. 2000; (6)2: 68–80; Reeves KD, Hassanein K. Randomized, prospective, placebo-controlled, double-blind study of dextrose prolotherapy for osteoarthritis thumb and finger (DIP, PIP and trapeziometacarpal) joints: Evidence of clinical efficacy. *Journal of Alternative and Complementary Medicine*. 2000; (6)4: 311–320.

[19] Rabago D, Nourani B. Prolotherapy for osteoarthritis and tendinopathy: A descriptive review. *Current Rheumatology Reports*. 2017; 19(6): 34.

[20] Hauser R. The regeneration of articular cartilage with prolotherapy. *Journal of Prolotherapy*. 2009; 1(1): 39–44.

[21] Hauser RA, Cukla JJ. Standard clinical x-ray studies document cartilage regeneration in five degenerated knees after prolotherapy. *Journal of Prolotherapy*. 2009; 1(1): 22–28 [cited 2017 May 17] http://journalofprolotherapy.com/standard-clinical-x-ray-studies-document-cartilage-regeneration-in-five-degenerated-knees-after-prolotherapy/; Reeves KD, Hassanein K. Randomized prospective double-blind placebo-controlled study of dextrose prolotherapy

for knee osteoarthritis with or without ACL laxity. *Alternative Therapies in Health and Medicine.* 2000; 6(2): 68.

[22] Topol GA, Podesta LA, Reeves KD, Giraldo MM, Johnson LL, Grasso R, Jamín A, Clark T, Rabago D. Chondrogenic effect of intra-articular hypertonic-dextrose (prolotherapy) in severe knee osteoarthritis. *PM&R.* 2016; 8(11): 1072–1082.

[23] Hung CY, Hsiao MY, Chang KV, Han DS, Wang TG. Comparative effectiveness of dextrose prolotherapy versus control injections and exercise in the management of osteoarthritis pain: A systematic review and meta-analysis. *Journal of Pain Research.* 2016; 9: 847–857.

[24] Lai L, Stitik T, Foye P, Georgy JS, Patibanda V, Chen B. Use of platelet-rich plasma in intra-articular knee injections for osteoarthritis: A systematic review. *PM&R.* 2015; 7(6): 637–648.

[25] Raeissadat SA, Rayegani SM, Hassanabadi H, Fathi M, Ghorbani E, Babaee M, Azma K. Knee osteoarthritis injection choices: Platelet-rich plasma (PRP) versus hyaluronic acid (a one-year randomized clinical trial). *Clinical Medicine Insights. Arthritis and Musculoskeletal Disorders.* 2015; 8: 1–8.

[26] Shen L, Yuan T, Chen S, Xie X, Zhang C. The temporal effect of platelet-rich plasma on pain and physical function in the treatment of knee osteoarthritis: systematic review and meta-analysis of randomized controlled trials. *Journal of Orthopaedic Surgery and Research.* 2017 Dec 1; 12(1): 16.

[27] Sampson S, Reed M, Silvers H, Meng M, Mandelbaum B. Injection of platelet-rich plasma in patients with primary and secondary knee osteoarthritis: A pilot study. *American Journal of Physical Medicine & Rehabilitation.* 2010; 89: 961–969; Wang-Saegusa A, Cugat R, Ares O, Seijas R, Cusco X, Garcia-Balletbo M. Infiltration of plasma rich in growth factors for osteoarthritis of the knee short term effects on function and quality of life. *Archives of Orthopaedic and Trauma Surgery.* 2011;131: 311–317; Filardo G, Kon E, Buda R, Timoncini A, Di Martino A, Cenacchi A, Fornasari PM, Giannini S, Marcacci M. Platelet-rich plasma intraarticular knee injections for the treatment of degenerative cartilage lesions and osteoarthritis. *Knee Surgery, Sports Traumatology, Arthroscopy.* 2011; 19: 528–35.

[28] Kadam R, Agrawal A, Chhallani A, Pandhare S, Gupta A, Sawant R. To assess the effects of platelet rich plasma application on pain in osteoarthritis knee. *International Journal of Research in Orthopaedics*. 2017; Apr 25; 3(3): 436–439; Dhillon MS, Patel S, John R. PRP in OA knee–update, current confusions and future options. *SICOT-J*. 2017; 3:27.

[29] Mei-Dan O, Carmont MR, Laver L, Mann G, Maffulli N, Nyska M. Platelet-rich plasma or hyaluronate in the management of osteochondral lesions of the talus. *American Journal of Sports Medicine*. 2012; 40(3): 534–541.

[30] Repetto I, Biti B, Cerruti P, Trentini R, Felli L. Conservative Treatment of Ankle Osteoarthritis: Can Platelet-Rich Plasma Effectively Postpone Surgery? *Journal of Foot and Ankle Surgery*. 2017 Apr 30; 56(2): 362–365.

[31] Sanchez M, Guadilla J, Fiz N, Andia I. Ultrasound-guided platelet-rich plasma injections for the treatment of osteoarthritis of the hip. *Rheumatology*. 2012; 51: 144–150; Dallari D, Stagni C, Rani N, Sabbioni G, Pelotti P, Torricelli P, Tschon M, Giavaresi G. Ultrasound-guided injection of platelet-rich plasma and hyaluronic acid, separately and in combination for hip osteoarthritis: A randomized controlled study. *American Journal of Sports Medicine*. 2016 Mar; 44(3): 664–671.

[32] Hegab AF, Ali HE, Elmasry M, Khallaf MG. Platelet-rich plasma injection as an effective treatment for temporomandibular joint osteoarthritis. *Journal of Oral and Maxillofacial Surgery*. September 2015; 73(9): 1706–1713.

[33] Chang KV, Hung CY, Aliwarga F, Wang TG, Han DS, Chen WS. Comparative effectiveness of platelet-rich plasma injections for treating knee joint cartilage degenerative pathology: A systematic review and meta-analysis. *Archives of Physical Medicine and Rehabilitation*. 2014; 95(3): 562–575.

[34] Görmeli G, Görmeli CA, Ataoglu B, Çolak C, Aslantürk O, Ertem K. Multiple PRP injections are more effective than single injections and hyaluronic acid in knees with early osteoarthritis: A randomized, double-blind, placebo-controlled trial. *Knee Surgery, Sports Traumatology, Arthroscopy*. 2017; 25(3): 958–965; Filardo G, Kon E, Ruiz MT, Vaccaro F, Guitaldi R, Di Martino A, Cenacchi A, Fornasari PM, Marcacci M. Platelet-rich plasma

intra-articular injections for cartilage degeneration and osteoarthritis: Single- versus double-spinning approach. *Knee Surgery, Sports Traumatology, Arthroscopy.* 2012; 20(10): 2082–2091.

[35] Hauser R, Hauser M. PRP Prolotherapy Injection Technique. *Journal of Prolotherapy.* 2009; 1(3): 12 [cited 2017 May 19] http://www.jour nalofprolotherapy.com/pdfs/issue_03/issue_03_12_platelet_rich_plasma.pdf.

[36] Singh A, Goel SC, Gupta KK, Kumar M, Arun GR, Patil H, Kumaraswamy V, Jha S. The role of stem cells in osteoarthritis. *Bone & Joint Research.* 2014 Feb 1; 3(2): 32–37.

[37] Perdisa F, Gostyn'ska N, Roffi A, Filardo G, Marcacci M, Kon E. Adipose-derived mesenchymal stem cells for the treatment of articular cartilage: A systematic review on preclinical and clinical evidence. *Stem Cells International.* 2015 Jul 9 [cited 2017 October 1] https://www.hindawi.com/journals/sci/2015/597652/cta/; Jang Y, Koh YG, Choi YJ, Kim SH, Yoon DS, Lee M, Lee JW. Characterization of adipose tissue-derived stromal vascular fraction for clinical application to cartilage regeneration. *Vitro Cellular & Developmental Biology-Animal.* 2015 Feb 1; 51(2): 142–150.

[38] Pham PV, Bui KHT, Duong TD, Nguyen NT, Nguyen TD, Le VT, Mai VT, Phan NLC, Le DM, Ngoc NK. Symptomatic knee osteoarthritis treatment using autologous adipose derived stem cells and platelet-rich plasma: A clinical study. *Biomedical Research and Therapy.* 2014; 1(1): 2–8.

[39] Striano RD, Chen H, Bilbool N, Azatullah K, Hilado J, Horan K. Non-responsive knee pain with osteoarthritis and concurrent meniscal disease treated with autologous micro-fragmented adipose tissue under continuous ultrasound guidance. *CellR4.* 2015; 3(5): e1690 [cited 2017 October 1] http://www.cellr4.org/wp-content/uploads/sites/2/2015/10/CellR4-P.M.-2906-Richard-David-Striano.pdf,

[40] Adriani E, Moio M, Di Paola B, Salustri W, Alfieri A, Parisi P, Ruggiero M, Borab Z, Carlesimo B. Percutaneous Fat Transfer to Treat Knee Osteoarthritis Symptoms: Preliminary Results. *Joints.* 2017 Jun; 5(02): 089–092.

[41] Yokota N, Yamakawa M, Shirata T, Kimura T, Kaneshima H. Clinical results following intra-articular injection of

Free Yourself from Chronic Pain & Sports Injuries

adipose-derived stromal vascular fraction cells in patients with osteoarthritis of the knee. *Regenerative Therapy.* 2017 Jun 30; 6: 108–112.

[42] Koh YG, Choi YJ, Kwon SK, Kim YS, Yeo JE. Clinical results and second-look arthroscopic findings after treatment with adipose-derived stem cells for knee osteoarthritis. *Knee Surgery, Sports Traumatology, Arthroscopy.* 2015; 23(5): 1308–1316.

[43] Koh YG, Jo SB, Kwon OR, Suh DS, Lee SW, Park SH, Choi YJ. Mesenchymal stem cell injections improve symptoms of knee osteoarthritis. *Arthroscopy.* 2013; 29(4): 748–755; Pak J. Regeneration of human bones in hip osteonecrosis and human cartilage in knee osteoarthritis with autologous adipose-tissue-derived stem cells: A case series. *Journal of Medical Case Reports.* 2011; 5: 296; Pham PV, Bui KHT, Duong TD, Nguyen NT, Nguyen TD, Le VT, Mai VT, Phan NLC, Le DM, Ngoc NK. Symptomatic knee osteoarthritis treatment using autologous adipose derived stem cells and platelet-rich plasma: A clinical study. *Biomedical Research and Therapy.* 2014; 1(1): 2–8.

[44] Perdisa F, Gostyn'ska N, Roffi A, Filardo G, Marcacci M, Kon E. Adipose-derived mesenchymal stem cells for the treatment of articular cartilage: A systematic review on preclinical and clinical evidence. *Stem Cells International* [cited 2017 October 1] https://www.hindawi.com/journals/sci/2015/597652/cta/.

[45] Centeno CJ, Al-Sayegh H, Bashir J, Goodyear S, Freeman M.D.. A prospective multi-site registry study of a specific protocol of autologous bone marrow concentrate for the treatment of shoulder rotator cuff tears and osteoarthritis. *Journal of Pain Research.* 2015; 2015(8): 269–276.

[46] Hauser RA, Ostergaard S. Direct bone marrow injections for avascular necrosis of the talus. *Journal of Prolotherapy.* 2012; 4: e891–e894; Hauser RA, Woldin B. Treating osteoarthritic joints using dextrose prolotherapy and direct bone marrow aspirate injection therapy. *Open Arthritis Journal.* 2014; 7(1): 1–9.

[47] Bert JM. Abandoning microfracture of the knee: Has the time come? *Arthroscopy.* 2015; 31(3): 501–505.

[48] Kim YS, Park EH, Kim YC, Koh YG. Clinical outcomes of mesenchymal stem cell injection with arthroscopic treatment in older

414

patients with osteochondral lesions of the talus. *American Journal of Sports Medicine*. 2013; 41(5): 1090–1099.

[49] Seijas R, Ares O, Alvarez P, Cusco X, Garcia-Balletbo M, Cugat R. Platelet-rich plasma for calcific tendinitis of the shoulder: a case report. *Journal of Orthopaedic Surgery*. 2012 Apr; 20(1): 126–130.

[50] Hauser RA. Cartilage regeneration in knees. *Journal of Prolotherapy*. 2009; 1: 22–28; Kon E, Filardo G, Delcogliano M, Presti ML, Russo A, Bondi A, Di Martino A, Cenacchi A, Fornasari PM, Marcacci M. Platelet-rich plasma: new clinical application: A pilot study for treatment of jumper's knee. *Injury*. 2009; 40(6): 598–603; Pak J. Lee JH, Park KS, Park M, Kang LW, Lee SH. Current use of autologous adipose tissue-derived stromal vascular fraction cells for orthopedic applications. *Journal of Biomedical Science*. 2017; 24(1): 9.

Chapter 14: Prolotherapy Regenerative Medicine for Low Back Pain and Sciatica

[1] Patrick N, Emanski E, Knaub MA. Acute and chronic low back pain. *Medical Clinics of North America*. 2016 Jan 31; 100(1):169–181; Frymoyer JW, Cats-Baril WL. An overview of the incidences and costs of low back pain. *Orthopedic Clinics of North America*. 1991; 22(2): 263–271; Rubin DI. Epidemiology and risk factors for spine pain. *Neurologic Clinics*. 2007; 25(2): 353–371.

[2] Hoy D, March L, Brooks P, Blyth F, Woolf A, Bain C, Williams G, Smith E, Vos T, Barendregt J, Murray C, Burstein R, Buchbinder R. The global burden of low back pain: Estimates from the Global Burden of Disease 2010 study. *Annals of the Rheumatic Diseases*. 2014; 73: 968–974.

[3] World Health Organization 2014: Priority diseases and reasons for inclusion: Low Back Pain [2017 April 1] http://www.who.int/medicines/areas/priority_medicines/Ch6_24LBP.pdf.

[4] Hoy D, Brooks P, Blyth F, Buchbinder R. The epidemiology of low back pain. *Best Practice & Research Clinical Rheumatology*. 2010; 24(6): 769–781; Manchikanti L, Singh V, Falco FJE, Benyamin RM, Hirsch JA. Epidemiology of low back pain in adults. *Neuromodulation: Technology at the Neural Interface*. 2014; 17(S2): 3–10.

[5] Freburger JK, Holmes GM, Agans RP, Jackman AM, Darter JD, Wallace AS, Castel LD, Kalsbeek WD, Carey TS. The rising

prevalence of chronic low back pain. *Archives of Internal Medicine.* 2009; 169(3): 251–258.

[6] Frymoyer JW, Cats-Baril WL. An overview of the incidences and costs of low back pain. *Orthopedic Clinics of North America.* 1991; 22(2): 263–271.

[7] Freburger JK, Holmes GM, Agans RP, Jackman AM, Darter JD, Wallace AS, Castel LD, Kalsbeek WD, Carey TS. The rising prevalence of chronic low back pain. *Archives of Internal Medicine.* 2009 Feb 9; 169(3): 251–258.

[8] Drezner JA, Herring SA, Harmon K, Rubin A. Managing low-back pain: steps to optimize function and hasten return to activity. *The Physician and Sportsmedicine.* 2001 Aug 1; 29(8): 37–43.

[9] Braddom RL. Perils and pointers in the evaluation and management of back pain. *Seminars in Neurology.* 1998; 18: 197–210.

[10]Golightly YM, Goode AP, Cleveland RJ, Nelson AE, Hannan MT, Hillstrom HJ, Kraus VB, Schwartz TA, Renner JB, Jordan JM. FRI0598 relationship of joint hypermobility with low back pain and lumbar spine osteoarthritis: A cohort study. *Annals of the Rheumatic Diseases.* 2016; 75(2): 659–659.

[11] Heneweer H, Vanhees L, Picavet HS. Physical activity and low back pain: A u-shaped relation? *Pain.* 2009 May 31; 143(1): 21–25.

[12] Borenstein DG. Chronic low back pain. *Rheumatological Disease Clinics of North America.* 1996; 22(3): 439–456.

[13] Zelle BA, Gruen GS, Brown S, George S. Sacroiliac joint dysfunction: Evaluation and management. *Clinical Journal of Pain.* 2005; 21(5): 446–455.

[14]Samini F, Gharedaghi M, Khajavi M, Samini M. The etiologies of low back pain in patients with lumbar disk herniation. *Iranian Red Crescent Medical Journal.* 2014; 16(10): Article ID15670, 5 pages

[15] Goldthwait JE, Osgood RB. A consideration of the pelvic articulations from an anatomical, pathological and clinical standpoint. *Boston Medical and Surgical Journal.* 1905; 152(21): 593–601.

[16] Mixter WJ, Barr JS. Rupture of the intervertebral disc with involvement of the spinal canal. *New England Journal of Medicine.* 1934; 211: 210.

[17] Ombregt B, Bisschop P, Ter Veer HJ. *A System of Orthopaedic Medicine*, 2nd ed (p. 739). London, England: Churchill Livingstone, 2003.

[18] Hills EC, Wieting JM. Mechanical low back pain. 20014 Nov 21 [cited 2017 July 5] http://www.emedicine.com/pmr/topic73.htm.

[19] Ombregt B, Bisschop P, Ter Veer HJ. *A System of Orthopaedic Medicine*, 2nd ed. (p. 775). London, England: Churchill Livingstone, 2003.

[20] Alpers BJ. The problem of sciatica. *Medical Clinics of North America.* 1953; 37:503 [cited 2017 July 5] https://www.ncbi.nlm.nih.gov/pmc/articles/PMC1822278/pdf/canmedaj00671-0040.pdf.

[21] Bernard TN Jr, Kirkaldy-Willis WH. Recognizing specific characteristics of nonspecific low back pain. *Clinical Orthopaedics and Related Research.* 1987; 217: 266–280.

[22] Samini F, Gharedaghi M, Khajavi M, Samini M. The etiologies of low back pain in patients with lumbar disk herniation. *Iranian Red Crescent Medical Journal.* 2014; 16(10): Article ID15670, 5 pages.

[23] Saal JA, Saal JS. Nonoperative treatment of herniated lumbar intervertebral disc with radiculopathy: An outcome study. *Spine.* 1989; 14(4): 431–437.

[24] Zelle BA, Gruen GS, Brown S, George S. Sacroiliac joint dysfunction: Evaluation and management. *Clinical Journal of Pain.* 2005; 21(5): 446–455.

[25] Cohen SP. Sacroiliac joint pain: A comprehensive review of anatomy, diagnosis, and treatment. *Anesthesia & Analgesia.* 2005; 101(5): 1440–1453.

[26] Slipman CW, Jackson HB, Lipetz JS, Chan KT, Lenrow D, Vresilovic EJ. Sacroiliac joint pain referral zones. *Archives of Physical Medicine and Rehabilitation.* 2000; 81(3): 334–338.

[27] Buijs E, Visser L, Groen G. Sciatica and the sacroiliac joint: a forgotten concept. *British journal of Anaesthesia.* 2007; 99(5): 713–716; Fortin JD, Vilensky JA, Merkel GJ. Can the sacroiliac joint cause sciatica? *Pain Physician.* 2003; 6(3): 269–272.

[28] Bernard TN Jr, Kirkaldy-Willis WH. Recognizing specific characteristics of nonspecific low back pain. *Clinical Orthopaedics and Related Research.* 1987; 217: 266–280.

[29] Merriman J. Prolotherapy versus operative fusion in the treatment of joint instability of the spine and pelvis. *Journal of the International College of Surgeons.* 1964; 42(2): 150–159.

[30] Hackett GS, Huang TC. Prolotherapy for sciatica from weak pelvic ligaments and bone dystrophy. *Clinical Medicine.* 1961 Dec; 8: 2301; Myers AB. Prolotherapy treatment of low back pain and sciatica. *Bull Hosp Joint Disease.* 1961 Apr 1; 22: 48–55.

[31] Bernard TN Jr, Kirkaldy-Willis WH. Recognizing specific characteristics of nonspecific low back pain. *Clinical Orthopaedics and Related Research.* 1987; 217: 266–280.

[32] Mennell J. *Back Pain, Diagnosing and Treating Using Manipulative Techniques* (p. 51). Boston, Massachusetts: Little, Brown and Company, 1960.

[33] Fortin JD, Falco FJE. The Fortin finger test: an indicator of sacroiliac pain. *American Journal of Orthopedics.* 1997; 26: 477–480.

[34] Kim WM, Lee HG, Won Jeong C, Kim CM, Yoon MH. A randomized controlled trial of intra-articular prolotherapy versus steroid injection for sacroiliac joint pain. *Journal of Alternative and Complementary Medicine.* 2010 Dec 1; 16(12): 1285–1290; Cusi M, Saunders J, Hungerford B, Wisbey-Roth T, Lucas P, Wilson S. The use of prolotherapy in the sacroiliac joint. *British Journal of Sports Medicine.* 2010 Feb 1; 44(2): 100–104. Mitchell B, Barnard A. Prolotherapy for sacroiliac joint pain. *Journal of Science and Medicine in Sport.* 2012 Dec 31; 15: S336; Rose R, Barnard A. Efficacy of prolotherapy treatment for sacroiliac joint instability and pain. *Journal of Science and Medicine in Sport.* 2015 Dec 1; 19: e70; Mitchell B, Rose R, Barnard A. Prolotherapy for sacroiliac joint pain-12 months outcomes. *Journal of Science and Medicine in Sport.* 2014 Dec 1; 18: e90; Ko GD, Mindra S, Lawson GE, Whitmore S, Arseneau L. Case series of ultrasound-guided platelet-rich plasma injections for sacroiliac joint dysfunction. *Journal of Back and Musculoskeletal Rehabilitation.* 2017; 30(2): 363–370.

[35] Castellvi AE, Goldstein LA, Chan DP. Lumbosacral transitional vertebrae and their relationship with lumbar extradural defects. *Spine.* 1984; 9(5): 493–495.

[36] Quinlan JF, Ryan M, Eustace S. Bertolotti's syndrome a cause of back pain in young people. *Orthopaedic Proceedings.* 2006; 88(2): 285–285.

[37] Apazidis A, Ricart PA, Diefenbach CM, Spivak JM. The prevalence of transitional vertebrae in the lumbar spine. *Spine Journal.* 2011 Sep 30; 11(9): 858–862.

[38] Vergauwen S, Parizel PM, Van Breusegem L, Van Goethem JW, Nackaerts Y, Van den Hauwe L, De Schepper AM. Distribution and incidence of degenerative spine changes in patients with a lumbo-sacral transitional vertebra. *European Spine Journal.* 1997; 6(3): 168–172.

[39] Olofin MU, Noronha C, Okanlawon A. Incidence of lumbosacral transitional vertebrae in low back pain patients. *West African Journal of Radiology.* 2001; 8: 1–6.

[40] Illeez OG, Atıcı A, Ulger EB, Kulcu DG, Ozkan FU, Aktas I. The transitional vertebra and sacroiliac joint dysfunction association. *European Spine Journal.* 2016 Nov 18: 1–7.

[41] Hauser RA. Lackner JB, Steilen-Matias D, Harris DK. A systematic review of dextrose prolotherapy for chronic musculoskeletal pain. *Clinical Medicine Insights. Arthritis and Musculoskeletal Disorders.* 2016; 9: 139; Cusi M, Saunders J, Hungerford B, Wisbey-Roth T, Lucas P, Wilson S. The use of prolotherapy in the sacroiliac joint. *British Journal of Sports Medicine.* 2010 Feb 1; 44(2): 100–104; Hackett GS. Prolotherapy in whiplash and low back pain. *Postgraduate Medicine.* 1960 Feb 1; 27(2): 214–219; Ongley M, Dorman T, Klein R, Eek B, Hubert L. A new approach to the treatment of chronic low back pain. *The Lancet.* 1987 Jul 18; 330(8551): 143–146; Hackett GS, Huang TC. Prolotherapy for sciatica from weak pelvic ligaments and bone dystrophy. *Clinical Medicine.* 1961 Dec; 8: 2301–2316.

[42] Ko GD, Mindra S, Lawson GE, Whitmore S, Arseneau L. Case series of ultrasound-guided platelet-rich plasma injections for sacroiliac joint dysfunction. *Journal of Back and Musculoskeletal Rehabilitation.* 2017; 30(2): 363–370.

[43] Kirchner F, Anitua E. Intradiscal and intra-articular facet infiltrations with plasma rich in growth factors reduce pain in patients with chronic low back pain. *Journal of Craniovertebral Junction & Spine.* 2016 Mar 2; 7(4): 250–256.

[44] Hussein M, Hussein T. Effect of autologous platelet leukocyte rich plasma injections on atrophied lumbar multifidus muscle in

low back pain patients with monosegmental degenerative disc disease. *SICOT-J.* 2016 Mar 22: Article ID 2016002, 7 pages.

[45] Wu J, Zhou J, Liu C, Zhang J, Xiong W, Lv Y, Liu R, Wang R, Du Z, Zhang G, Liu Q. A prospective study comparing platelet-rich plasma and local anesthetic (LA)/corticosteroid in intra-articular injection for the treatment of lumbar face joint. *Pain Practice.* 2017; 17(7): 914–924; Singla V, Batra YK, Bharti N, Goni VG, Marwaha N. Steroid vs. Platelet-Rich Plasma in Ultrasound-Guided Sacroiliac Joint Injection for Chronic Low Back Pain. *Pain Practice.* 2017 Jul 1; 17(6): 782–791.

[46] Hunt CL, Eldrige JS, Mauck WD, van Wijnen AJ, Qu W. Poster 124: Office-Based Stem Cell Therapies for Painful Degenerative Facetogenic and Sacroiliac Joint Disease: A Case Series. PM&R. 2017 Sep 30; 9(9): S174–5; Pettine K. Suzuki R, Sand T, Murphy M. Treatment of discogenic back pain with autologous bone marrow concentrate injection with minimum two year follow-up. *International Orthopaedics.* 2016; 40(1): 135–140.

Chapter 15: Prolotherapy Regenerative Medicine for Disc Disease

[1] Naylor A. Intervertebral disc prolapse and degeneration: The biomechanical and biophysical approach. *Spine.* 1976; 1(2): 108–114.

[2] Powell MC, Wilson M, Szypryt S, Symonds EM. Prevalence of lumbar disc degeneration observed by magnetic resonance in symptomless women. *The Lancet.* 1986 Dec 13; 328(8520): 1366–1367.

[3] Ombregt L. *A System of Orthopaedic Medicine.* 3rd ed. London, England: Churchill Livingstone Elsevier, 2013.

[4] Hackett GS, Hemwall GA, Montgomery GA. *Ligament and Tendon Relaxation Treated by Prolotherapy.* 5th ed. (p. 9), commenting on work of Newman PH). Oak Brook, Illinois: Institute in Basic Life Principles, 1991.

[5] Acarpglu ER, Iatridis JC, Setton LA, Foster RJ, Mow VC, Weidenbaum M. Degeneration and aging affect the tensile behavior of human lumbar annulus fibrosus. *Spine.* 1995; 20(24): 2690–2701.

[6] Krag MH, Seroussi RE, Wilder DG, Pope MH. Thoracic and lumbar internal disc displacement distribution from in vitro loading of human spinal motion segments: Experimental results

and theoretical predictions. *Spine.* 1987; 12: 1001–1007; Ombregt, L. *A System of Orthopaedic Medicine.* 3rd ed., London, England: Churchill Livingstone Elsevier, 2013.

[7] Ombregt, L. *A System of Orthopaedic Medicine.* 3rd ed. London, England: Churchill Livingstone Elsevier, 2013.

[8] Nachemson A. Advances in low back pain. *Clinical Orthopaedics and Related Research.* 1985 Nov 1; 200: 266-278; Paster RZ. Nonpharmacologic management of low back pain. *Family Practice Recertification Management of Chronic Low Back Pain Special Supplement.* 1999 Jun; 21(7): 6–9.

[9] Buschbacher R. *Practical Guide to Musculoskeletal Disorders: Diagnosis and Rehabilitation,* 2nd ed. (p. 100). Boston, Massachusetts: Butterworth Heinemann, 2002; Cyriax JH. *Illustrated Manual of Orthopaedic Medicine,* 2nd ed. (p. 199). Oxford, England: Butterworth-Heineman, 1998.

[10] Hakelius A. Prognosis in sciatica: A clinical follow-up of surgical and nonsurgical treatment. *Acta Orthopaedica Scandinavica.* 1970; 41(Sup 129): 1–16; Nashold BS, Hrubec Z. *Lumbar Disc Disease: A Twenty-Year Clinical Follow-Up Study.* St. Louis, Missouri: Mosby, 1971.

[11] Alaranta H. A prospective study of patients with sciatica. *Spine.* 1990; 15: 1345–1349.

[12] Panagopoulos J, Hush J, Steffens D, Hancock MJ. Do MRI findings change over a period of up to 1 year in patients with low back pain and/or sciatica? A systematic review. *Spine.* 2017; 42(7): 504–512.

[13] Cook CE, Arnold PM, Passias PG, Frempong-Boadu AK, Radcliff K, Isaacs R. Predictors of pain and disability outcomes in one thousand, one hundred and eight patients who underwent lumbar discectomy surgery. *International Orthopaedics.* 2015; 39(11): 2143–2151.

[14] Bush K, Cowan N, Katz DE, Gishen P. The natural history of sciatica associated with disc pathology. *Spine.* 1992; 17(10): 1205–1222; Delauche-Cavalier MC, Budet C, Laredo JD, Debie B, Wybier M, Dorfmann H, Ballner I. Lumbar disc herniation: Computed tomography scan changes after conservative treatment of nerve root compression. *Spine.* 1992; 17(8): 927–933; Matsubara Y, Kato F,

Mimatsu K, Kajino G, Nakamura S, Nitta H. Serial changes on MRI in lumbar disc herniations treated conservatively. *Neuroradiology.* 1995; 37: 378–383.

[15] Borenstein D. Etiology of low back pain. *Family Practice Recertification Management of Chronic Low Back Pain Special Supplement.* 1999; 21(7): 6.

[16] Altun I, Yüksel KZ. Lumbar herniated disc: Spontaneous regression. *Korean Journal of Pain.* 2017; 30(1): 44–50.

[17] Cameron JA, Thielen KM. Autologous platelet rich plasma for neck and lower back pain secondary to spinal disc herniation: Midterm results. *Spine Research.* 2017 Aug 30; 3(2): Article ID 100030, 5 pages.

[18] Monfett M, Harrison J, Boachie-Adjei K, Lutz G. Intradiscal platelet-rich plasma (PRP) injections for discogenic low back pain: An update. *International Orthopaedics.* 2016; 40(6): 1321–1328.

[19] Tuakli-Wosornu YA. Terry A, Boachie-Adjei K, Harrison JR, Gribbin CK, LaSalle EE, Nguyen JT, Solomon JL, Lutz GE. Lumbar intradiskal platelet-rich plasma (PRP) injections: A prospective, double-blind, randomized controlled study. *PM&R.* 2016; 8(1): 1–10; Basso M, Cavagnaro L, Zanirato A, Divano S, Formica C, Formica M. What is the clinical evidence on regenerative medicine in intervertebral disc degeneration? *Musculoskeletal Surgery.* 2017: 1–12.

[20] Lumbar intradiscal platelet rich plasma injections- a multicenter, prospective study in patients with disc disruption; IRB Number: 2015-716. 2016 Aug [2017 May 14] https://www.hss.edu/clinical-trials_lumbar-intradiscal-prp-platelet-injections-disc-disruption.asp,

[21] Orozco L, Soler R, Morera C, Alberca M, Sánchez A, García-Sancho J. Intervertebral disc repair by autologous mesenchymal bone marrow cells: A pilot study. *Transplantation.* 2011; 92(7): 822–828; Pettine KA, Murphy MB, Suzuki RK, Sand TT. Percutaneous injection of autologous bone marrow concentrate cells significantly reduces lumbar discogenic pain through 12 months. *Stem Cells.* 2015; 33(1): 146–156.

[22] Kristin C, Robert S, Michelle P. Effects of the intradiscal implantation of stromal vascular fraction plus platelet rich plasma in patients with degenerative disc disease. *Journal of Translational Medicine.* 2017; 15:12.

[23] Navani A, Ambach MA, Wei JJ, Gupta D. Biologic therapies for intervertebral degenerative disc disease: A review of novel applications. *Journal of Stem Cell Research, Reviews, & Reports.* 2017; 4(1): Article ID 1023, 9 pages; Zeckser J, Wolff M, Tucker J, Goodwin J. Multipotent mesenchymal stem cell treatment for discogenic low back pain and disc degeneration. *Stem Cells International.* 2016: Article ID 3908389, 13 pages.

Chapter 16: Prolotherapy Regenerative Medicine for Sports Injuries: Returning the Athlete Safely to His/Her Sport

[1] Owens BD. Return to Play Following Musculoskeletal Injury, *An Issue of Clinics in Sports Medicine*, E-Book. Philadelphia, Pennsylvania: Elsevier Health Sciences, 2016.

[2] Reeves KD, Fullerton BD, Topol G. Evidence-based regenerative injection therapy (prolotherapy) in sports medicine. In *The Sports Medicine Resource Manual* (pp. 611–619). Philadelphia, Pennsylvania: Saunders (Elsevier), 2008.

[3] Rompe JD, Nafe B, Furia JP, Maffulli N. Eccentric loading shockwave treatment, or a wait-and-see policy for tendinopathy of the main body of tendo achillis: A randomized controlled trial. *American Journal of Sports Medicine.* 2007; 35(3): 374–383.

[4] Bernuzzi G, Petraglia F, Pedrini MF, De Filippo M, Pogliacomi F, Verdano MA, Costantino C. Use of platelet-rich plasma in the care of sports injuries: Our experience with ultrasound-guided injection. *Blood Transfusion.* 2014 Jan; 12(Suppl 1): s229.

[5] Paoloni JA, Orchard JW. 1. The use of therapeutic medications for soft-tissue injuries in sports medicine. *Medical Journal of Australia.* 2005 Oct 3; 183(7): 384.

[6] McAlindon TE, LaValley MP, Harvey WF, Price LL, Driban JB, Zhang M, Ward RJ. Effect of intra-articular triamcinolone vs saline on knee cartilage volume and pain in patients with knee osteoarthritis: a randomized clinical trial. *Journal of the American Medical Association.* 2017; 317(19): 1967–1975.

[7] Soliman DMI. Advantages of dextrose, platelet rich plasma and stem cells over the traditional conventional methods in treatment of sports injuries and joint osteoarthritis. *Journal of Sports Science.* 2017; 5: 113–118.

[8] Topol GA, Reeves KD, Hassanein K. Efficacy of dextrose pro-lotherapy in elite male kicking-sport athletes with chronic groin pain. *Archives Physical Medicine and Rehabilitation*. 2005; 86(4): 697–702.

[9] Seven MM, Ersen O, Akpancar S, Ozkan H, Turkkan S, Yıldız Y, Koca K. Effectiveness of prolotherapy in the treatment of chronic rotator cuff lesions. *Orthopaedics & Traumatology: Surgery & Research*. 2017; 103(3): 427–433.

[10] Maxwell NJ, Ryan MB, Taunton JE, Gillies JH, Wong AD. Sonographically guided intratendinous injection of hyperosmolar dextrose to treat chronic tendinosis of the Achilles tendon: a pilot study. *American Journal of Roentgenology*. 2007; 189(4): W215–W220.

[11] Topol GA, Reeves KD. Regenerative injection of elite athletes with career-altering chronic groin pain who fail conservative treatment: A consecutive case series. *American Journal of Physical Medicine and Rehabilitation*. 2008; 87(11): 890–902.

[12] Khan SA, Kumar A, Varshney MK, Trikha V, Yadav CS. Dextrose prolotherapy for recalcitrant coccydynia. *Journal of Orthopaedic Surgery*. 2008; 16(1): 27–29.

[13] Alderman DD. Prolotherapy for golfer's elbow and pain. *Practical Pain Management*. June 2008. 8(5): 56–64

[14] Hauser RA, Hauser MA. *Prolo Your Sports Injuries Away*. Oak Park, Illinois: Beulah Land Press, 2001.

[15] World Anti-Doping Agency. 2013 prohibited list [cited 2017 February 28] https://www.wada-ama.org/en/questions-answers /2013-prohibited-list#item-361.

[16] Platelet-rich plasma therapy big with athletes. *Fox News*. 2012 Jul 3 [cited 2017 May 28] http://www.foxsports.com/other/story/ platelet-rich-plasma-therapy-big-with-athletes-070312; Zanon G, Combi A, Benazzo F, Bargagliotti M. The use of PRP in athletes with muscular lesions. In *Bio-Orthopaedics: A New Approach* (239–245). Berlin Heidelberg: Springer, 2017.

[17] Randelli PS. Fossati C, Menon A, Ragone V, D'Ambrosi R, Cabitza P, De Girolamo L. Use of PRP in sports medicine 56. *Arthroscopy and Sport Injuries: Applications in High-level Athletes*. 2016: 439; Hernandez D. Several Dodgers have used platelet rich plasma. *LA Times*. 2013 Mar 13 [cited 2017 July 4] http://articles.latimes.

com/2013/mar/13/sports/la-sp-0314-dodgers-prp-20130314; Zanon G, Combi F, Combi A, Perticarini L, Sammarchi L, Benazzo F. Platelet-rich plasma in the treatment of acute hamstring injuries in professional football players. *Joints*. 2016 Jan–Mar; 4(1): 17–12.

[18] Dines JS, Williams PN, El Attrache N, Conte S, Tomczyk T, Osbahr DC, Dines DM, Bradley J, Ahmad CS. Platelet-rich plasma can be used to successfully treat elbow ulnar collateral ligament insufficiency in high-level throwers. *American Journal of Orthopedics*. 2016; 45(5): 296–300.

[19] Laver L, Carmont MR, McConkey MO, Palmanovich E, Yaacobi E, Mann G, Nyska M, Kots E, Mei-Dan O. Plasma rich in growth factors (PRGF) as a treatment for high ankle sprain in elite athletes: A randomized control trial. *Knee Surgery, Sports Traumatology, Arthroscopy*. 2015 Nov 1; 23(11): 3383–3392.

[20] Bernuzzi G, Petraglia F, Pedrini MF, De Filippo M, Pogliacomi F, Verdano MA, Costantino C. Use of platelet-rich plasma in the care of sports injuries: Our experience with ultrasound-guided injection. *Blood Transfusion*. 2014; 12(1): s229.

[21] Sanli I, Morgan B, van Tilborg F, Funk L, Gosens T. Single injection of platelet-rich plasma (PRP) for the treatment of refractory distal biceps tendonitis: Long-term results of a prospective multi-center cohort study. *Knee Surgery, Sports Traumatology, Arthroscopy*. 2016; 24(7): 2308–2312.

[22] Dragoo JL. Wasterlain AS, Braun HJ, Nead KT. Platelet-rich plasma as a treatment for patellar tendinopathy: A double-blind, randomized controlled trial. *American Journal of Sports Medicine*. 2014; 42(3): 610–618.

[23] Pearl J. Professional Athletes and Platelet Rich Plasma Injections. 2015 Jun [cited 2017 May 28] https://www.mortonsneuroma.com/professional-athletes-and-platelet-rich-plasma-injections/; Devine D. Steph Curry had platelet rich plasma treatment on his right knee. *Yahoo Sports*. 2016 May 4 [cited 2017 July 4] https://sports.yahoo.com/blogs/nba-ball-dont-lie/stephen-curry-had-platelet-rich-plasma-treatment-on-his-right-knee-182950035.html.

[24] Matthews KRW, Cuchiara ML. US National Football League athletes seeking unproven stem cell treatments. *Stem Cells and Development*. 2014; 23(S1): 60–64.

[25] Stem cell treatment: out from the shadows, onto the cutting edge. *Sports Illustrated*. 2014 Jul 30 [cited 2017 May 28] http://mmqb.si.com/2014/07/30/stem-cell-treatment-nfl-sports-medicine; Moen MH, Pas HI. Stem cell treatment? Please answer these simple questions first.*British Journal of Sports Medicine* 2017; 51:1512–1513.

[26] Albano JJ, Alexander RW. Autologous fat grafting as a mesenchymal stem cell source and living bioscaffold in a patellar tendon tear. *Clinical Journal of Sport Medicine*. 2011 Jul 1; 21(4): 359–361.

[27] Hernigou P, Lachaniette CH, Delambre J, Zilber S, Duffiet P, Chevallier N, Rouard H. Biologic augmentation of rotator cuff repair with mesenchymal stem cells during arthroscopy improves healing and prevents further tears: a case-controlled study. *International Orthopaedics*. 2014 Sep 1; 38(9): 1811–1818.

Chapter 17: Frequently Asked Questions

[1] Governor Signs Emerging Therapies Act of 2017 [cited 2017 October 1] http://www.prnewswire.com/news-releases/governor-signs-emerging-therapies-act-of-2017-with-strongside-solutions-300439103.html.

[2] Topol GA, Podesta LA, Reeves KD, Giraldo M, Johnson LL, Grasso R, Jamín A, Clark T, Rabago D. Chondrogenic effect of intra-articular hypertonic-dextrose (prolotherapy) in severe knee osteoarthritis. *PM&R*. 2016; 8(11): 1072–1082.

[3] Durant TJS, Dwyer CR, McCarthy MBR, Cote MP, Bradley JP, Mazzocca AD. Protective nature of platelet-rich plasma against chondrocyte death when combined with corticosteroids or local anesthetics. *American Journal of Sports Medicine*. 2017; 45(1): 218–225.

[4] Sakata R, Reddi AH. Platelet-rich plasma modulates actions on articular cartilage lubrication and regeneration. *Tissue Engineering Part B: Reviews*. 2016; 22(5): 408–419.

[5] Wang M, Yuan Z, Ma N, Hao C, Guo W, Zou G, Zhang Y, Chen M, Gao S, Peng J, Wang A, Wang Y, Sui X, Xu W, Lu S, Liu S, Guo Q. Advances and prospects in stem cells for cartilage regeneration. *Stem Cells International*. 2017: Article ID 4130607, 16 pages.

[6] Bausset O, Magalon J, Giraudo L, Louis ML, Serratrice N, Frere C, Magalon G, Dignat-George F, Sabatier F. Impact of local anesthetics and needle calibres used for painless PRP injections on platelet

functionality. *MLTJ Muscles, Ligaments and Tendons Journal*. 2014; 4(1): 18–23; Carofino B, Chowaniec DM, McCarthy MB, Bradley JP, Delaronde S, Beitzel K, Cote MP, Arciero RA, Mazzocca AD. Corticosteroids and local anesthetics decrease positive effects of platelet-rich plasma: An in vitro study on human tendon cells. *Arthroscopy: The Journal of Arthroscopic & Related Surgery*. 2012; 28(5): 711–719.

[7] Rahnama R, Wang M, Dang AC, Kim HT, Kuo AC. Cytotoxicity of local anesthetics on human mesenchymal stem cells. *Journal of Bone and Joint Surgery*. 2013; 95(2): 132–137.

[8] Orthokine (definition) [cited 2017 August 5] https://en.wikipedia.org/wiki/Orthokine.

[9] Anitua E, Troya M, Zalduendo MM, Orive G. The effect of different drugs on the preparation and biological outcomes of plasma rich in growth factors. *Annals of Anatomy-Anatomischer Anzeiger*. 2014; 196(6): 423–429; Anitua E, Troya M, Zalduendo M, Orive G. Effects of anti-aggregant, anti-inflammatory and anti-coagulant drug consumption on the preparation and therapeutic potential of plasma rich in growth factors (PRGF). *Growth Factors*. 2015; 33(1): 57–64.

[10] Ramsook RR, Danesh H. Timing of platelet rich plasma injections during antithrombotic therapy. *Pain Physician*. 2016; 19(7): E1055.

Chapter 19: Joint Pain: The Nutrition Connection

[1] Seaman DR. The diet-induced proinflammatory state: A cause of chronic pain and other degenerative diseases? *Journal of Manipulative and Physiological Therapeutics*. 2002 Apr 30; 25(3): 168–179.

[2] Ross J. Amino acids and diet in chronic pain management. *Practical Pain Management Journal*. 2012 [cited 2017 August 21] https://www.practicalpainmanagement.com/treatments/nutraceutical/amino-acids-diet-chronic-pain-management.

[3] Advincula de Araújo L, Addor F, Campos PMBGM. Use of silicon for skin and hair care: An approach of chemical forms available and efficacy. *Anais Brasileiros de Dermatologia*. 2016; 91(3): 331–335.

[4] Reffitt DM, Ogston N, Jugdaohsingh R, Cheung HFJ, Evans BAJ, Thompson RPH, Powell JJ, Hampson GN. Orthosilicic acid

stimulates collagen type 1 synthesis and osteoblastic differentiation in human osteoblast-like cells in vitro. *Bone.* 2003; 32(2): 127–135.

[5] Martin KR. The chemistry of silica and its potential health benefits. *Journal of Nutrition, Health & Aging.* 2007 Mar-Apr; 11(2): 94-97.

[6] Barel A, Calomme M, Timchenko A, De Paepe K, Demeester N, Rogiers V, Clarys P, Berghe DV. Effect of oral intake of choline-stabilized orthosilicic acid on skin, nails and hair in women with photodamaged skin. *Archives of Dermatological Research.* 2005 Oct 1; 297(4): 147–153.

[7] Reffitt DM, Ogston N, Jugdaohsingh R, Cheung HFJ, Evans BAJ, Thompson RPH, Powell JJ, Hampson GN. Orthosilicic acid stimulates collagen type 1 synthesis and osteoblastic differentiation in human osteoblast-like cells in vitro. *Bone.* 2003; 32(2): 127–135; Martin KR. The chemistry of silica and its potential health benefits. *Journal of Nutrition, Health & Aging.* 2007 Mar-Apr; 11(2): 94–97; Geusens P, Pavelka K, Rovensky J, Vanhoof J, Demeester N, Calomme M, Vanden Berghe D. A 12-week randomized, double-blind, placebo-controlled multicenter study of choline-stabilized orthosilicic acid in patients with symptomatic knee osteoarthritis. *BMC Musculoskeletal Disorders.* 2017; 18(1): 2.

[8] Jurkić LM, Cepanec I, Pavelić SK, Pavelić K. Biological and therapeutic effects of ortho-silicic acid and some ortho-silicic acid-releasing compounds: New perspectives for therapy. *Nutrition & Metabolism.* 2013; 10(1): 2.

[9] Ross J. Amino acids and diet in chronic pain management. *Practical Pain Management Journal.* 2012 [cited 2017 August 21] https://www.practicalpainmanagement.com/treatments/nutraceutical/amino-acids-diet-chronic-pain-management.

[10] https://en.wikipedia.org/wiki/Endorphins [cited 2017 August 25].

[11] Juhl JH. Fibromyalgia and the serotonin pathway. *Alternative Medicine Review.* 1998 Oct; 3: 367–375.

[12] Ehrenpreis S, Balagot RC, Myles S, Advocate C, Comaty JE. Further studies on the analgesic activity of D-Phenylalanine in mice and humans. In *Endogenous and Exogenous Opiate Agonists and Antagonists: Procedures of the International Narcotics Research Club*

Convention (pp. 379–382). Philadelphia, Pennsylvania: Elsevier, 1979.

[13] https://store.lidtke.com/products/endorphigen-60capsules.

[14] Sampson HA. Food allergy. *Journal of the American Medical Association.* 1997; 278(22): 1888–1894; Van de Laar MA, van de Korst JK. Food intolerance in rheumatoid arthritis: A double blind controlled trial of the clinical effects of elimination of milk allergens and azo dyes. *Annuals of Rheumatological Diseases.* 1992 Mar 1; 51(3): 298–302.

[15] Cotter N. Diet and Pain. In *Integrative Pain Management* (p. 255). New York, New York: Oxford University Press, 2016.

[16] Sapone A, Bai JC, Ciacci C, Dolinsek J, Green PHR, Hadjivassiliou M, Kaukinen K, Rostami K, Sanders DS. Schumann M, Ullrich R, Villalta D, Volta U, Catassi C, Fasano A. Spectrum of gluten-related disorders: Consensus on new nomenclature and classification. *BMC Medicine.* 2012; 10(1): 13.

[17] Lubrano E, Ciacci C, Ames PRJ, Mazzacca G, Ordente P, Scarpa R. The arthritis of coeliac disease: Prevalence and pattern in 200 adult patients. *Rheumatology.* 1996; 35(12): 1314–1318.

[18] Usai P, Francesa M, Piga M, Cacace E, Lai MA, Beccaris A, Piras E, Nasa GL, Mulargia M, Balestrieri A. Adult celiac disease is frequently associated with sacroiliitis. *Digestive Diseases and Sciences.* 1995; 40(9): 1906–1908.

[19] Zipser RD, Patel S, Yahya KZ, Baisch DW, Monarch E. Presentations of adult celiac disease in a nationwide patient support group. *Digestive Diseases and Sciences.* 2003; 48(4): 761–764.

[20] Lynd FT et al. The Naalehu disease (in Hawaii). *American Journal of Veterinary Research.* 1965; 26: 1344–1349; Krook L, Wasserman RH, McEntee K, Brokken TD, Teigland MB. Cestrum diurnum poisoning in Florida cattle. *Cornell Veterinarian.* 1975; 65(10): 557–575.

[21] Childers NF, Margoles MS. An apparent relation of nightshades (solanaceae) to arthritis. *Journal of Neurological and Orthopedic Medical Surgery.* 1993; 12: 227–231.

[22] Childers NF. *Arthritis-Childer's Diet to Stop It: Nightshades, Aging and Ill Health*, 4th ed. Florida: Horticultural Publications, 1993.

[23] Reginster JY, Deroisy R, Rovati LC, Lee RL, Lejeune E, Bruyere O, Giacovelli G, Henrotin Y, Dacre JE, Gossett C. Long-term effects of glucosamine sulphate on osteoarthritis progression: A randomized, placebo-controlled clinical trial. *The Lancet*. 2001; 357 (9252): 251–256.

[24] Runhaar J, Rozendaal R, van Middelkoop M, Bijlsma JW, Doherty M, Dziedzic K, Lohmander LS, McAlindon T, Zhang W, Bierma-Zeinstra SM. No treatment effects of oral glucosamine for subgroups of knee and hip osteoarthritis patients: An individual patient data meta-analysis from the OA trial bank. *Osteoarthritis and Cartilage*. 2017; 25: S408–S409.

[25] Hochberg MC. Martel-Pelletier J, Monfort J, Möller I, Castillo JR, Arden N, Berenbaum F, Blanco FJ, Conaghan PG, Domenech G, Henrotin Y, Pap T, Richette P, Sawitzke A, du Souich P, Pelletier JP. Combined chondroitin sulfate and glucosamine for painful knee osteoarthritis: A multicentre, randomized, double-blind, non-inferiority trial versus celecoxib. *Annals of the Rheumatic Diseases*. 2015 Feb 13 [cited 2017 October 1] http://ard.bmj.com/content/early/2015/02/13/annrheumdis-2014-206792.info.

[26] Diehl HW, May EL. Cetyl myristoleate isolated from Swiss albino mice: An apparent protective agent against adjuvant arthritis in rat. *Journal of Pharmaceutical Science*. 1994; 83: 296–299.

[27] Siemandi H et al. Arthritic episodes in patients with various auto-immune diseases characterized by the common terminology "arthritis" and "psoriasis": A randomized clinical trial. *Townsend Letter*. Second quarter; 1997.

[28] Whitehouse MW, Macrides TA, Kalafatis N, Betts WH, Haynes DR, Broadbent J. Anti-inflammatory activity of a lipid fraction (Lyprinol) from the NZ green-lipped mussel. *Inflammopharmacology*. 1997; 5: 237–246.

[29] Lau CS, Chiu PKY, Chu EMY, Cheng IYW, Tang WM, Man RYK, Halpern GM. Treatment of knee osteoarthritis with Lyprinol®, lipid extract of the green-lipped mussel—a double-blind placebo-controlled study. *Progress in Nutrition*. 2004; 6(1): 17–31.

[30] Caruso I, Pietrogrande V. Italian double-blind multicenter study comparing S-adenosyl methionine, naproxen and placebo in the treatment of degenerative joint disease. *American Journal of Medicine*. 1987; 83(5A): 66–71.

[31] Muller-Fassbender H. Double-blind clinical trial of S-adenosyl methionine versus ibuprofen in the treatment of osteoarthritis. *American Journal of Medicine*. 1987; 83(5A): 81–83.

[32] Soeken KL, Lee WL, Bausell RB, Agelli M, Berman BM. Safety and efficacy of S-adenosyl methionine (SAMe) for osteoarthritis. *Journal of Family Practice*. 2002; 51(5): 425–430.

[33] Maroon J, Bost J, Baughman J. Results of omega-3 EFA for spine pain. Presented at the *American Association Neurological Surgeons Annual Meeting*, New Orleans, April 18, 2005.

[34] Phillipson BE, Rothrock DW, Connor WE, Harris WS, Illingworth DR. Reduction of plasma lipids, lipoproteins, and apoproteins by dietary fish oils in patients with hypertriglyceridemia. *New England Journal of Medicine*. 1985; 312(19): 1210–1216.

[35] Appel LJ, Miller ER, Seidler AJ, Whelton PK. Does supplementation of diet with "fish oil" reduce blood pressure? A meta analysis of controlled clinical trials. *Archives of Internal Medicine*. 1993; 153(12): 1429–1438.

[36] Issa AM, Mojica WA. The efficacy of omega-3 fatty acids on cognitive function in aging and dementia: A systematic review. *Dementia and Geriatric Cognitive Disorders*. 2006; 21(2): 88–96.

Chapter 20: Conclusion: The Road You Walk

[1] Baker AD. Abnormal magnetic-resonance scans of the lumbar spine in asymptomatic subjects. A prospective investigation. In *Classic Papers in Orthopaedics*. 2014 (pp. 245–247). London, England: Springer; Brinjikji W, Luetmer PH, Comstock B, Bresnahan BW, Chen LE, Deyo RA, Halabi S, Turner JA, Avins AL, James K, Wald JT. Systematic literature review of imaging features of spinal degeneration in asymptomatic populations. *American Journal of Neuroradiology*. 2015 Apr 1; 36(4): 811–816; Jensen, M. Magnetic resonance imaging of the lumbar spine in people without back pain. *New England Journal of Medicine*. 1994; 331(2): 69–73.

INDEX

Page references in *italics* refer to figures and photos.